Handbook of Learning Disabilities
Volume III: Programs and Practices

Handbook of Learning Disabilities

Volume III: Programs and Practices

Kenneth A. Kavale, Ph.D.
Professor and Chair
Division of Special Education
The University of Iowa
Iowa City, Iowa

Steven R. Forness, Ed.D.
Director of Mental Retardation and
Developmental Disabilities Program
Principal, Neuropsychiatric Hospital School
Professor of Psychiatry and Biobehavioral Sciences
UCLA School of Medicine
Los Angeles, California

Michael Bender, Ed.D.
Vice President of Educational Programs
The Kennedy Institute
Professor of Education
The Johns Hopkins University
Joint Appointment, Department of Pediatrics
The Johns Hopkins School of Medicine
Baltimore, Maryland

A College-Hill Publication
Little, Brown and Company
Boston/Toronto/San Diego

College-Hill Press
A Division of
Little, Brown and Company (Inc.)
34 Beacon Street
Boston, Massachusetts 02108

Library of Congress Cataloging in Publication Data
Main entry under title:

(Revised for volume 3)

Handbook of learning disabilities.

    Bibliography: v. 1.
    Includes index.
    Contents: v. 1. Dimensions and diagnosis — —
v. 3. Programs and practices.
    1. Learning disabilities — Handbooks, manuals, etc.
2. Special education — Handbooks, manuals, etc.
3. Remedial teaching — Handbooks, manuals, etc.
I. Kavale, Kenneth A., 1946–   II. Forness,
Steven R., 1939–   III. Bender, Michael, 1943–
[DNLM: 1. Learning Disorders — handbooks. WS 39 H236]
LC4704.H365   1987   371.9   86-26396
ISBN 0-316-48368-0 (pbk.: v. 1)

ISBN 0-316-48374-5

Contents

Preface

Over the past twenty five years, the field of learning disabilities (LD) has witnessed amazing growth. From modest beginnings, it has become the special education category serving by far the most individuals. Accompanying this unprecedented growth has been a significant increase in the literature available about all aspects of LD. Consequently, it has become a challenge for even the most dedicated professional to keep abreast of the latest information. The many books now available tend to be either texts, providing basic information but little critical evaluation, or highly technical publications focusing on specific topics.

The *Handbook of Learning Disabilities* volumes are intended to occupy a place between these two extremes. The comprehensive coverage of these three books will provide the basic information, as well as a more in-depth critical evaluation. Our main goal is to provide students and practitioners with ready access to the essentials for understanding and treating LD.

Our thesis is that, although an individual with learning disabilities may have an underlying neurologic processing difficulty that may indeed have had something to do with the development of the learning disability, the documentation of such problems is only necessary to the extent that federally or locally mandated procedures now call for such evidence in determination of eligibility for services. Such information has not proven critical in determining which approaches need to be used or in planning remedial programs. Therefore, there are no chapters on visual processing or sensory–motor integration, since these areas have not been shown to be areas of prime importance to remediation; nor are there separate chapters on attention and memory or on information processing, since these areas are still inchoate and have not yet led to specific remedial strategies. Each of these areas is discussed, however, and possible principles or guidelines that can be gleaned from existing evidence are suggested. There is a focus on direct instruction of academic skills, on language strategies to the extent that these are integrated into the reading lesson or taught as skills valuable unto themselves, on increasing the time the child actually spends in reading instruction or in the experience of reading, and on related matters such as social functioning, family issues, and maturational outcomes.

It is clear that learning disabilities is a field fraught with controversy, even in terms of its most basic diagnostic criteria and remedial methods.

The focus of these *Handbooks* is on a balanced evaluation of these issues and on what can reasonably be deduced, from existing knowledge, about the nature of LD, the diagnostic process, and the basic strategies of remediation. Our purpose is not an extensive review of controversial ideas, although these will be presented periodically throughout as preambles to specific procedures or approaches.

These volumes stand somewhere between "edited" and "authored" texts; most contributed chapters were first published as papers in *Learning Disabilities: An Interdisciplinary Journal,* but they have been substantially updated and adapted in collaboration with the original authors. In these chapters, we have credited the original author(s) on the first page of the chapter. However, it should be understood that we made editorial changes and additions to the original material in every case. Other chapters were written by us expressly for these volumes. Our primary goal throughout has been to provide the best and most recent information possible for understanding, assessing, and treating individuals with learning disabilities.

Introduction

The LD field possesses a wide variety of options for providing programs and practices and this volume of the *Handbook of Learning Disabilities* provides an overview of those options. The previous two volumes focused on diagnostic and treatment issues in LD. The purpose of this volume is to place those issues in an overall context. Methods and interventions are delivered in a variety of frameworks, and the goal of this volume is to show the possible choices with respect to program and practice options.

What type of program is best for the LD student? The many possible choices developed over time by the LD field make this a difficult question. No single option is either correct or appropriate but is contingent upon the particular needs of the LD student. Once decisions about methods and interventions are made, it is necessary to determine the most efficacious means for delivery of those remedial techniques. This means that decisions about programs and practices need to be made, but first it is necessary to know the choices available. With this knowledge, the LD professional can make rational decisions about the best way to provide for the needs of an LD student.

The volume is divided into four parts. The first part deals with the foundations for programming. Specifically, curriculum is the focus and the means by which programs and practices can be structured. The second part explores possible programmatic areas as well as an overview of possible service arrangements. The third part deals with the role of technology in service delivery to the LD student. Specifically, the use of computers in management and remediation is explored. The fourth part deals with LD beyond the elementary school years. The chapters review the possibilities for postsecondary education and explore the long-term consequences of LD. The goal is to provide perspective on the LD condition that may be useful in decisions about programmatic alternatives.

The third volume of the *Handbook of Learning Disabilities* deals with the context for remediation. Besides a variety of methods and interventions, the LD field has also developed an assortment of program and service arrangements. This volume presents an overview beginning with basic curriculum matters and ending with the adult outcomes of LD. The goal is to provide a comprehensive perspective about the programmatic possibilities in order to allow the LD professional to make the best choices for an LD student.

Contributors

Donn E. Brolin, Ph.D.
Professor
Department of Educational and
  Counseling Psychology
University of Missouri — Columbia
Columbia, Missouri

Gregory Church, M.S.
Computer Coordinator
Special Education Division
The Kennedy Institute
Baltimore, Maryland

James R. Corcoran, Ph.D.
Counseling Psychologist
St. Mary Hospital
Quincy, Illinois

Timothy R. Elliott, Ph.D.
Assistant Professor
Department of Psychology
Virginia Commonwealth University
Richmond, Virginia

David L. Hayden, Ph.D.
Branch Chief
Information Management Branch
Division of Special Education
Maryland State Department of
  Education
Baltimore, Maryland

M. E. B. Lewis, Ed.D.
Principal
The Kennedy School
The Kennedy Institute
Baltimore, Maryland

Charles T. Mangrum, Ed.D.
Professor of Education
Chairman, Graduate Program in
  Reading and Learning Disabilities
University of Miami
Coral Gables, Florida

David S. Mark, M.Ed.
Human Resources Officer
Signet Bank
Baltimore, Maryland

Gale M. Morrison, Ph.D.
Associate Professor
Graduate School of Education
University of California
Santa Barbara, California

Lois T. Pommer, Ed.D.
Psychology Associate
Psychological Sciences Institute
Baltimore, Maryland

Gary M. Sasso, Ph.D.
Assistant Professor
Division of Special Education
College of Education
University of Iowa
Iowa City, Iowa

Stuart J. Schleien, Ph.D.
Associate Professor
Division of Recreation, Park, and
  Leisure Studies
University of Minnesota
Minneapolis, Minnesota

Stephen S. Strichart, Ph.D.
Professor, College of Education
Department of Curriculum and
  Instruction
University Park Campus
Florida International University
Miami, Florida

The Foundations for Programming

The chapters in Part I lay the groundwork for LD programming. Before anything can be done, there must be insight into the question of what needs to be done. This need is often determined specifically from the diagnostic information obtained and more generally from the curriculum. The two chapters in Part I explore the issue of curriculum. Chapter 1 explores the question of curriculum development with respect to building a broad framework that includes not only an academic emphasis, but also elements aimed at social and career education. What is the relationship among academic, social, and career curricula in planning for LD students? This is the primary question addressed in the first chapter. The second chapter discusses curriculum planning with respect to philosophical and psychological conceptions. A thematic approach is suggested wherein instruction is reflected through a common theme for all subjects.

The chapters in Part I present a framework for programming. Programs and practices should not be haphazard activities, but rather a process delivered through a rational structure. These chapters provide that structure and allow for the initiation of appropriate and meaningful programming.

CHAPTER I

Curriculum Development

G. M. Morrison

A t one point it might have been a simple task to define the curricular focus for LD students: enhancing academic skills. Although the improvement of academic performance remains a primary goal, recent insights about the nature of LD and individual student needs suggest that a broader view of curriculum is required for educating LD students. The need for social and career education is now evident, but a major question must be answered: What is the relationship among academic, social, and career education in program planning for LD students?

The relative emphasis each component should receive and how that emphasis should be determined are basically curricular questions. Rather than focusing on how to teach, curriculum provides a framework for decisions about what to teach and the manner in which individual components are best combined.

Definitions of curriculum vary in nature and scope. One very broad definition is that "curriculum is what a learner experiences in a learning situation" (Meyen & Horner, 1976, p. 268). In further explicating what it is that a learner experiences, we encounter a myriad of complex influences on a child's learning experience. A narrower definition of curriculum has

Portions of this chapter originally appeared in **G. M. Morrison**, Relationship among academic, social, and career education in programming for handicapped students, in M. C. Wang, M. C. Reynolds, & H. J. Walberg (Eds.), *Handbook of special education: Research and practice.* Oxford England: Pergamon Press, in press.

been chosen to guide discussion in this chapter. Curriculum is defined as "a series of planned, systematic learning experiences organized around a particular rationale or philosophy of education (Wood & Hurley, 1977) that includes goals and objectives in particular content areas (i.e., language, cognitive, perceptual, etc.)" (Mori & Neisworth, 1983, p. 2). By considering curriculum as a blueprint for *content,* we are able to examine curricula, curriculum models, and strategies for curriculum decision making to illuminate the relationship between content areas and how decisions are made in reference to this relationship. Thus, the focus of discussions about curricula is on "what to teach" instead of on "how to teach," or on content instead of on instructional strategies.

CURRICULUM SOURCES

The focus, then, is on the "what" of programming because, as suggested by Poplin (1979), in many respects we do not know what is being taught in special education. It must be understood that curriculum decisions emanate from many sources. For example, philosophical trends influence decisions about curriculum. The recent emphasis on teaching the basics affects decisions about what to teach and how to prioritize offerings for LD students.

Government policies also affect the nature of the curriculum offered to LD students. The least restrictive environment mandate of Public Law 94-142 has affected where these children are educated, which ultimately has an effect on *what* they are taught. The individualized educational program mandate has resulted in a specific process for determining the content of individual programs that involves input from both school personnel and parents of disabled children. The appropriate education aspect of the law has implied that there are certain qualitative standards of education that must be met.

Certain historical developments in the field of education of disabled individuals have had a great impact on classroom practices. In terms of curriculum development, the use of the unit method in classes for the mentally retarded (Ingram, 1935; Meyen, 1972) provides a guide for teachers in content and skill areas. This method was very popular in the beginning years of the special day class arrangement. Even as the administrative structures of special education have changed, this method has provided a structure for curriculum in classrooms for disabled children.

DETERMINING GOAL PRIORITIES

The determination of curriculum content typically has been made with three major considerations: (1) consideration of the characteristics and needs of the students who will be exposed to the curriculum, (2) determination of "useful" content for these individuals, and (3) examination of the needs and values of the society in which these individuals will be participating (Klein, Pasch, & Frew, 1979; Willoughby–Herb, 1983). The third of these is perhaps the most complex and, potentially, the most influential. Societal influences can include the input of parents, concerned citizens, teachers, and other educational personnel who have a vested interest in the education of LD children. The values and biases of these parties must be considered in the curriculum development process, despite the fact that the biases may often be in conflict. For example, Elkind (1983) described the potential discrepancy between content-centered and child-centered curriculum. The curriculum that experts agree on (content-centered) may differ from that preferred by teachers (child-centered) who interact with children daily. However, some overall agreement on curriculum parameters is essential.

Perhaps the place to look for agreement is at the level of general goals for disabled individuals. Stemming from the *Report of the National Commission on Excellence in Education* in 1983 and subsequent discussions of this document (CEC Ad Hoc Committee, 1983; Will, 1984), the consensus seems to be that goals for disabled children should be the same as those for children without disabilities: students should be allowed to develop, to the maximum degree possible, those skills that will enable them to be productive adults. Although this goal seems straightforward, the various means to achieve it are certainly topics for debate. For example, which content areas should be mastered, and to what degree, to enable students to reach this goal?

Reynolds and Birch (1982) described the distinction between cultural imperatives and cultural electives in the consideration of educational programming. Cultural imperatives are those skills that should be required of all students, whereas cultural electives are those skills that are not absolutely essential. Cultural imperatives include (1) speaking, listening, comprehending, reading, and writing for every day personal and social needs, (2) those basic math skills required in the marketplace for daily life, (3) the knowledge of self-care, health, and protection for community living, (4) social skills for acceptable behavior in citizenship and in group life, and (5) career education to prepare for employment, an economically useful life, and other life roles.

Of the above areas, those involving academic subjects traditionally have received greater emphasis in curriculum plans (Polloway, Payne, Patton, & Payne, 1985). As exemplified in *Lau v. Nichols* (1977), parents, in particular, want their children to be prepared to compete successfully in the society in which they live. Academic skills are considered critical in gaining this success. Smith and Dexter (1980) defined basic academics as "those fundamental skills which are considered prerequisite for the effective functioning of any individual in the every day life of our society" (p. 72). However, given this broad definition of basic academics, social and career education become keys to "effective functioning" for LD individuals.

Historical Influences

The degree of emphasis placed on the acquistion of academic skills changes with time and the zeitgeist of the era. For example, the movement of the 1920s and 1930s to place mildly mentally retarded individuals in special classrooms was, in part, intended to remove them from high expectations for academic achievement and to provide a more "well-rounded" program, including social and vocational skill training. As a result of a philosophical movement away from the potentially stigmatizing effects of segregating these students and a failure to document the academic benefits of special class placement (Kirk, 1964), a range of less restrictive placement alternatives became available. Two of these alternatives, placement in regular classrooms and placement in resource room programs, represent returns to an emphasis on academic skill training.

Although program emphasis is not always clearly delineated, efficacy studies do not always match program priorities with the weighting of emphasis on outcome variables (MacMillan & Semmel, 1977). However, the main point is that prioritization of content goals of curricula for LD students is influenced significantly by the programming philosophies of the time. The LD field faces a debate about curricular content emphasis, especially with respect to the relative contributions of academic goals and social or vocational objectives.

Philosophical Influences

In support of emphasizing the teaching of cognitive skills, Elkind (1983) encouraged giving up the "clinical bifurcation" of cognitive and affective instruction. He believed that a good curriculum does not need an affective component. Learning, if properly arranged, is naturally socially motivated. However, some professionals believe that social and affective development in disabled children cannot be taken for granted, given the extra challenges these individuals face in adapting to their life settings (Dil, 1983; Strain, Cooke, & Apolloni, 1976). These professionals emphasize understanding disabled children as they function cognitively *and* socially in environments inside and outside of school. This more ecological view of the child recognizes that progression or regression in one realm (cognitive or social) of a child's functioning affects functioning in the other realm. However, acceptance of teaching social and affective skills has been slow, perhaps because of the generally sensitive and inherently more complex nature of these skills (Childs, 1979).

Although the struggle in prioritization more commonly takes place between the academic and social areas of the curriculum, advocates for vocational and career education have been more vocal in the last 10 years (Brolin, 1982). Some support an emphasis on vocational skills in educational planning for LD students, especially during adolescent years as these individuals prepare to enter the job market or postschool job placements (Greenan, 1982; Muraski, 1982). Others support the incorporation of career educational goals and objectives throughout students' tenure in the educational system (Brolin, 1982; Mori, 1982; Muenster, 1982). This more comprehensive view of career education defines a "lifelong developmental process that allows individuals to acquire the attitudes, habits, values, and skills to prepare for a successful and personally satisfactory work life" (Mori, 1982, p. 41). This kind of curriculum incorporates academic and social skills as part of the preparation for the work world. Career education does not imply a concentration on one content area at the expense of another, but advocates the integration of all content areas toward the achievement of career success.

THE ROLE OF POLICY IN CURRICULUM DECISIONS

The intent of Public Law 94-142 is to provide an "appropriate" education for all handicapped children. Providing an "appropriate" education requires decisions about curriculum and programming. Two major components of Public Law 94-142 (least restrictive environment and individualized educational program) affect the content of special education programming.

Appropriate Education

The question of appropriate education has been the focus of several landmark cases in the United States. Early cases such as the *Pennsylvania Association for Retarded Children v. the Secretary of Education, PA* (1972) stated that education is a basic right that cannot be denied nonhandicapped *or* handicapped individuals. Given this basic right, the *content* of education and treatment came into focus with *Wyatt v. Stickney* (1972), which ensured a "realistic opportunity to lead a more useful and meaningful life and return to society"; the Pennhurst (1981) standards of "appropriate habilitation in the least restrictive environment"; and the *Youngberg v. Romeo* (1982) decision that ensured "minimally adequate training." The interpretation of these decisions is related to content issues because they indicate a level of quality that must be adhered to. The courts have found it necessary to specify not only the right to education but what might be construed to be the right to a certain quality of education. The implications of the latter involvement could have significant effects on what is to be taught to LD individuals.

Least Restrictive Environment

The least restrictive environment component of PL 94-142 specified that the LD child must be educated, to the maximum extent appropriate, with children who are not disabled. The major vehicle for compliance with this mandate has been the availability of a continuum of placements for LD students that vary with the extent of restrictiveness (Deno, 1970). Although basically administrative in nature, these placements have a critical impact on the nature of the curriculum offered to students (Meyen & Horner, 1976). Meyen and Horner (1976) described the curricular consequences of alternative models for placement as they vary according to (a) the teacher who has responsibility for instruction, (b) the amount of time a child spends in each setting, (c) the focus of the total instructional program, (d) the locus of administrative control (regular or special education), and (e) the heterogeneity of pupil characteristics.

The balance of content offerings vary in different settings. A resource room arrangement usually offers instruction in specific academic areas to a child for a few hours per day. LD students who are in this setting might receive social and vocational instruction in their regular classroom settings. Alternatively, in a special day class setting, the LD child is offered a total and, it is hoped, well-rounded program encompassing all educational needs. Curricular emphases are likely to vary vastly from setting to setting for LD children, as are the desired individual outcomes for these children (Morrison & MacMillan, 1983). Meyen and Horner (1976) warned that "unless the curriculum dimension of mainstreaming is successfully dealt with, like the special class, mainstreaming will become an additional administrative model rather than an instructional delivery system" (p. 268).

Individualized Educational Programs

The mandate for Individualized Educational Programs (IEPs) for all handicapped children has greatly affected the nature of curriculum decision making. Decisions about the goals and objectives of a program for an individual child must be made with the input of a multidisciplinary team that includes child's parents and, when appropriate, the child. Institutionalization of the IEP team has made parental input more influential than it was in the past. Although the amount of influence that parents have on an IEP team has been questioned (Yoshida, Fenton, Maxwell, & Kaufman, 1978), the opportunity exists for parents to directly affect the prioritization of goals and objectives for their child.

Acknowledging the impact that the IEP mandate has had on programming for disabled children, the distinction should be made between individualized programming and comprehensive programming. Individualized programming is defined by Mercer and Mercer (1981) as "an instructional program in which the student works on appropriate tasks over time under conditions that are motivating. It may occur within various instructional arrangements . . . ." (p. 4). In contrast, comprehensive programming, as used in this chapter, refers to the consideration of curriculum decisions in the context of constructing an overall program for disabled students as groups. The danger that exists in special education today is ignoring comprehensive programming in lieu of the creation of numerous individual plans.

ORGANIZATION AND EMPHASIS OF CURRICULUM CONTENT

The "what to teach" decisions in curriculum planning for LD students are generally focused on three broad areas: academic, social, and vocational. Selection of specific skills within these areas and emphasis placed on skills differ according to the age of the target students, the nature of their LD conditions, and the general philosophy and values of those in decision-making positions (parents, teachers, and other pertinent school personnel).

The following examples demonstrate how curriculum content is organized and emphasized primarily for the mildly mentally retarded. The LD field has not devoted similar efforts to the structuring of curriculum, but these examples illustrate how the process is conceptualized and may be, at least, partly applicable to planning for LD students.

Age and Content Interaction

Campbell (1968) graphically captured the relationship between age (level of schooling) and instructional emphasis for various content areas and nature of disablity (Figure 1-1). Content areas are charted according to the degree of instructional emphasis at different academic levels. It should be noted that the chart represents a program as it would be presented in a special day class format. Skill emphasis would be expected to change according to the administrative arrangement associated with content presentation.

Perhaps the greatest utility of a model that charts changes across age levels for instructional emphasis is as a guide for curriculum development efforts. Similar models have been used for emotionally disturbed children (McDowell & Brown, 1978) and for demonstrating the developmental aspects of career education (Muenster, 1982). This model could also be

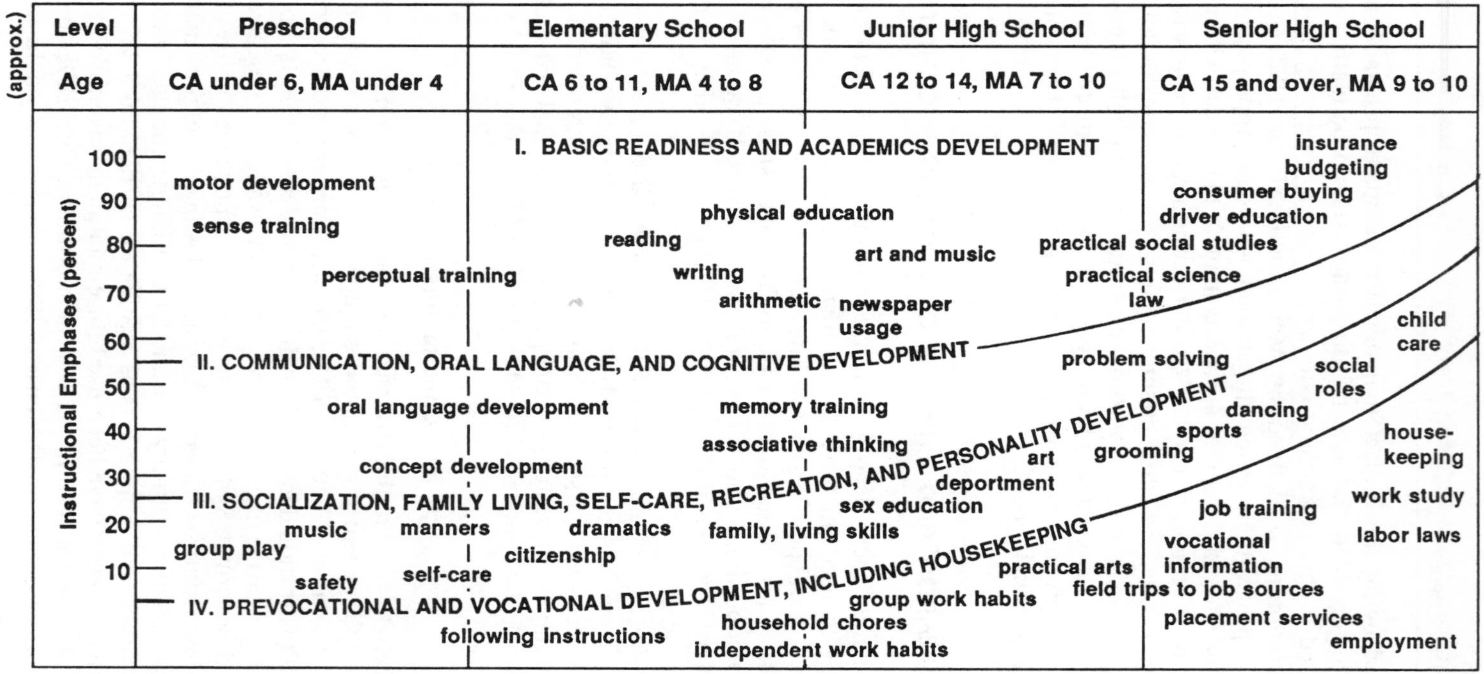

Level	Preschool	Elementary School	Junior High School	Senior High School
Age	CA under 6, MA under 4	CA 6 to 11, MA 4 to 8	CA 12 to 14, MA 7 to 10	CA 15 and over, MA 9 to 10

Instructional Emphases (percent) (approx.): 100, 90, 80, 70, 60, 50, 40, 30, 20, 10

I. BASIC READINESS AND ACADEMICS DEVELOPMENT

II. COMMUNICATION, ORAL LANGUAGE, AND COGNITIVE DEVELOPMENT

III. SOCIALIZATION, FAMILY LIVING, SELF-CARE, RECREATION, AND PERSONALITY DEVELOPMENT

IV. PREVOCATIONAL AND VOCATIONAL DEVELOPMENT, INCLUDING HOUSEKEEPING

- motor development
- sense training
- perceptual training
- oral language development
- concept development
- group play
- music
- manners
- safety
- self-care
- reading
- physical education
- writing
- arithmetic
- memory training
- associative thinking
- dramatics
- family, living skills
- citizenship
- following instructions
- household chores
- independent work habits
- art and music
- newspaper usage
- sex education
- art
- deportment
- group work habits
- practical arts
- field trips to job sources
- insurance
- budgeting
- consumer buying
- driver education
- practical social studies
- practical science
- law
- problem solving
- dancing
- sports
- grooming
- social roles
- child care
- house-keeping
- job training
- vocational information
- work study
- labor laws
- placement services
- employment

FIGURE 1–1

Curricular content areas by organizational levels in EMR programs. Adapted from L. W. Campbell, *Study of Curriculum Planning* (1965). California State Department of Education. Sacramento, California.

used as a guide for critiquing and adjusting existing programs, such as those represented by the curriculum guides described in the following section.

Cautions are necessary, however, in the uncritical use of this kind of model. First, empirical verification of changing emphases across age levels is nonexistent. Although one could argue convincingly that empirical verification may not be as critical as agreement by experts and consumers (parents and children), documentation is usually lacking about the latter as well. For example, Figure 1-1 shows a definite decrease in the emphasis of academic development. Despite the fact that most professionals might agree with that trend, some individuals (parents or professionals still looking for a cure) might strongly question the merit of "giving up" on academics at any stage. Therefore, the assumptions and philosophies behind the use of any guide should be examined for pertinence to the ultimate consumers of the resulting curriculum.

CURRICULUM GUIDES

A similar organization of content is available in less succinct and more detailed form in the array of curriculum guides throughout local school systems. The development of these guides was especially prevalent during the initial days of special day classes for disabled children, when the assumption of a different set of goals was new. However, as a survey conducted by Cegelka (1978) indicated, the majority of available curriculum guides have been developed specifically for use with mildly and moderately retarded students at the primary and intermediate levels.

In an evaluation of 250 curriculum guides, Simches and Bohn (1963) found that most were merely a "rephrasing and reemphasizing of available courses of study used for normal children that do not even have the benefit of form, structure, and sequence connected with standard curriculum development" (p. 115). Their objections were partly based on their contention that although mentally retarded children were originally put in special classrooms to provide them with a distinct curriculum, they were usually presented with a "watered-down" version of curricula encountered in regular classroom settings.

One of the more popular guides, developed by Goldstein and Siegle (1958), was the *Illinois Curriculum Guide,* which emphasized social and vocational skills. Basic tool subjects were presented in a context similar to that in which students would be expected to apply the skills. Cegelka's (1978) analysis of curriculum guides revealed a content redundancy based on the *Illinois Curriculum Guide* and noted that this content reflected the 1940s pioneering work in special education.

Although representing extensive efforts by professionals to compile recommended scope and sequences of tasks to teach mentally retarded children, the resulting guides need to be critically examined and updated in light of recent developments in instructional technology as well as in changing philosophies of what to teach these students. Periodic review of existing school district guides for curriculum is critical, not only to insure that there is some coherence in what students are taught, but to give teachers, and others involved in the educational system, the sense that they are active contributors to the decision-making process as well as participants in the implementation of curriculum goals.

Unit Method

The unit method is a curricular approach that emphasizes content that has been utilized mainly for mentally retarded students in special class settings. In this approach, content is structured or organized in units, which are based on areas of interest of retarded children. Skill areas are incorporated into activities that reflect these areas of interest. Reading, writing, language, arithmetic, social studies, and other skills are taught in the context of a unit topic such as "Playing House" or "Life on a Farm." Basic tool subjects are taught in situations in which actual applications can be made. Ingram (1935) suggested a number of criteria for effective units of experience. Units should include a variety of experiences that span the settings in which a student is expected to function (school, home, community). Units should emphasize activities that utilize tool subjects as well as provide opportunities for the development of social participation skills. Finally, unit selection should be based on the intended students' level of mental, social, and physical functioning.

Thorsell (1961) criticized unit topics as haphazard selections from regular education. Other criticisms of the unit method have included the isolation of individual units, lack of developmental sequence of concepts and content, and lack of uniqueness of content for problems of the mentally retarded.

In response to some of these criticisms, Meyen (1972) developed an organizational framework within which units can be developed. His "Life Experience Unit" approach is based on six core areas of learning experiences: arithmetic concepts, communication skills, social competencies, safety, health, and vocational skills. Skills and concepts from all core areas are included in each unit. Meyen outlined developmental steps and guidelines for writing Life Experience Units to ensure that units are comprehensive, integrated, and teach necessary academic and social skills. The unit approach presents content in an integrated manner to accommodate the special learning characteristics of the intended consumers, mentally retarded students. Emphasis is placed on teaching functional life skills, which necessitates the inclusion of skills from academic, social, and vocational areas. Skill selection is based on the usefulness of each skill for the life functioning of the students. The unit method might be seen as the forerunner of more recent efforts in the career development area.

Curriculum Development Projects

Before 1965 there were few major efforts to systematically develop curricula for disabled children. Curricular efforts were mainly reflected in curriculum guidelines compiled by state and local agencies. Meyen and Horner (1976) attributed this lack of emphasis on systematic curriculum development to several factors. First, despite the original reason for separating special education students (to provide them with a specialized curriculum), emphasis was placed on other aspects of special education, such as assessment of student characteristics and evaluation of the efficacy of administrative arrangements. Curriculum development often followed the latest trends in conceptualizing disabilities. For example, Strauss and Lehtinen (1947) recommended curricular modifications according to the etiology of learning problems (brain injury). This led to an approach developed according to a perceptual model. The mainstreaming movement also represented a movement motivated by philosophical, conceptual, and political reasons that had vast implications for curriculum planning. Again, curriculum played an accommodating rather than a leading role.

Another reason for lack of emphasis on formal curriculum development was the paucity of special educators trained in curriculum development for special education. This lack of professional commitment accompanied minimal availability of funds to develop a systematic curricula. However, to reverse this trend, there was an increased commitment of federal monies in the 1970s specifically for the purpose of curriculum designed for the mentally retarded.

A major contribution of the curriculum projects that came out of the 1970s was their example of how curricula could be constructed in a systematic and scholarly manner. Meyen and Horner (1976) presented a model of the influences that should be systematically used in the curriculum development process. The model emphasized child variability, material, institutional setting, and teacher characteristics as critical influences on curriculum. Consideration of these variables in the context of curriculum development follows certain stages: (a) specification of target population, needs, and objectives, (b) description of rationale and instructional design, (c) development and testing, (d) evaluation and revision, and (e) dissemination and implementation. The curriculum development process has been described in detail by Mayer (1982) and others associated with the projects described below. The process of curriculum development can be complex if quality products are to be produced, a fact not always appreciated by local school systems attempting to develop their own curricula. School districts must weigh the trade-off between having a well developed curriculum that local professionals do not feel ownership of versus one that they can relate to that is not appropriately documented or tested.

An example of an early curriculum project is the Social Learning Curriculum (Goldstein, 1975), which has been described as one of the most comprehensive curriculum design efforts. The focus of the curriculum is on the development of social competence in primary-level children. Integrated into the instructional experiences are emphases on skills and concepts related to language, math, and motor development. Development of this curriculum was based on models representing a child's need areas (physical, social, and psychological) and expanding environment (self, home and family, neighborhood, and community). The overall scheme of the curriculum is represented in phase books covering the following topics: perceiving individuality, recognizing the environment, recognizing interdependence, recognizing the body, recognizing and reacting to emotions, recognizing what senses do, communicating with others, getting along with others, identifying helpers, and maintaining body functions. The design of activities in these books encourages the use of inductive teaching strategies. This curriculum represents an effort to integrate critical content areas into a topical presentation of material.

Career Education Programs

Advocates for the implementation of a comprehensive career education program argue convincingly that career education can become a vehicle for teaching academic and social skills as well as vocational skills (Brolin, 1982; Leggett, 1978; Muenster, 1982). Leggett (1978) described the significant overlap of special education and career education programming goals. Overlapping characteristics include (a) the development of self-awareness in terms of interests, attitudes, and capabilities; (b) a commitment to the development of the whole child, capitalizing on strengths and remediating deficits; (c) the development of an awareness of others and ways of facilitating interpersonal interactions; and (d) an awareness of careers and the competencies necessary to succeed in those careers. Leggett called for the expansion of the "friendship of commitment" into a true partnership of special and career education.

The Council for Exceptional Children (1978) defined career education as

the totality of experiences through which one learns to live a meaningful, satisfying work life... providing the opportunity to learn, in the least restrictive environment possible, the academic, daily living, personal-social, and occupational knowledges and skills necessary for attaining their highest levels of economic, personal, and social fulfillment. This can be obtained through work (both paid and unpaid) and in a variety of other societal roles and personal life styles ... student, citizen, volunteer, family member, and participant in meaningful leisure-time activities. (Brolin, 1982, p. 3)

Brolin (1982) described a Life Centered Career Education (LCCE) model developed to combine the goals of special and career education. LCCE is designed to promote the acquisition of three major categories of competencies (daily, personal-social, and occupational skills) throughout four stages of career development (awareness, exploration, preparation, and placement, follow-up, and continuing education) starting early in elementary school and spanning a student's educational career. The teaching of target skills takes place within the contexts of a student's school, family, and community. Brolin emphasized that "career education is not intended to replace traditional education but, rather, to redirect it to be more relevant and meaningful for the student and to result in the acquisition of attitudes, knowledges, and skills one needs for successful community living and working" (p. 3).

Although career education offers a seemingly logical organizaton and weighting of competencies in academic, social, and vocational areas, such programs have not been adopted extensively. Burton and Bero (1984) surveyed junior and senior high school teachers and local employers and found that there were large gaps in teacher and employer perceptions of what skills and abilities are necessary to prepare students for life and work. Teachers focused on isolated job-related tasks and basic academic skills, whereas employers emphasized the need for personal, social, and coping skills. There was little recognition of the relationship between academics and career education competencies outlined in programs such as that of Brolin (1982). The viability of a career education method of integrating content depends on educational personnel recognizing its compatibiity with existing programming (see Ellington & Winskoff, 1982) and its potential for offering a comprehensive, relevant organization of curriculum content.

CONTENT DECISIONS

The models and orientation described thus far all contribute to the final decisions concerning program content. If one of these models and the accompanying products or guides for products is not adopted intact by a consumer group, decisions regarding curriculum content will be critically influenced by the decision-making process itself. Meyen (1982) described curriculum development as a process and a legacy, noting the "startling lack of papers dealing with curriculum development" (p. 1). The documentation of a decision-making process in the development of a curriculum may be a more valuable contribution, in the long run, than the curriculum product itself. Although personal and professional philosophies and state-of-the-art knowledge change with time, decision-making models can always be adapted for use in new curriculum development efforts.

Prioritizing Goals and Objectives

Although comprehensive curriculum development models have been described in the literature (see Mayer, 1982), few of these deal specifically with the process of weighting the emphasis of content areas. Isolated attempts have been made to prioritize the importance of teaching skills to specified groups of disabled children. For example, Geiger, Brownsmith, and Forgnone (1978) surveyed 122 teachers to determine the relative importance of 550 skills and 26 skill areas in the instructional process. Teachers ranked these skills on a 5-point rating scale that ranged from "essential" to "very unimportant." There was strong agreement between the relative rankings of general skills and specific skills, despite the fact that these rankings were done independently. The authors emphasized the importance of this consensus of skill importance as a first step in improving the quality of programming.

The preceding example of prioritizing goals (Geiger et al., 1978) focused on the input of teachers. Input should also be considered from parents, community members, and other professionals who are concerned about quality education for LD children. A system could conceivably be constructed to include and weight input from these other sources.

Matching Goals and Objectives to Individual Needs

The decision-making processes described thus far have been concerned with the prioritization of goals and objectives for groups of disabled youngsters. A key to making any curricular approach relevant and effective is to match it to the critical characteristics of the consumers, that is, the disabled children themselves. Poplin and Gray (1980) noted

> The danger of using a predetermined curriculum as the basis for assessment and instructional programming, no matter how sound its rationale, is that the curriculum becomes the master; the child's needs are seen only in terms of what the curriculum has to offer. The only content suitable as a basis for effective assessment and instruction results from a comparison of the child's present abilities and the

abilities and understanding necessary for a satisfying and self-fulfilling life. (p. 78)

This passage reinforces the need to link a child's characteristics with the determination and prioritization of specific goals and objectives. This theme is realized in the mandate of PL 94-142 for Individualized Educational Programs (IEPs). The requirements of the IEPs themselves and the process surrounding their construction insures the link between a child's characteristics and program goals.

Dardig and Heward (1981) described a procedure for prioritizing IEP goals. The procedure includes listing and discussing many possible goals, determining criteria for prioritizing goals, individual team member ratings, synthesizing individual responses, and producing a prioritized list of annual goals. They suggested the following criteria for prioritizing annual goals:

- Will the child be able to use the skill in the immediate environment?
- Is it a functional, useful skill?
- Will the child be able to use the skill often?
- Has the child demonstrated an interest in learning this skill?
- Is success in teaching this skill likely?
- Is the skill a prerequisite for learning more complex skills?
- Will the child become more independent as a result of learning this skill?
- Will the skill allow the child to qualify for improved or additional services, or services in a less restrictive environment?
- Is it important to modify this behavior because it is dangerous to the child or others?

Each team member rates the list of goals according to each criterion (1 = lowest priority, 5 = highest priority). The ratings of each team member are synthesized into a group rating, which serves as the final prioritization. The suggested procedure provides a systematic process of goal prioritization that should contribute to the productivity and ease of working of IEP teams. Additionally, it provides a sound basis for decisions about the emphasis of various content areas for individual LD students.

Poplin (1979) outlined a three-step procedure for coordinating curriculum and IEP development, emphasizing a more traditional approach: (1) delineate goals or constructs of a given special education area (e.g., academics or self-help), (2) delineate general objectives, and (3) reduce general objectives to short-term instructional goals. The resulting curricular maps are used as a source for selection of goals and objectives as well as a structure for monitoring and evaluating student progress. Poplin emphasized that "special educators should never be forced to use a set of curriculum objectives that they have not had an active part in developing" (p. 5). Poplin also noted that the disadvantages of the time-consuming processes were outweighed by the advantages of having an original and relevant set of curriculum objectives.

The decision-making procedures previously outlined represent considerations of disabled children as members of groups and as individuals. Voeltz, Evans, Freedland, and Donellon (1982) analyzed the decision-making patterns of teachers in the process of prioritizing goals for educational programming. These investigators found that teachers considered both general professional education practices *and* the individual characteristics of disabled children. It is likely that group and individual perspectives for prioritizing content areas are both necessary considerations in the provision of appropriate programs for LD students.

Integrating Academic, Social, and Career Education

Recognizing the numerous historical, philosophical, theoretical, empirical, and policy influences that affect programs for disabled children is a first step in answering questions about the relationship among academic, social, and career content emphases. With the advent of PL 94-142 and its mandates (least restrictive environment, individualized educational programs, due process, and nondiscriminatory assessment), process has become a critical variable in the determination of educational programming. That is, a structure has been established for making decisions about the education of disabled children. The process remains constant for all children, but the content of what is recommended for each child differs as a result of the contributors to the process. In other words, contributors to the construction of overall curriculum patterns in the past, such as parents and educational personnel, are now determining similar patterns at individual levels.

From one perspective, it makes sense to define process variables for the determination of content presentation because process variables are more general than specific patterns of curricular content matched with individual characteristics. Process variables can also be expected to last, in contrast to content emphasis that may vary according to current trends.

However, there are dangers in relying too heavily on process guidelines for the determination of *what* to teach LD students. One danger is that a focus on individual decision making might devalue the development of an overall curricular plan for disabled children as a group. Despite the variability within this group, these individuals have certain needs in common that can be addressed by a systematic, organized approach to the prioritization and presentation of content. Further, a single individualized approach cannot take advantage of the accumulated knowledge that has been amassed on how best to educate children with certain characteristics.

Therefore, it seems wise to recommend a balance between the individualized approach inherent in the IEP process and a global approach guided by verified practices.

Another trend that will influence future programming efforts in the education of disabled children is that of accountability. Accountability is critical at all levels, from research and development projects to the implementation of individual programs. The underlying intent of the push for accountability is to provide proven practices for use in the education of disabled children.

Focus for Research and Development

Questions about the relationship among academic, social, and career goals for programming effectiveness have not been satisfactorily answered. Should one content area be preferred above the others? What should the order of prioritization be? Are content areas best taught in concert in an integrated curriculum? Of course, the answers to these questions will vary according to students' disabilities and age levels.

Although the logical impulse is to say that these questions need to be answered through vigorous and well-controlled research studies, several cautions should be noted. First, we may be asking the wrong questions. A parallel situation can be found in the classic question, "Does mainstreaming work?" The error is primarily in asking a simplistic question for a complex situation. However, as Forness and Kavale (1984) suggested, the question of proven procedures has been confused with a question of policy. The question of prioritization of curriculum content areas might be answered if there were agreement on what the desired outcomes should be. However, given the necessity of considering the opinions of many individuals, it is unlikely that an agreement on preferred outcomes could be obtained. Therefore, research documented answers to these questions would be accepted as valid by some but not others ... and we are once again in the fact versus philosophy bind.

Inherent conflicts of interest between researchers and practitioners further complicate the issue of programming effectiveness. For example, educators who are working with children in the schools need answers and solutions right now. The questions to which they need answers are broad and involve numerous variables. They need answers to these questions within the contingencies of administrative systems that cannot change for the sake of a well-controlled study. On the other hand, researchers are committed to answering questions according to certain methods to get valid and reliable answers. The nature of many methodologies typically used in the social sciences requires that questions be answered in small bits and pieces, ideally with as much control over the environment as possible. Therefore, educational research is usually reduced to how much control can be compromised to answer some of the pressing questions related to practice (or how "loose" can this study be and still get published?). In order to change these inherent conflicts between research and practice, further examination of both systems will be needed to identify where compromises can most effectively be made.

Despite conflicts, there are avenues in which research and development efforts could provide leadership. These efforts could focus on decision-making processes and how different patterns of influence within these processes affect educational outcomes for disabled children. Morrison, MacMillan, and Kavale (1985) noted that the procedures utilized in referral, assessment, and identification processes significantly affect a child's placement and, therefore, the overall program focus. Ysseldyke and Algozzine (1982) and others (Yoshida et al., 1978) have documented the numerous influences that determine decisions made by multidisciplinary teams. If these processes are a major factor in the determination of educational programming for disabled children, then the development of effective, exemplary practice is critical.

Ultimately, educational programming for disabled children should include consideration of the relationship of programming to the larger context of schools, in general, or regular education, in particular. Quality education for disabled students would be more likely if this relationship were clearly defined. Perhaps the vehicle for considering this larger issue is one in which regular education is now heavily involved, the effective schools movement (Averch, Carroll, Donaldson, Kiesling, & Pincus, 1984). Some of the indicators of effective schools are clear school mission, instructional leadership, high expectations, emphasis on academics, frequent monitoring of student progress and its utilization in curriculum planning, and home-school relations. These variables are logically related to effective programming for disabled children as well. Many questions must be considered: How does school-wide curriculum relate to that specifically geared to disabled children? Are the same sets of goals and objectives pertinent for disabled children? How do they vary? In what way are they the same? What is the responsibility of school-wide personnel for involvement in the education of disabled children? What is the administrative and instructional relationship between regular and special education?

Perhaps the most critical component in the curriculum development process is the individual teacher. The teacher must be aware of exemplary practices and must be a critical consumer about what is available. As the person who plans and implements programs for LD students at a very basic level, the teacher must be in a position to make informed decisions.

For example, the availability of "canned" curricula is increasing. Professionals who are potential consumers of these curricula need to be able to decide which packages are quality programs. Meyen and Horner (1975) recommended the following questions to guide the review of a curriculum:

- What was the project's organizational structure?
- What individuals were responsible for conducting the curriculum development activities?
- What model or body of research formed the basis for the curriculum?
- What curriculum products have been produced, and how are they being disseminated?
- Who are the individuals who are expected to use the curriculum products?
- Who are the individuals who are expected to be taught with the curriculum products?
- Does the curriculum design specify a particular organizational structure (i.e., classroom, resource room, one-to-one, etc.)?
- What is the content of the curriculum products?
- Does the curriculum specify a particular teaching format?
- What procedure was used to evaluate the curriculum products? (p. 271)

As implementors of programs for LD children, teachers hold a great deal of power, as well as responsibility, in guiding the planning of effective programs.

In addition to being critical consumers of existing curricula, teachers should also have the competencies and motivation to become more personally involved in curriculum development efforts. As Poplin (1979) emphasized, this involvement has the advantage of facilitating increased teacher competence and confidence as well as increasing the effectiveness of educational programming. Fergason noted that without the effort of teachers of severely handicapped children to implement the "spirit" of policy-backed philosophy of training functional skills, reform and development efforts in this area are threatened. Teacher involvement and commitment may be critical not only in the implementation, but in the development of programming structure and guidelines. One way of facilitating this process is to provide some level of training in curriculum development at the preservice level.

Another of the key competencies that a teacher should have for curriculum development is the ability to collaborate with other professionals. Teacher training has typically focused on teaching skills to work with disabled children as opposed to working with other adults. An investigation by Morrison, Lieber, and Morrison (in press) revealed that regular and special education teachers viewed situations in which they needed to meet with other teachers and professionals as anxiety-provoking events for which they were ill-equipped. Thus, group process and leadership skills might be an important target for emphasis in future training efforts. If, as suggested earlier in this chapter, decision-making processes are critical to the development of effective programming, then training key personnel in these processes is one step to insuring effective programs for LD children.

SUMMARY

This chapter has described major influences on what is taught to LD students. It should be noted that some of the contributing factors were dated in terms of their major impact. Further, none of the avenues to development of curriculum approaches were systematic or comprehensive. It is obvious that LD professionals must renew their interest in and commitment to the development of a strong curricular structure. Any efforts in this direction should include a careful examination of the many factors that insure a sound, cohesive structure for LD students.

CHAPTER 2

Curriculum Planning

M. E. B. Lewis

C urriculum is intended to be a series of activities providing introduction, exercise, and application of skills necessary to perform specific learning tasks. The sequence is an infinite spiral projection, formalized in an academic setting, carrying the student toward independent learning. The generation of such curriculum usually reflects the educational philosophy of its creators. One approach to creating a scheme of learning activities is the *thematic approach,* a humanistic approach presenting developmental instructional tasks in a limited format. The format relates all stimulae to one central idea. The ideas should be relevant to the current experiences and settings of the students. Through a year-long projection of themes, skills, and media an innovative, evaluative, and controllable product emerges. This chapter explores the curricular mode, the instructional setting, the specific population, the applicability of results, and a related *caveat.*

A BRIEF HISTORY

Curriculum is by nature sequential, assisting an individual along a continuum of learning, providing experiences and reasoned objectives for

This chapter originally appeared as an article by **M. E. B. Lewis** in *Learning Disabiities: An Interdisciplinary Journal* (Vol. I (3), 25–33, 1982) and was adapted by permission of Grune & Stratton for inclusion in this *Handbook.*

learning new things. By building on prerequisite skills brought to the new learning task by the student, teachers can challenge students to solve problems by using what they know and, it is hoped, by helping them toward independent thinking and diminished reluctance to approach the unknown.

There are both philosophical and psychological models for generating curriculum (McNeil, 1976). These relate to beliefs about the nature of learning, the purpose of learning, and the nature and purpose of the learner (Pratt, 1980; Rubin, 1977). These beliefs range from idealistic notions about the intrinsic values of education as expressed in Greek and Roman cultures to realistic and pragmatic theories of modern pedagogical and psychological theorists. It has only been in this century that the mass production of reading matter and mandated opportunities for individuals to pursue an education and to learn have flourished.

Ancient civilizations believed that learning and the formal process of education were purposeful arts, disciplining the mind and spirit to reason and govern. They were not intended for general consumption. This elitist posture continued to the Renaissance and Reformation, when mere discipline and mental exercise were replaced with notions of feeding the inner and outer man so that he might understand and enjoy science, nature, literature and serve God and man as well. This preindustrial European expansion of learning caused some to wonder about what was to be learned. Mere mental calisthenics would no longer suffice. In the twelfth century, Peter of Blois queried:

> What does it profit a student to spend his days in these things which neither in the Army, nor in the cloister, nor in politics, nor in the church, nor anywhere else are any good to anyone — except in the schools. (Pratt, 1980, p. 20)

Variety and versatility characterized the Renaissance, but today's mass education mandate requires a new approach. With compulsory education comes a varied population to educate — the gifted, the able, the disabled, the unable. Creative curricula must emerge to solve the problem of stimulating and challenging all learners to their potential for achievement, mindful of the affective as well as the cognitive domain.

Modern curriculum developers, therefore, design their products with philosophies in mind (McNeil, 1976). These include *perennialism,* the belief that the purpose of education is unchanging, that is, perennial. Verbal ability is stressed, and liberal education (as opposed to vocational education) is considered the best means for generating a fully intellectually developed individual. The drawbacks to such a model are obvious.

Revelance or social reconstructionism stresses society's need for the services of the individual over any considerations for the individual's needs within the society. Effecting community change through analysis of problems is the objective of training. An underlying assumption is made about the innate potential and strength of the learner. A value system consistent among those who will be trained and the maintenance of such a value system are implied. There is an advantage to such a system, however, in that problem solving, a high level skill (Bloom, 1976; Gagne, 1965), is the target.

A conservative and American belief about education underlies the third philosophy, *essentialism*. Schools are for basic learning, the so-called 3R's. Thorough grounding in basics is all that is necessary. No intrinsic values. No proposed outcomes. A good foundation. The rest is extraneous. The implied beliefs of the work ethic are here. Modern competency-based curriculum has its roots in this philosophy. There are indeed values to good grounding in the basics for sound education. The drawbacks to competency-based education, however, include the trap of a minimum competency setting. Aiming for the minimum instead of the maximum can reduce student motivation to achieve.

Cognitivism is a psychological exercise in problem solving to avoid repeated error. Organizational skill is developed throughout the individual's educational career to allow problem solving in the most productive and efficient manner. In this era of proficiency measurement, this theory has its merits. Its technological edge precludes affective development to any great extent. Value is placed on analysis and conceptualization.

Conversely, the affective domain is given a place in the *self-actualization* model of curriculum development. The objectives of education and of learning are independence and contentment. A fulfilled individual is often a more productive member of society and, hence, is more likely to approach the potential to achieve "Wholeness" is a concern of the curriculum developer because, as educators, we have an obligation to the whole student. Provided that a balance between affect and cognition is maintained, this philosophy provides a foundation for thematic development of curriculum.

Philosophical models mesh with certain psychological conceptions about learning. Four factors must be considered in the development of any curriculum — the task, the learner, the sequence, and the means of evaluating the complete process.

The application of the thematic approach outlined in this chapter reflects considerations of the psychological factors and adherences to elements of perennialism, essentialism, and self-actualization.

APPLICATION

When an LD program is thematic, instruction is reflected through a common theme approach to all subjects taught in the course of a given period of time. Instruction can be implemented through multisensory activities, VAKT, Fernald language experience, structural and phonetic analysis, whole group instruction, small group instruction, one-to-one instruction, peer learning, and most recently, the use of personal computers, including the programming of those computers.

Certain assumptions underlie the implementation of any curriculum with a homogeneous population of severely learning disabled children. Typically, such students have experienced up to 5 years of school failure and have certain fears and long held personal perceptions that often have to be clarified before meaningful instruction can begin. Further explanation of this is discussed in the rationale of one of the sample thematic units found at the end of this chapter. The assumptions held for implementing thematic instruction with the learning disabled can include:

- LD students are normal people.
- LD students require a great deal of structure in their programs of instruction, in their learning environment, and in the management of their behavior.
- Learning is a multisensory process.
- Students learn best that which they can react to and experience directly.
- Skills taught in isolation have a transient rather than a permanent effect.
- Language skills cannot be divorced from content skills.
- Repetition of concepts and procedures is essential to internalization.
- A history of school failure recommends new and different approaches over the standard task hierarchy presentation of material and curriculum.

Kubie (1964) expressed the view that there is a distinction between discipline and freedom that the mere polarity of their placement in educational theory indicates. Writing during the turbulent decade when a good part of the current educational rhetoric and technology emerged, Kubie indicated that merely programming teachers to sequence behaviors and give tools to students does not serve their avowed pedagogical duties —they must discipline students enough to think and apply their thoughts as they will, freely. Educators have not been distinguished by their embrace of what goes on outside the classroom. Only recent minimum competency standard settings and functional literacy requirements have bought educators into the real world.

The National Council of Teachers of English publishes an annual collection of thematic language arts units to encourage English and reading teachers at the secondary level to recognize that instruction revolving around a cogent and relevant theme motivates students to be more creative, organized, and sensitive. Themes such as growing old, humor, death, advertising, sports, careers, feminism, and politics arouse teachers and students to meet a multisensory challenge. Such themes also give a needed incentive to teachers still clinging to the ideas of genre (the novel, poetry, drama) and skill (spelling, letter writing, grammar) as curricular ends in themselves, rather than as means of implementing instruction within a more global intercurricular theme.

There is a paucity of research and literature on the thematic approach in curriculum. Its values in application at the secondary level are traditionally known in the isolated application of a single content area.

Themes can be decided on in advance for the entire academic year. For example:

September: Who Am I? — introduction to individuals and their limitations.

October: Mystery — observation and inferential thinking skills.

November: Sports — a kinesthetic motivational unit for demonstrating power and learning socialization.

December: Money — planning a budget reading advertisements, making decisions.

January: Travel — an exploration of the world, including cultures, money, traditions, religions, map reading, schedule reading, cooking.

February: Politics — issues, debate, expression of opinions, reading and listening to the news.

March: Entertainment — media, live performance, writing.

April: Animals — sex education, wild life throughout the world, survival, evolution, keeping a pet responsibly.

May: Local Geographic Area — ethnic groups, historical sights, cooking local attractions and problems.

All instruction revolves around the theme. Everything the students read, write, hear, discuss, calculate, all social concepts, all scientific concepts, all elective applications that can be made (e.g., art, music) are based on the theme. This allows students to see a connection among the isolated periods of the day. Classes need not be self-contained. Students can be grouped primarily by ability and secondarily by level of maturity. Their schedule can be varied and yet structured. The applications for these themes are demonstrated in the sample curricular outlines included at the end of this chapter in Appendix 2-1.

ASSUMPTIONS ABOUT LEARNING

LD students are normal people LD students are active, inquisitive youngsters who often have a desire to learn but have experienced frustraation from years of failure in regular elementary schools. They do not wish to be treated as different or as unable to grasp whatever their age peers can grasp. The application of the thematic approach, then, is one that is not necessarily a special education procedure. Relating curriculum to student need and experience is not the domain of any special education area.

LD students require a great deal of structure in their programs of instruction. LD students are often described as students who have "fallen between the cracks" in educational programming. They are students who require strong organizational measures to establish tasks and to provide a channel for accomplishment of those tasks. Thematic instruction provides connection among the academic and nonacademic subjects of the day, giving students the means for establishing the relationship between information covered in a morning social studies and an assignment in an afternoon writing class. All learning should be purposeful (Pratt, 1980; Gorman, 1974) but purpose must be concretely established for the disabled learner to appreciate such purpose.

All activities in a curriculum for LD students must be structured for accountability. Does the instruction reflect teacher awareness of the student's special needs? Does such instruction reflect understanding and value of the student's strengths? Development of units of instruction relevant to students' experiences assists accountability. For example, in a population that is mostly male city dwellers, sports works well and offers variety in programming. A unit on humor or satire may not work as well, since humor requires a high level of verbal skills that some LD students may not have acquired. Such a unit would reflect the planners lack of awareness of student characteristics.

LD students require a great deal of structure in their learning environment. Among the identifying characteristics of LD students are concentration and attention deficits. Creating the appropriate physical setting for learning takes care, time, and creativity. A classroom with too many distracting posters, bulletin boards, and equipment will serve to confuse students and to confound the teacher's purpose. The learning environment also reflects the way teachers conceive the nature of learning. A classroom set up with the teacher's desk in the center front, looking out over rows of desks, presents the teacher as the center of instruction, the source of all information. Conversely, a total learning center arrangement, with independent stations set up around the room, belies an assumption of maturity, self-motivation, and ability on the part of students that may not be present. Ideally, students should work for part of each period on an independent assignment and for the rest of the period in group instruction. Distraction should be minimized. Posters and bulletin boadrs should be relevant to the theme and strategically placed in the room.

LD students require a great deal of structure in the management of their behavior. The best conceived and programmed curriculum, the most innovative instruction, is worthless without responsible behavior from the learner. A history of school failures produces frustration and related behavior. One system of behavior management is a nontangible point system. For example, criteria of performance can be used and applied ten times during the day. Under such a system, students are encouraged to assume responsibility for a standard of behavior by timing themselves out, ignoring distracting behaviors from others, and gaining privileges. This enhances an ability to remain on task.

Learning is a multisensory process. Educators have an obligation to educate the whole child in the most appropriate manner. We know that some individuals respond more readily to visual stimulation than to auditory stimulation. Recognizing that, we have an obligation to stimulate all sensory channels. Materials should be presented in as varied a manner as possible. The effects of reinforcement are acute and the fact that students can choose the manner in which they will learn a particular new skill assists them in becoming more responsible and more satisfied that they have a role in their education.

Bombardment with printed material is unfair to the LD student, whose problems with learning may stem from a language-processing problem or a visual-processing problem. The world has much printed material, but a large amount of what stimulates the adult is in other sensory modes. News is reported orally as well as visually. We become informed outside of school in more ways than books, papers, and worksheets.

Students learn best that which they can relate to and experience directly. Abstract concepts, prolonged debate of esoteric issues, and manipulation of foreign objects do not work well as a foundation for teaching the learning disabled. The thematic approach is founded on principles of pragmatism — what can the student do with what he or she is learning? Topics of interest are generated out of what is known about the daily experiences of the student. Sports, money, and travel can be quite motivating. It's vital that themes include direct experiences such as films, field trips, and artifacts.

Skills taught in isolation have a transient rather than a permanent effect. Spelling today, grammar tomorrow, and comprehension questions the next day present valuable information in an unconnected manner. If learning is indeed a continuum, the links between skills must be made plain to the learner. Meaningful application comes through repetition and fresh application of skills in a content area.

Language skills cannot be divorced from content skills. The language arts classroom is the domain of reading, spelling, grammar, usage, writing, vocabulary development, and oral language skills. Mathematics, social studies, science, art, music, physical education, industrial arts, and drama each have a vocabulary. The correct spelling of terms is essential to expressive writing in any content area. The appropriate application of terminology to projects, to assignments, and to giving and receiving directions is part of all content study. Needless to say, reading is vital, and therefore, adequate comprehension of materials and the ability to organize information must be demonstrated. The application of language skills is not taught in the English class alone. Content teachers must organize their instruction to cover language skills as well as content knowledge.

Repetition of concepts and procedures is essential to internalization. The development of any curriculum for LD students requires provisions for repetition of concepts and procedures. The thematic curriculum presents introduction and reinforcement of skills throughout the year. When skills are isolated and not reinforced through other thematic applications, confusion can result. Continued connection and usage strengthens the possibility of future independent learning and application.

A history of school failures recommends new and different approaches over the standard task hierarchy presentation of material and curriculum. A student who has experienced years of school failure and the resulting frustration is testimony to the lack of success that traditional skill hierarchies can generate. A more subtle, enriching, and applicable set of goals and objectives, utilizing multisensory materials, including computers, is required. Language experience, oral presentation, field trips, cooking, and role-play often elicit a more positive response on the part of students who would otherwise become bored.

SUMMARY

The thematic approach has been successfully applied in instructional programs for the learning disabled. It is not an approach that is limited to a special education population. Such a consistent and purposeful presentation of curriculum activities can and has been implemented in the regular school curriculum. The reason is that good planning and teaching are common components of any good system of instruction.

Teachers are poor copies of each other. Programs are also problematic when replicated without consideration for the individual population with which such a program will be used. The warning that must be issued with such a program is this: Make it your own. Expand here, condense there. The format is workable but must reflect the population for which it was developed. Remember, this is an *approach* to curriculum development, not a curriculum in itself.

APPENDIX 2-1

Curricular Outline #1: Who Am I?

Rationale

A self discovery unit starts the year because students enter school as strangers to one another. Introducing oneself requires self-awareness skills. This unit assists students in establishing who they are, where they come from, why they are in a special school or class, and what they want to do in the future.

Many severely disabled students believe that they are more handicapped than they actually are. The thematic unit, Who Am I?, allows them to explore their bodies and minds and draw some independent conclusions.

All learning activities reflect the theme. Reading, writing, speaking, and listening and social studies, science, and electives are conducted in a format that relates to self awareness and permits students to explore and domonstrate what they learn about themselves. A multisensory instructional setting is utilized.

Disruptive behaviors can be addressed in this format. Anger, frustration, depression, withdrawal, and constant talking can be symptoms of greater problems. The compensating behaviors a student has employed in response to the demands made through years of school failure must be reduced for meaningful remediation to take place.

Objectives

This unit is designed to elicit the following behaviors from students:

- ability to articulate their perceptions of themselves as individuals, members of families, members of communities, citizens of a nation or of the world
- ability to recognize and identify disabling conditions in themselves and others
- ability to identify traits of character and personality that generate both positive and negative reactions in themselves.
- ability to appropriately use the vocabulary of personality in oral and written projections
- ability to identify their current and possible future roles — child, parent, consumer, worker, friend, etc.

Sample Activities

LANGUAGE ARTS

- keep a journal of daily activities and feelings
- participate in Magic Circle or Class Meeting discussions on a topic of pertinence: How I Pick a Friend, Why I Admire _____, The Nicest Thing About Me Is . . .
- read selections about people who overcame various disabilities

- prepare a class newspaper about who makes news in the class and what issues are of concern to the individuals in the class.
- interview a relative or friend on tape
- play This is Your Life

MATHEMATICS

- calculate and compare populations: family, community, city, state, country
- observe someone — note number of various movements (blinking, raising an arm, opening mouth, etc.)
- add up the bones of the body and classify them into groups (arm, head, torsos, etc.)
- note and compare differences in height, weight, coloring, etc. for members of your class, family, school — calculate percentages of brunettes, blue-eyed students, people over five feet tall, etc.
- create a mathematical profile of yourself, your family, or school

SOCIAL STUDIES, SCIENCES

- locate your street, community, city, state, country, and continent on a map
- participate in a sensory deprivation experiment — blindfolded, with cotton in your ears, in a wheelchair, or one hand taped — then articulate the experience in writing or on tape
- identify areas of the brain and explain what parts of the body are controlled by the identified areas
- define and explain your learning disablilty as if to a stranger
- learn and use the Manual Alphabet for one period per week
- create a family tree

ELECTIVE AREAS

- make a personal crest or coat of arms (art)
- cast your hand, foot, or face in clay (art)
- compose your own theme music or select a signature tune (music)
- make a keychain with your initials (industrial arts)
- make a memory box (industrial arts)

MULTISENSORY APPLICATIONS

- personal computer
- language master
- cassette recorder
- record player
- projectors: movie, filmstrip, opaque, overhead

Curricular Outline #2: Travel

Rationale

LD students often have difficulty seeing themselves as individuals within a locale — family, community, city, state, country, continent, hemisphere, and planet.

This unit is designed to introduce and reinforce geographical concepts such as the relation of places to each other, scale, map reading, map making, directionality, and cultural differences.

It is also an excellent opportunity to provide a series of multisensory experiences — field trips, movies, filmstrips, map skills via a computer, and sampling of cultural distinctions via food, costume, and language.

Objectives

This unit is designed to elicit the following behaviors from students:

- ability to locate their street and community on a map
- ability to locate their city and state on a map
- ability to locate their country and continent on a map
- ability to name the languages of different countries when the name of the country is presented orally or in print
- ability to name the inhabitants of different countries when the name of the country is presented orally or in print
- ability to calculate mileage according to scale on a map
- ability to convert distance from English to metric units
- ability to interpret a train, plane, and bus schedule
- ability to name the currency of a variety of countries when presented with the name of the country orally or in print
- ability to follow directions to get from one location to another
- ability to give directions to another in such a way that that individual arrives at a predetermined location

Sample Activities

LANGUAGE ARTS

- prepare language experience stories from field trips
- relate vocabulary/spelling to the names of countries and their inhabitants
- learn a vocabulary for travelers (plane, train, suitcase, jet, ticket, first class, coach, pilot, conductor, engineer, reservation, etc.)
- keep a travel diary
- prepare language experience stories from vacations
- make a travelogue

MATHEMATICS

- relate vocabulary/spelling to the currency of different countries
- relate vocabulary/spelling to English/metric conversion
- calculate mileage
- calculate scale mileage
- convert from English to metric units
- calculate space travel distance between planets
- calculate differences in various currencies

SOCIAL STUDIES

- locate small areas on a map using a map index
- locate cities, states, countries, and continents on maps
- follow directions in a simple to complex progression to get from one location to another
- make a map of the school
- make a map of the community
- make a map of the city
- give directions in a simple to complex progression of steps for another student to follow
- create a treasure hunt

ELECTIVE AREAS

- recognize the national anthems of various countries (music)
- record music that will be used in the class travelogue (music)
- create travel posters (art)
- make frames for travel posters (industrial arts)

MULTISENSORY APPLICATIONS

- personal computer
- language master
- cassette recorder
- record player
- projectors: movies, filmstrip, opaque, overhead

Curricular Outline #3: Money

Rationale

Using money is among the most functional of skills and is utilized throughout a lifetime. For many states, proficiency measures must be mastered for a student to be promoted or to graduate. These include functional mathematics skills and monetary concepts.

December can be used as the time for the money unit theme because of the abundance of stimulus materials — brochures, sale notices, and advertisements for Christmas goods. The manipulation of financial concepts and the implementation of a budget is a skill that can be introduced at the elementary level.

The opportunity for lab exercises is extensive and the multisensory activities of this season are especially motivating. Money concepts are reinforced in the travel unit.

Objectives

This unit is designed to elicit the following behaviors from students:

- ability to identify a variety of coins
- ability to identify the value of coins

- ability to identify the relative value of coins (five pennies equal one nickel, two quarters equal one half dollar)
- ability to recognize and identify relative values of currency
- ability to write a check
- ability to demonstrate comparison shopping techniques
- ability to prepare and follow a budget for two weeks
- ability to interpret an advertisement in print or an advertisement heard on the radio or television
- ability to name three propaganda devices
- ability to name the currency of a variety of countries
- ability to write a commercial selling a product
- ability to present a commercial orally
- ability to balance a checkbook

Sample Activities

LANGUAGE ARTS

- learn vocabulary/spelling of financial terms
- prepare language experience stories about money — "If I won the lottery," "What would I do with a million dollars?"
- study careers in finance — banker, tax collector, stock broker, etc.
- participate in class discussions about future plans and what it costs to live as an adult
- role play an adult situation of living alone or with a roommate
- plan a budget
- read advertisements and identify the propaganda devices used to convince the buyer
- role play commercial situations: salesperson/customer, bank teller/depositor, etc.

MATHEMATICS

- make change from various coins and currency
- run a class store for purchasing school supplies
- keep an inventory for the class store
- keep a mock bank account for the month
- balance a checkbook for the month
- prepare and follow a budget for two weeks
- calculate inflation rates for various amounts
- calculate tax rates for various amounts of income
- complete a tax form
- complete a W-2 form
- accurately use a vocabulary for financial terms — coin, currency, inflation, credit, interest, deposit, withdrawal, etc.

SOCIAL STUDIES

- identify the currency of various countries
- locate the countries whose currencies are under study

- interpret news articles about inflation
- appropriately use a vocabulary of finance
- sequence countries in order of inflation rates
- go on a shopping trip and spend a predetermined amount of money on as many gift articles as possible

ELECTIVE AREAS

- make objects to sell at a school bazaar (industrial arts)
- conduct a school bazaar (career awareness)

MULTISENSORY APPLICATIONS

- personal computer
- field trips
- audio/visuals

PART II

Program Options and Service Delivery

T he first two chapters in Part II deal with two types of education: career and leisure. Chapter 3 discusses career education for LD students. With the possibility that LD may produce long-term negative consequences, it is important to transcend only an academic focus for intervention and encompass the totality of an LD student's experience, of which productive work activity is an important part. To prepare for work, career development should include four stages: awareness, exploration, preparation, and placement. These stages are included in a Life-Centered Career Education Model that possesses the overall goal of providing skills needed to function as a responsible adult. With the growing amount of free time available in our society, it is important to make that discretionary time both enjoyable and useful. Chapter 4 discusses research that shows how it is possible to instruct LD students in ways that make their free time more constructive and more socially acceptable.

Once it is determined how we should intervene with an LD student, a question remains about where an LD student should be placed. What is the best service delivery arrangement for an LD student? Chapter 5 explores that question by examining the "efficacy" question in terms of the effectiveness of regular classes, special classes, and resource rooms for delivering instruction to LD students. Using the Cascade Model as a framework, service arrangements are evaluated with respect to five methodological concerns. Generally, setting is viewed as a macrovariable that is an important consideration in terms of structure, but not primary in an instructional sense since instruction is influenced by many microvariables that have a more direct affect on the achievements of an LD student.

CHAPTER 3

Career Education

Donn E. Brolin
Timothy R. Elliott
James R. Corcoran

In 1971, the U.S. Office of Education gave top priority to career education as a critical educational need for all children attending American
schools. Education officials were vitally concerned about the large number
of students (over a million) who dropped out of school every year and the
many who only remained to get their diploma but learned very little. It was
believed that the introduction of career education would bring greater
relevance and meaning to being in school and that students would become
more aware of themselves, their potential, and the type of career that they
could assume as responsible adults.

Many years have passed since the introduction of the career education
concept (Marland, 1971) at a national conference of school officials.
Although many believed career education was just another short-term educational reform, the concept is still alive. In many respects, it is even more
widely adopted than during the period of state and federal promotion
when legislation and funds were readily available for its widespread
development and implementation.

This chapter originally appeared as an article by **Donn E. Brolin, Timothy R. Elliott,** and
James R. Corcoran in *Learning Disabilities: An Interdisciplinary Journal* (Vol. III (1), 1-14, 1984)
and was adapted by permission of Grune & Stratton for inclusion in this *Handbook.*

This chapter is intended to present the concept of career education as an important curricular and instructional approach for individuals with learning disabilities. The chapter includes a description of the basic tenets of career education, an explanation of how career education can address the problems of LD students, and a description of a life-centered, competency-based model that we believe is appropriate to implement for these individuals.

As with the term "learning disabilities," there is no one universally accepted definition of "career education." Kenneth B. Hoyt, the first and only director of the former U.S. Office of Career Education is most often quoted for his definitions. At the Helen Keller Centennial Conference, Hoyt (1980) described career education as:

> ... making *work* a personally meaningful and productive part of the total lifestyle of all persons ... that *work* as used in career education, is defined as "conscious effort, other than that aimed at coping or relaxation, to produce benefits for oneself and/or for oneself and others." Furthermore, the word "career" as used in career education, is defined as "the totality of work one does in his/her lifetime." (p. 2)

Two important concepts about career education are apparent in Hoyt's description: (a) that it is a focus on productive work activity and (b) that career is more than an occupation, it is all the various kinds of work engaged in throughout a lifetime. It is important to note that career education proponents do not conceive this to be the only education students receive but rather a substantial part of education. Career education is intended to re-direct some teaching activity around a career development theme for more relevant and meaningful learning (Hines & Hohenshil, 1985). Figure 3-1 illustrates the provision of career education from kindergarten through adulthood.

In Figure 3-1, general education and continuing education consist of learning about the world in which we live, basic academic skills, esthetic appreciation, physical education, and the like. Specific vocational programming consists of vocational counseling, vocational assessment, vocational education and training, job placement, and follow-up. Career education, on the other hand, adds a third important dimension that is often missing in a comprehensive educational program. The three components are not necessarily discrete entities to be taught separately, but rather reflect the major thrust of what is being taught. In other words, when certain academic skills are being taught, instruction should have a career development perspective, as described in the following paragraphs.

Career education is a total educational concept (Brolin, 1985). The following constitute some of its major important tenets:

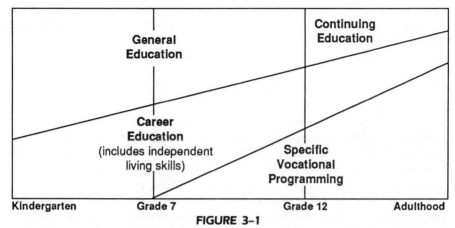

FIGURE 3-1
Illustration of the major components of a comprehensive educational program.
Note: from Brolin, D. (1982) *Vocational preparation of persons with handicaps,* p. 75.
Reproduced with permission from Charles E. Merrill Publishing Co., Columbus, OH.

- It begins in early childhood and continues through the retirement years.
- It encompasses the total school curriculum and provides a unified approach to education for life.
- It focuses on the various life roles, settings, and events that are important in the productive work life of the individual.
- It encourages all members of the school community to have a shared responsibility and a mutual cooperative relationship among various disciplines.
- It includes learning in the home, in private-public agencies, and in the employment community, as well as in the school.
- It encourages all teachers to relate their subject matter to career implications.
- It recognizes the need for basic education, citizenship, family responsibility, and other important educational objectives.
- It provides for career awareness, career exploration, and skills development at all levels and ages.
- It provides a balance of content and experiential learning with substantial hands-on activities.
- It provides a personal framework to help individuals plan their lives through carefully conceived career decision making.
- It promotes the opportunity for students to acquire a marketable entry-level occupational skill before leaving school.
- It actively involves parents in all phases of education.

- It actively involves the community in all phases of education.
- It requires a lifelong education based on principles related to total individual development. (Brolin & Kokaska, 1979, p. 104)

CAREER DEVELOPMENT

Four distinct stages or levels of career development are generally considered critical for developing a successful work personality. The first stage is *career awareness,* which should begin in the early elementary years and continue throughout the individual's educational program and beyond. Young students must begin to learn what kinds of paid and unpaid work people do, the work habits and skills needed for various kinds of work, the positive aspects of work, and how they can someday become successful workers.

During the late elementary or junior high school years, the second stage of career development, *career exploration,* should be initiated. This is a hands-on stage that gives students the opportunity to explore occupations, avocations, volunteer, and other productive work activities, and the responsibilities of home and family life. Community resources must be utilized so real world requirements can be explored and incorporated into learning. Students can begin to assess their interests, abilities, and needs in relation to their future work roles as adults.

Career preparation is the third stage of career development and generally begins in high school. If students have been given adequate career awareness and exploration opportunities, they should be able to engage in logical, tentative career decision making about courses appropriate to interests, abilities, and needs. This would include not only vocational courses but those that relate to other areas of career development and adult function.

The last stage of career development is *career placement, follow-up, and continuing education.* Learning does not end at graduation and careers are not defined solely by the first or last job acquired. Individuals must be provided lifelong learning opportunities so that successful post-school adjustment will occur and continue not only in a job but in family, civic, avocational, and productive leisure activities. A joint effort among educators, community agencies, and the family is of utmost importance because career education cannot be accomplished solely by educators.

Meyen and White (1980) noted that career education content does not fall into a precise developmental sequence or hierarchy. They also noted that evaluation is difficult because there is no normative base for comparing individuals on concepts and skills and few good evaluation procedures and instruments.

The career education approach is not a specific service or separate programming option, as many seem to believe. It requires the integration or *infusion* of career education concepts into the content of various subject matter

(Burton & Bero, 1984). It attempts " ... to assist students in perceiving the relationship between educational subject matter and the larger world outside the classroom" (Lamkin, 1980, p. 11) so individuals can be prepared for a wide variety of productive social, personal, economic, avocational, and leisure-time roles (Smith, 1983). Educators must find ways to facilitate the career development process so that the student develops a healthy work personality.

Career education then, is a sequence of carefully planned educational activities designed to assist individuals acquire the knowledge, skills, and attitudes needed to engage in the various life roles and settings that require productive work activity. Educational activities should be purposeful, developmental, and planned to prepare the individual for the productive work roles of student, homemaker, family member, citizen, volunteer, employee, recreator, and retiree.

CAREER EDUCATION AND LEARNING DISABILITIES

Although the problems that complicate the academic performance of students with learning disabilities have received considerable attention, few have recognized the relationship of these problems to career development (Mori, 1980). Recently, the connection between the academic deficiences of LD students and their postschool career adjustment has been recognized. Learning disabilities do affect the quality of life for these persons after they leave the traditional school system (White, Alley, Deshler, Shumaker, Warner, & Clark, 1982). Many problem areas and deficiences of the learning disabled impede both academic performance and career development.

Basic Academic Deficiencies

Students may possess a diverse range of specific learning disabilities in areas of reading, oral and written communication, and arithmetic ability (Wallace & McLoughlin, 1979). Consequently, most LD individuals develop idiosyncratic styles of learning and communication as they progress through the traditional school systems (Deshler, et al., 1982). As adults, the mechanisms that enabled the LD person to cope in the educational setting become liabilities in the work world, impeding tasks such as completing job application forms, listening attentively, comprehending oral and written instruction from supervisors, and actively soliciting guidance and assistance when a problem is recognized on the job. The didactic approach that commonly pervades traditional instructional methods provides little preparation for the world of work. Basic literacy and communication skills are essential for adequate job performance (Gillet, 1978).

Auditory and Visual Deficiencies

Many students with learning disabilities exhibit deficiencies in retaining and perceiving information acquired through auditory and visual senses. Instructions that are communicated in this way may soon be forgotten in the work environment. Blalock (1982b) has observed that auditory and visual deficiencies interfere in communicating within a noisy workplace, understanding telephone messages, enunciating unfamiliar and polysyllabic words, and comprehending directions and technical terms. Recall is sometimes impaired, and individuals may stammer while trying to complete a thought, which can result in staccato, interrupted speech. The decreased self-esteem and reluctance to seek assistance and clarification from supervisors that often ensues is understandable in light of these deficiencies (Blalock, 1982b; Deshler et al., 1982).

Social-Perceptual Difficulties

Goldman and Hardin (1982), recognizing the complex process by which a person receives, integrates, and expresses information acquired through social interaction, found the ability of social perception to be a distinguishing variable between LD children and non-LD children. This characteristic can be manifested in various degrees, but is usually observed as social immaturity, clumsiness, improper social judgments, naivety of social cues and nonverbal expression, impulsivity, and difficulties in interpreting societal mores and nuances within context (Gillet, 1981; Blalock, 1982a). Many LD students lack self-confidence, and some research has indicated that students with learning disabilities may make negative first impressions on casual observers, more so than non-LD peers (T. Bryan, Pearl, Donahue, J. Bryan, & Pflaum, 1983). Problems such as these can hamper effective interaction in all aspects of life.

White and colleagues (White, Deshler, Schumaker, Warner, Alley, & Clark, 1983) noted that schools have not adequately equipped LD students with the abilities to handle many of the social and affective aspects of life and have not sufficiently furnished realistic expectations of life outside the classroom. Deshler and associates (1982) reported that many adolescents and former students with learning disabilities express dissatisfaction with their quality of life. They indicate less involvement in social and recreational activities than students classified as "normal" during the school years.

Poor Vocational Adjustment

Several studies from the University of Kansas Institute for Research in Learning Disabilities have contributed substantially to our awareness of problems experienced by adults previously diagnosed as learning disabled

(Alley, Deshler, Clark, Schumaker, & Warner, 1983; Deshler, et al., 1982; White, et al., 1982, 1983). Although these studies report young adults seem to be doing as well as non-LD peers in getting a job, maintaining the position, and having friends, the jobs they acquire typically are of less social status. They appear to be adjusting vocationally, but many state they are dissatisfied with their employment and fault their school training. The discrepancy between the ability to acquire and maintain a job and the voiced dissatisfaction with the obtained job suggests that these young adults tax their survival skills to the utmost. Lacking some basic academic skills and perhaps uncomfortable in social situations that might expose their inability to perceive social cues, these adults may have sought jobs that would not necessitate the completion of detailed job application forms, an extensive interview with a prospective employer, or require social perception and interaction.

Two additional areas of concern are the inadequate training opportunities and limited higher education opportunities for persons with learning disabilities. Problems in these areas complicate the lives of LD individuals and often hinder their transition into productive adult roles.

Certain postsecondary training opportunities may be open to persons with learning disabilities. With the efforts of vocational rehabilitation to extend services to LD individuals, researchers have analyzed the implications of residual learning disabilities in the rehabilitative process (Blalock, 1982a; Crimando & Nichols, 1982; Geist & McGrath, 1983; Thomas, 1981). Other enterprises, like career development centers and vocational schools, have attempted to accommodate persons with learning disabilities by offering an array of services (Siefferman, 1983). However, these agencies do not necessarily attempt to address the multidimensional career needs of a person with a learning disability, nor do they provide these services throughout a person's lifespan. Vocational rehabilitation, for example, provides services that assist individuals in accommodating their disabilities. The diagnosis of learning disability alone does not automatically qualify a person to be eligible for vocational rehabilitation services: it is incumbent upon a rehabilitation counselor and client with a learning disability to first demonstrate how the impairment poses a vocational handicap before an agreement is entered. Vocational rehabilitation criteria for determining the severity and eligibility of a learning disability differ somewhat from those of the educational system and may vary from state to state. The primary aim of vocational rehabilitation is gainful employment for the client; services focus on this goal. Obviously, many adults with learning disabilities may be ineligible for such services or have career development needs beyond the occupational roles that vocational rehabilitation emphasizes.

Most institutes of higher education are chiefly concerned with the provision of advanced learning experiences. This lofty philosophy may not be appropriate for some adults with learning disabilities, and others may not meet admission requirements. Some prospective students with learning disabilities may qualify and aspire to an academic education but may come from families that cannot afford the spiraling expenses accompanying higher learning. Student services have tried to meet the career needs of students with disabilities in a variety of novel ways, including workshops (Egelman, 1981), special courses (Evenson & Evenson, 1983), and plans to enhance cooperation between college counseling centers and vocational rehabilitation (Perry, 1981). Nevertheless, Lopez and Clyde-Snyder (1983) reviewed existing models of service to disabled students and found none geared to the needs of students with learning disabilities. Service models were primarily confined to separate, distinct aspects of student life, such as counseling, social or vocational skills, or academic remediation. The researchers noted the lack of a comprehensive support system (academic or otherwise) to assist students with learning disabilities pursuing degrees in higher education. Universities are typically not equipped to address the intricate career development needs of persons with disablities other than isolated, specific areas that are related to the academic setting, and what services are available are reserved to enrolled students.

CAREER EDUCATION INSTRUCTION

Recent evidence provides more impetus for the recognition of the career development stages of LD students. Mori (1982a) studied career attitudes and job knowledge among special education, regular, and academically talented students. He found that students who were classified as learning disabled were one of two subgroups that were markedly lower than other groups in terms of career development. The other groups appeared to be experiencing normal career development on the scales employed, whereas LD students appeared career immature. Mori strongly recommended the immediate inclusion of career education from kindergarten to high school to offset what he considered regrettable, if not irreversible, impairments to students' career development. Hardin (1978) suggested that the needs of LD individuals must be looked at in relation to the different work environments that they must function in — home, community, school, and employment. This seems to support the case for career education as a viable instructional strategy for persons with learning disabilities.

This section will identify and describe important instructional aspects and services from a career education perspective. The discussion will focus on the stages of career development at four academic levels: elementary, junior high, senior high, and postsecondary.

Elementary Level: Career Awareness

The early educational experiences of the LD child should provide a sound basis conducive to future learning and personal growth. In order for this to transpire, areas of concern can be addressed in the classroom before they develop into problems for each student.

Elementary students are typically considered to be in the developmental stage of career awareness. It is vital for the student to begin visualizing and understanding the roles people assume in our society, the occupational world , and the worth of personal traits and attributes. This necessitates self-awareness and growth of a positive self-image. In turn, effective interpersonal communication skills can be fostered with a respect for others. With this knowledge of self and others, the student is sufficiently prepared to engage in career fantasy and role-play, and to make tentative career choices.

Initial perceptions of the world of work begin with career awareness. The student with a learning disability is not unlike any other student, becoming interested in what people do at home, at work, and at leisure. Children observe the activities adults undertake and may inquire why adults engage in such activities. Quite often children fantasize about being involved in work situations and may role-play such fantasies, mimicking the behavior of adults (Gillet, 1980). At any early elementary age, students with learning disabilities may already have certain options squelched if they are discouraged or deterred from such productive imagery by those who perceive the student as lacking potential to pursue some goal. Students should be encouraged to act out their perceptions of self in occupational and social roles, "trying-on" images. In essence, a work personality begins to take root during this stage.

Productive career fantasy hinges on the ability to process and explore options. This developmental stage should provide each LD child with an opportunity to "try-on-for-size" the perceptions and stereotypes of future roles as a parent, co-worker, and hobbyist. Since the previous learning experiences of LD children may be slanted by perceptual deficiencies, it is crucial that they receive ample opportunities to gain awareness of other roles and options outside their existing range of experiences.

Junior High Level: Career Exploration

The junior-high school level is typically considered to mark the onset of genuine career exploration. Role-play now acquires more solemn undertones as students seriously begin to examine their abilities and the practicality of their images and fantasies of adult roles. Casual, leisurely experiences now evolve into part-time jobs, hobbies, and extracurricular activities. These experiences slowly hone a student's interests and abilities. Yet, the career development and attitudes of LD students may be stunted in comparison to their non-LD peers at the junior high level (Mori, 1982a). Bingham (1978) observed differences between the career attitudes and maturity of LD students and their peers, and remarked that this may obstruct their career choice process in the junior-high years. Unless substantial career-related experiences have been provided earlier, instructors at the junior high level will have to carefully implement plans to create learning situations conducive to career awareness to counter some immaturity that the LD student may have.

This transitional stage is especially crucial for the LD student. Exploration exerts perceptual, cognitive, and affective abilities. Due to their differing styles of learning, LD students may misinterpret relevant information that would be beneficial in making tentative career choices. Misinformation gathered through distorted perceptions may result in unrealistic choices or a restricted range of options for exploration. Feelings of selfworth may also be negatively affected. A history of frustration and learned helplessness in previous school experiences may contribute to an inability to tolerate ambiguity, tension, reflection, and uncertainty. Impulsive, impatient, uncooperative behavior may ensue (Bingham, 1981).

During this time, it is important to encourage the development of selfconfidence. Abilities and assets should be highlighted and emphasized to facilitate healthy exploration. Vocational assessment is important. Abilities, interests, and aptitudes can be uncovered in a thorough career/vocational assessment, and subsequent education can focus on these assets, developing them to the utmost. Evaluation should acquaint the student with a broader range of occupational and personal options, not restrict or confine options. Hands-on experiences in the community can familiarize students with those options in which they have interest and aptitude.

Senior High Level: Career Preparation

Most LD students find secondary education complex and their capacity for skill development often plateaus at this time (Schumaker et al., 1983). If satisfactory career awareness and career exploration are accomplished, the high school student is ready to embark on career preparation and eventual placement. The temptation to connect career development solely with job-related experiences must be resisted. During this period of development, time should be given to the other roles adolescents will be assuming in the future, roles that include family, community, avocational, and personal-social responsibilities.

Ideally, LD students should understand their personal abilities and interests by the time they enter high school. This self-awareness is imperative for the meaningful, productive experiences that should be provided at this level of career development. Coursework should not sidestep the pragmatic aspects of education; direct hands-on experiences are indispensable. For many LD students, this translates into vocational education. For others who aspire to training in postsecondary settings, attention should be paid to the unique coping and study skills LD students may need. An excellent model implementing career education for LD high school students is the *Experience Based Career Education* program developed by Larson and associates (1981).

Postsecondary Level: Career Placement, Follow-up, and Continuing Education

The stage of career placement, follow-up, and continuing education, which is often neglectted, clearly illustrates the ongoing nature of career education. Learning does not end at graduation, and careers are not defined solely by the first or last job acquired. Individuals must be engaged in lifelong learning, and educators are not bereft of duties once the last course is taught. Placement into an occupational arrangement should transpire near the end of the last semester of schooling. Although this is not always possible, it can be facilitated by a joint effort among the educators, the school counselor, and community contacts. If further training is needed, certain community agencies, such as state vocational rehabilitation (VR) offices, may be of valuable assistance in procuring job-training opportunities.

Placement into postschool training or a job position is accompanied by new responsibilities in family, civic, avocation, and leisure/recreational roles. The capability to adjust and effectively fulfill these new assumed roles is dependent on the LD student's mastery of competencies in daily living, personal-social, and occupational skills. The student should be performing at a level appropriate for adults in our society. By concentrating on the development of these skills in school, the student can merge into society with confidence and ability. Such competencies do not come naturally; they must be taught, learned, and practiced.

The key to efficient postsecondary intervention for adults with learning disabilities is in community services (Hines & Bruno, 1985). Persons who are sponsored by vocational rehabilitation and students who are able to engage in university or trade school programs obviously maximize their potential on the job, in the community, and in the home. Still, adults with learning disabilities need a service delivery system that can attend to their lifelong career development (Brolin & Carver, 1982).

Many young adults with learning disabilities are not proceeding through the various stages of career development as described above. Adult services have to begin at the career awareness and exploration stages.

Unfortunately, for many it is too late! They have not developed the work personality (values, habits, interests, motivations, goals, and general skills) needed to be successful employees, homemakers, citizens, and participants in meaningful avocational, recreational, and interpersonal relationships. Personalities become established early in life and the work personality is no exception.

What can be done to thwart the irreversible effects of inadequate early career preparation? Obviously, we believe the answer lies in substantial and systematic career education curriculum effort that extends from kindergarten through postsecondary education. Students need to learn and be able to perform certain critical career skills for living and working in this society. A competency-based curriculum approach that integrates career development into its design is what we believe is necessary. Such a model is described in the next section (Brolin, 1983).

THE LIFE-CENTERED CAREER EDUCATION MODEL

Several models have been proposed to meet the career needs of students with disabilities at all levels of their development. The school-based career education model adapted by Clark (1979) and the experience-based career education model (EBCE) adapted by Larson (1981) are two good examples of career education models. Another is the life-centered career education (LCCE) model devised by Brolin, McKay, and West (1978). All three of these particular models can be comfortably assimilated by a school district to provide a comprehensive approach promising the maximum benefits to students. The LCCE model will be presented at length since it is a competency-based approach developed by one of the authors and illustrates the full breadth and impact of an extensive curriculum method of career education, kindergarten through adulthood.

Since career education encompasses the diverse learning environments and roles individuals assume in our society, a curriculum model must be broad in scope to provide students with the opportunity to acquire skills for functioning in different areas. The life-centered career education (LCCE) model is one such approach. LCCE was developed in a series of studies and is available in publications by the Council for Exceptional Children (CEC), *Life-Centered Career Education: A Competency-Based Approach* (Brolin, 1978, 1983) and *Trainer's guide for Life Centered Career Education* (Brolin, McKay, & West, 1978). This model currently exists in several school systems and adult programs nationwide and is a comprehensive approach that can be used to meet the career development needs of all disabled students, including those with learning disabilities.

The LCCE curriculum is composed of 22 major competencies to be acquired by each student in the categories of daily living, personal-social, and occupational skills. These competencies are interfaced with two crucial dimensions of career education: (a) school, family, and community experiences, and (b) the four stages of career development — awareness, exploration, preparation, and placement, follow-up, and continuing education.

Table 14-1 delineates the 22 competencies, categorized into the curriculum areas of daily living, personal-social, and occupational skills. Accompanying these major competencies are 102 subcompetencies that reflect the basic outcomes that should be achieved for a student to be adept at the corresponding competency. LCCE is viewed as a channel for coordinating all elements and environments of an individual's life to facilitate growth by integrating school, family, and community components to make education meaningful and to realize the individual's potential.

The Competencies

The 22 competencies and adjacent subcompetencies were developed in a grant-funded project (Brolin, 1978) to establish a competency-based curriculum. The project involved 12 school districts across the nation and over 300 school personnel. Designed initially to meet the career needs of students with mental impairments, the Council for Exceptional Children (CEC) later assisted in the extension of the model for the education of students with other disabilities. These competencies have been subjected to stringent review by hundreds of school personnel and have received unqualified endorsement. As these competencies have been applied to students and adults with various disabilities, this model can be interfaced with current strategies to promote career education for students with learning disabilities.

Daily Living Skills

The LCCE includes nine daily-living skills, which relate to the avocational, family, leisure, and civic work activities of each student. Forty-two subcompetencies cover skills essential for developing independent or semi-independent living status. The subcompetencies are designed to equip disabled students with the skills necessary to become independent citizens. These competencies may be developed to the extent that later occupational possibilities may emerge for the student who is particularly adept in one or more of these areas (Brolin, 1982).

Personal-Social Skills

Independence extends beyond the everyday, domestic abilities. People must also develop skills that enable them to interact effectively in a

TABLE 3–1

Life-Centered Career Education Competencies and Subcompetencies.

Competency	Subcompetencies		
Daily Living Skills			
1. Managing family finances	1. Identify money and make correct change	2. Make wise expenditures	3. Obtain and use bank and credit facilities
2. Selecting, managing, and maintaining a home	6. Select adequate housing	7. Maintain a home	8. Use basic appliances and tools
3. Caring for personal needs	10. Dress appropriately	11. Exhibit proper grooming and hygiene	12. Demonstrate knowledge of physical fitness, nutrition, & weight control
4. Raising children, enriching family living	14. Prepare for adjustment to marriage	15. Prepare for raising children (physical care)	16. Prepare for raising children (psychological care)
5. Buying and preparing food	18. Demonstrate appropriate eating skills	19. Plan balanced meals	20. Purchase food
6. Buying and caring for clothing	24. Wash clothing	25. Iron and store clothing	26. Perform simple mending
7. Engaging in civic activities	28. Generally understand local laws & government	20. Generally understand Federal Government	30. Understand citizenship rights and responsibilities
8. Utilizing Recreation and Leisure	34. Participate actively in group activities	35. Know activities and available community resources	36. Understand recreational values
9. Getting around the community (mobility)	40. Demonstrate knowledge of traffic rules and safety practices	41. Demonstrate knowledge & use of various means of transportation	42. Drive a car
Personal-Social Skills			
10. Achieving self awareness	43. Attain a sense of body	44. Identify interests and abilities	45. Identify emotions
11. Acquiring self confidence	48. Express feelings of worth	49. Tell how others see him/her	50. Accept praise
12. Achieving socially responsible behavior	53. Know character traits needed for acceptance	54. Know proper behavior in public places	55. Develop respect for the rights and properties of others

4. Keep basic financial records

5. Calculate and pay taxes

9. Maintain home exterior

13. Demonstrate knowledge of common illness prevention and treatment

17. Practice family safety in the home

21. Prepare meals

22. Clean food preparation areas

23. Store food

27. Purchase clothing

31. Understand registration and voting procedures

32. Understand Selective Service procedures

33. Understand civil rights & responsibilities when questioned by the law

37. Use recreational facilities in the community

38. Plan and choose activities wisely

39. Plan vacations

46. Identify needs

47. Understand the physical self

51. Accept criticism

52. Develop confidence in self

56. Recognize authority and follow instructions

57. Recognize personal roles

(continued)

TABLE 3-1 *(continued)*

Competency	Subcompetencies		

Personal-Social Skills (continued)

13. Maintaining good interpersonal skills	58. Know how to listen and respond	59. Know how to make & maintain friendships	60. Establish appropriate heterosexual relationships
14. Achieving independence	62. Understand impact of behaviors upon others	63. Understand self organization	64. Develop goal seeking behavior
15. Achieving problem solving skills	66. Differentiate bipolar concepts	67. Understand the need for goals	68. Look at alternatives
16. Communicating adequately with others	71. Recognize emergency situations	72. Read at level needed for future goals	73. Write at the level needed for future goals
17. Knowing & exploring occupational possibilities	76. Identify the personal values met through work	77. Identify the societal values met through work	78. Identify the remunerative aspects of work

Occupational Guidance and Preparation

18. Selecting & planning occupational choices	82. Identify major occupational needs	83. Identify major occupational interests	84. Identify occupational aptitudes
19. Exhibiting appropriate work habits & behaviors	87. Follow directions	88. Work with others	89. Work at a satisfactory rate
20. Exhibiting sufficient physical-manual skills	94. Demonstrate satisfactory balance and coordination	95. Demonstrate satisfactory manual dexterity	96. Demonstrate satisfactory stamina and endurance
21. Obtaining a specific occupational skill			
22. Seeking, securing and maintaining employment	98. Search for a job	99. Apply for a job	100. Interview for a job

*From D. Brolin, (1978), pp. 10–11.

61. Know how to
establish close
relationships

65. Strive toward
self
actualization

69. Anticipate
consequences

70. Know where to
find good
advice

74. Speak
adequately for
understanding

75. Understand the
subtleties of
communication

79. Understand
classification
of jobs into
different
occupational
systems

80. Identify
occupational
opportunities
available
locally

81. Identify sources
of occupational
information

85. Identify
requirements
of appropriate
and available
jobs

86. Make realistic
occupational
choices

90. Accept
supervision

91. Recognize the
importance of
attendance and
punctuality

92. Meet demands
for quality work

93. Demonstrate
occupational
safety

97. Demonstrate
satisfactory
sensory
discrimination

101. Adjust to
competitive
standards

102. Maintain
postschool
occupational
adjustment

plethora of personal and social contexts. Seven personal-social skills have been determined to be crucial to optimum functioning in family, community, and occupational settings. Thirty-two subcompetencies are designed to help students build confidence, solve problems, interact successfully with others, make decisions, conduct themselves properly in public, and communicate adequately with others. Acquisition of these skills facilitates adjustment in the community and productive interaction among relatives, peers, and co-workers. These abilities are critical to satisfying relationships and have dire consequences when absent in the work place.

Occupational Skills

Six competencies constitute this domain and are directed toward various stages of occupational preparation. The first two apply to basic concepts of the world of work and advance awareness of occupational opportunities, possibilities, and decision-making. The next three competencies pertain to the cultivation of specific occupational skills that may be appropriate to existing personal interests and predetermined abilities. The last competency refers to the process of seeking, procuring, and maintaining an occupational position. Twenty-seven subcompetencies are provided to assist in the attainment of these major competency areas.

Integrating the Competencies

Career education can be used as an instructional strategy to address many of the problems that have been associated with learning disabilities. The LCCE model furnishes a curriculum approach to implement career education. The competencies can guide instruction, channelling the education of each LD student toward a productive, realistic goal. Instructors must determine how they can integrate career education concepts and competencies into the content of various subject matter. In this manner, students will begin to understand the relationship between what is being taught and the real world.

A hypothetical example of "infusion" may be warranted at this point. Infusion refers to the process of integrating career education concepts into the subject matter of a regular or special class. Assume that competency #1/subcompetency #4 "Keep Basic Financial Records" (Table 3–1) is being taught in a math, vocational education, or special education class. Also assume that career awareness and exploration relative to this subcompetency have already occurred and now it is time to learn career preparation. Activities and strategies that can be infused into the instructional unit in relation to the various career roles of working in the home, on a job, in various avocational activities, and in community and volunteer projects follow.

- *Work in the home.* Students develop a tentative budget including all sources of expenditures (housing expenses, rent, food, bills, loans, etc). Parents are asked to help construct the family budget. A budget counselor from a local community agency demonstrates budgeting techniques.
- *Occupation.* Students select an occupation that requires keeping financial records. Speakers representing that occupation describe their job duties and help students perform some of their functions.
- *Avocation.* Students select an avocation that requires financial records. Parents and/or community representatives engaged in the avocation demonstrate how they perform this activity.
- *Community and volunteer projects.* Students select one volunteer project that interests them. Community representatives that need volunteers requiring this skill demonstrate how they perform this activity. Students then volunteer to work on the project.

The above example is, of course, simplified for ease of explanation. There are many other activities that can be used to teach this subcompetency. The educator may use a variety of instructional techniques and methods such as games, role play, puppetry, simulated businesses, occupational notebooks, careers of the month, field trips, learning packages, collages, job dictionaries, arts and crafts, card games, What's My Line?, occupational games, values clarification, guest speakers, job analysis activities, work samples, and special work assignments.

Not every student with a learning disability may overcome problems in basic reading comprehension or computation. The LCCE approach advocates the attainment of awareness and skill in these areas as they can be adapted and utilized in a career perspective. Practical limitations are considered; practical goals are set. Yet it is important for a citizen in our society to have some semblance of budgeting ability. This, of course, makes the teaching of basic arithmetic skills relevant and practical. In a similar fashion, a student will need to be able to recognize and complete an application for employment — an exercise that may prove to be an enjoyable homework assignment or, at the very least, an enlightening one.

Table 3-2 conveys the relationship that can exist in the attempt to resolve problems that often accompany learning disabilities. These problems are often characteristic of a learning disability and are addressed by one or more of the 22 major competencies. Tutoring in these competency units can, directly or indirectly, offer an avenue to circumvent some problem areas and surmount others.

The LCCE approach is an attempt to teach LD students and those with other disabilities the skills needed to function as responsible adults.

TABLE 3–2
Relation of LCCE Competency Units to Areas of Concern for Students With Learning Disabilities

Areas of Concern	Appropriate LCCE Competency
Basic Academic Deficiencies	
Arithmetic ability	1. Managing family finances
Reading ability	16. Communicating adequately with others
Oral and written communication	13. Maintaining good interpersonal skills
	16. Communicating adequately with others
Social Perceptual Difficulties	
Interpreting & understanding social cues in context	14. Achieving independence
	16. Communicating adequately with others
Social judgments	15. Achieving problem-solving skills
Social immaturity and "abrasiveness"	12. Achieving socially responsible behavior
Personal Social Adjustment	
Self-confidence	10. Achieving self-awareness
	11. Acquiring self-confidence
	14. Achieving independence
Use of Leisure Time	8. Utilizing recreation and leisure
Interpersonal Relationships	4. Rearing children, enriching family living
	13. Maintaining good interpersonal skills
Family Relationships	2. Selecting, managing, and maintaining a home
	4. Rearing children, enriching family living
	5. Buying and preparing food
	6. Buying and caring for clothing
	13. Maintaining good interpersonal skills
Awareness of Civic Responsibilities	7. Engaging in civic activities
	12. Achieving socially responsible behavior
Vocational Adjustment — Meaningful and satisfying employment	17. Knowing and exploring occupational possibilities
	18. Selecting and planning occupational choices
	19. Exhibiting appropriate work habits and behaviors
	20. Exhibiting sufficient physical-manual skills
	21. Obtaining a specific occupational skill
	22. Seeking, securing and maintaining employment

This can be accomplished by providing relevant learning experiences that are geared specifically to the needs of each student. The LCCE approach exemplifies how career education can provide the relevant, comprehensive educational experience needed by LD students.

SUMMARY

Although most career education personnel profess the goal of their educational efforts is to prepare their students for adult life, few attain this goal. The majority of students with disabilities are unemployed or underemployed as adults, and they have major social-personal-family problems (Alley et al., 1983; Department of Education, 1982; White et al., 1982).

The career education approach presented in this chapter is a total educational concept. It requires, as the President's Commissions on Excellence in Education and other study groups have recommended, a much closer relationship with the student's parents and the community's resources. It also requires the active involvement of all school disciplines in a truly cooperative and collaborative partnership so that ALL children can be adequately educated in ALL schools.

Career education provides an alternative to the educational needs and dilemmas posed by those with learning disabilities. First, it requires self-awareness experiences so that students can become more aware of their own unique interests, needs, values, aptitudes, goals, and potentials. Students with learning disabilities have many assets that they need to recognize and capitalize on throughout their educational program. They must become aware of the world of work and have the opportunity to explore areas of interest.

A second benefit of career education is its early attention to the world of work and its requirements. Students with learning disabilities will be able to make more realistic choices as the result of exposure to possibilities that are within their capabilities and interest areas. This earlier focus will give them the opportunity to improve those skills that can be improved so they can acquire the skills needed for career success. Career education must begin in the early elementary grades if LD students are to succeed in vocational and life skills education at the secondary and post-secondary levels.

A third value of career education is its emphasis on realistic, meaningful activities and experiences that relate to the requirements of the real world. Extensive use of community resource people, including those from business and industry, is an absolute requirement. This should be done inside and outside of the school environment and should utilize up-to-date "tools of the trade." This approach motivates students if they can relate the experiences to their interests, needs, special aptitudes, and skills. The involvement of parents as a resource will also reap benefits as they become more involved in providing career experiences in conjunction with the instructional program. In the process, parents can also get a more realistic assessment of their child's needs and potentials.

Another benefit of career education is its reliance on a variety of instructional strategies to meet learner needs. Since so many LD students need special considerations, the career education approach attempts to find how students can best learn important concepts and skills. In the process, many students with auditory and visual deficiencies will learn appropriate coping skills so they can follow instructions, respond to typical social and vocational cues, and recognize important signs and forms used in everyday living and working.

The LCCE approach described in this chapter adds one additional dimension to career education — competency or skill development. Every student is required to learn specific skills, including a marketable occupational skill — if it is humanly possible! The pride and self-confidence that results from this attainment proves to the LD student and to their parents, teachers, employers, and significant others that they are people who have many skills and potentials and, incidentally, have a learning disability.

Career education will not solve all the problems that are presented by LD students, but it can address many needs that are not currently being met. Society is becoming more demanding and complex. Educators must be willing to change and incorporate into their curriculum and instruction those methods and materials that work. Career education provides the opportunity for students to acquire those personal and career skills that are necessary for successful and satisfying work activities.

CHAPTER 4

Leisure Education

Stuart J. Schleien

During the 1970s and into the present decade, there was and continues to be a growing need for preparing and educating all people for leisure. Shorter workweeks, increased vacation time, earlier retirement, and a transition from a work-oriented to a leisure/work-oriented society have all contributed to greater amounts of unobligated leisure time (Howe, 1981).

In light of substantial increases in the amounts of free time for all persons (*U.S. News & World Report,* 1981), appropriate, enjoyable, and cooperative discretionary time use becomes a primary and magnified problem for learning disabled individuals. Children with learning disabilities are typically deficient in leisure skill activities and generally have not developed appropriate attitudes toward leisure. Learning disabled students do not usually use their free time in constructive, cooperative, and socially acceptable ways (Wehman, 1979). Self-initiated and independent recreational activities are not frequently part of their repertoires. Since involvement in leisure skill activities and play facilitates social, cognitive, adaptive, and gross and fine motor skill development (O'Morrow, 1976), it is critical that LD children learn to use their free time enjoyably and appropriately during their school-age years and beyond.

This chapter originally appeared as an article by **Stuart J. Schleien** in *Learning Disabilities: An Interdisciplinary Journal* (Vol. I (9), 105–122, 1982) and was adapted by permission of Grune & Stratton for inclusion in this *Handbook.*

LEISURE PROBLEMS

The problem of free time is compounded for LD children because they are faced with even greater amounts of leisure time than the average citizen. This may be due, in part, to less time spent in school, since the Office of Special Education and Rehabilitative Services (OSERS) only mandates a free and appropriate education for all children 3 to 21 years of age. Additionally, it has been reported that within the next few years, only 20% of all disabled individuals completing school at the secondary level will gain full-time employment or continue their education at the college level (Leisure Information Service, 1976).

Another reason why LD students are faced with many hours of unfulfilled discretionary time is directly related to the past development of their leisure repertoires. All too often, learning-disabled children progress through an educational or institutional program without ever receiving training or education in skills necessary to constructively and cooperatively use their free time (Swift & Lewis, 1985). Leisure skill curricular content has not been given sufficient attention, time, resources, or energy in most educational programs offered disabled students (Wehman & Schleien, 1981). Special education classroom teachers and regular educators have not been concerned about the nonschool and postschool recreation environments and leisure activities in which disabled students participate or might function in the future (Ford et al., 1980).

Even though educational and vocational training programs for special populations have been supported by society, this advocacy does not exist for leisure education programs. Most parents send their children to school to learn. The phrase "to learn" usually refers to the Three Rs, that is, reading, writing, and arithmetic, to the exclusion of the Fourth R, recreation. The term *to learn* has not traditionally meant *to play*. A disproportionate amount of unoccupied time results, with few available leisure resources and accessible facilities and programs to affect it (Beland, 1980).

Additionally, there seems to be a general societal view, accepted by educators, that recreation should occur primarily following school hours, during vacations, and on weekends, and valuable school time should be only indirectly devoted to such pursuits (Green, 1968). Consequently, the typical amount of time allotted to leisure education and activities during school hours is minimal in comparison to other curricular areas.

Although children with severe behavioral deficits have been trained in ball skills (Kazdin & Erickson, 1975; Whitman, Mercurio, & Caponigri, 1970), simple table games (Wehman, 1977), independent free play (Wehman, 1977), and social play (Paloutzian, Hasazi, Streitel, & Edgar, 1971; Strain, 1975) in public school classrooms, there is a relative paucity of literature focusing on leisure education programs for

LD children (Shulman, 1976). Parten (1932) reported that average school-age learners typically proceeded through developmental sequences of constructive and appropriate play. Additionally, it was discovered that hyperactive children with learning impairments continued to be more inappropriately active and less compliant than normal peers in both play and task-related settings (Cunningham & Barkley, 1979).

In the last 15 years, education of LD students has witnessed rapid growth, exhibiting versatility in the use of a broad range of teaching materials and methods (e.g., toys, recreation). An eclectic approach to the education of the youngster labeled *learning disabled* has evolved. Diagnosis and appropriate prescriptive programs to remediate learning disabilities are currently the approaches accepted by most educators. Although the fields of medicine, psychology, and optometry have had vested interests in learning disabilities, recreation professionals have continued to neglect this special population (Sabatino, 1976), as evidenced by the paucity of research and other material published in this area.

It is speculated that leisure education and recreation can play vital roles in the education of the school-age LD youngster. Besides the mastery of school learning, one of the normal tasks of preadolescence is the development of peer relationships. Preadolescents live in a world where game skills are very important. This age group enjoys participation, talking about adventures, and the previous evening's television programs. Few preadolescent youngsters are inner-directed (O'Morrow, 1976). To maintain self-esteem, these children require personal achievement along with recognition and love from adults and peers. Preadolescents feel good about themselves when meeting the developmental tasks of their own age (Ambrose, 1974; Piaget, 1951). Individuals will not experience feelings of self-worth if they are unprepared for adolescence (e.g., learning disabilities). However, adolescence will arrive, ready or not.

There are several steps educators and parents can take to support academic and normal growth of LD youngsters. Cruickshank, Morse, and Johns (1980) suggested encouraging students to engage in nonacademic activities. These activities may include sports, hobbies, and travel, or basically any activity that bypasses learning problems and offers youngsters a chance to consider themselves other than disabled.

Koppitz (1971) recommended after-school recreation activities and summer camp programs as parts of comprehensive special education programs for LD children. Additionally, according to her plan, all children would be screened to identify youngsters who are too immature or vulnerable to be able to benefit from a regular kindergarten program at the time of school entry. This screening procedure would evaluate a youngster's social, emotional, and mental development by observing the child in group free play.

Just as professionals from other allied disciplines recognized the need for the development of recreation, leisure, and cooperative play skills by LD children, so, too, is it time that the recreation profession develops, implements, and evaluates school-based leisure education programs for these youngsters.

SIGNIFICANCE OF LEISURE EDUCATION

With the passage of many state and federal laws (e.g., Public Law 94-142), and as a result of many judicial and educational actions, it is now the responsibility of educational practitioners in the United States to provide for the educational (including leisure education) development of disabled students. The propositions offered in this chapter are (a) not only do LD students have the right to be participating members of heterogeneous communities in a leisure context, but such participation is inherently good, and (b) it is now feasible to arrange educational service delivery systems in ways that maximize the probability of leisure participation. One way that LD and non-LD citizens will learn to live and play cooperatively and learn from each other as fully participating members of heterogeneous communities is through longitudinal interaction during their school years (Brannan, 1977; Ford et al., 1980). It is proposed, therefore, that LD youngsters be educated for leisure in settings that encourage and support extensive longitudinal interactions (i.e., the school).

Federal legislation (Coval, Gilhool, & Laski, 1977) and innovative recreational and educational programming techniques have encouraged therapeutic recreators and educators to begin providing appropriate leisure education services to LD youngsters in educational environments. Depriving many of these students of an education for leisure must not continue to be an educational alternative. It is the responsibility of all recreators to accept the challenge of developing and implementing leisure education delivery systems that maximize opportunities for LD students to learn leisure and cooperative play skills necessary for full participation in heterogeneous postschool communities.

With the recent influx of thousands of LD children into public school programs, there is an increased need for therapeutic recreation specialists and special education classroom teachers to participate in leisure education program planning, implementation, and evaluation. Inasmuch as play and recreation are critical parts of the socialization process of most children (Piers, 1972), the development of leisure and free play skills by LD students appears to be a critical instructional area in which therapeutic recreators and special educators could provide valuable assistance.

RATIONALE FOR LEISURE EDUCATION

Leisure education or therapeutic recreation may be defined as those experiences of a recreational nature having the potential of being therapeutic for all. Leisure education is concerned with enabling individuals with physical, mental, emotional, or social disabilities to acquire appropriate socioleisure life-styles (O'Morrow, 1976).

Unfortunately, in most localities throughout the nation, leisure education services and programs are either unavailable or completely lacking. Although most public school systems provide some form of physical education, mandated by Public Law 94-142, leisure education services are quite frequently inadequate. Results from a recent needs assessment survey of 316 public school, community recreation, and adult programs serving disabled individuals indicated an overwhelming need for more leisure skills services and improved leisure education programs (Schleien, Porter, & Wehman, 1979). Most returns indicated a lack of leisure education curriculum. Instructional difficulties in working with disabled individuals interfered with optimal delivery of recreation services.

Beland (1980) investigated the competencies needed by special education teachers and administrators to implement a school-based leisure education curriculum for LD students. It was determined that the teaching competencies ranking highest in role importance were (a) to integrate leisure education goals into disabled students' IEPs, and (b) to gain knowledge of what constitutes a comprehensive education program.

Written support for leisure education can be found in the educational literature. Historically, the impetus for and support of leisure education originated in the schools (Kraus, 1978). Additionally, the development of leisure education programs had been designated as educational responsibilities (Leisure Information Service, 1976). But when recreation and leisure activity goals were incorporated into public school programs, it was usually assumed that those responsible for the activities to meet student's goals needed special training from a recreation specialist. Thus, students did not receive the recreation-related services they needed (Gilhool, 1976).

Today, a growing interest in leisure education exists. An emphasis on the school to provide these services has been recognized (Mundy, 1975). Since play experiences contribute significantly to the socialization and life-long leisure skill repertoires of most children, the development of play and leisure skills would appear to be an important instructional area in which therapeutic recreation specialists could perform valuable program assistance (Gunn & Peterson, 1978). Similarly, Brannan, Chinn, and Verhoven (1981) stated that the child's use of free time and attitude toward recreation and play may determine the degree of success experienced through educational efforts. In working with severely disabled children, Wehman (1977) addressed the necessity of providing intensive structure and sequence in leisure skill development. This type of systematic programming will only occur in the schools. Brightbill (1961) insisted that intervention during the early years was regarded as the most critical time to effect learning, and, therefore, a leisure thrust during this period seems logical if basic development of attitudes and skills are to be acquired.

Since recreation as a related service, including assessment of leisure functioning, therapeutic recreation, recreation programs in schools and communities, and leisure education, was included in PL 94-142 and recognized in other legislation, the preparation for leisure as part of the special education curriculum for handicapped children was identified as an important programming need. According to the federal law, related services such as recreation and leisure education should be provided when a child can benefit from that particular programming discipline. When assessment data indicate such a need, recreation services are provided to assist the special child in school. Efforts to actually provide leisure education programs to school-age children, however, have been minimal and of low priority (Weiss, 1976).

A committee of the National Therapeutic Recreation Society, formulated to study the impact of PL 94-142 on recreation, initiated a national study to determine the involvement of therapeutic recreation and leisure education in state and local education agencies. In 93% of the states responding to the national survey, recreation services were not included in the interpretation of the state plans (Coyne, 1981).

LEISURE EDUCATION FOR LEARNING DISABLED CHILDREN

Since learning disabilities is the most recent formalized category of special education (Hallahan & Kauffman, 1976), it is not surprising to find a lack of experimental research and curricula regarding this population. Tarver and Hallahan (1976) noted that little experimental research has studied the characteristics (e.g., hyperactivity, disorders of attention) of children with learning disabilities.

Martin (1977) investigated 210 research reports concerning therapeutic recreation. This was the first effort to systematically examine and classify the available research related to therapeutic recreation. A content analysis using the data base of the TRIC system (Martin, 1971), a computerized retrieval system concerning recreation for special populations, was made to determine content areas of the data-based research. A majority of the research focused on the mentally retarded population (24%), with physical disabilities a close second (21%). Learning disabilities was not even mentioned as an area, making it clear that this special population was not receiving any attention from researchers. Other populations cited were general illness (20%), mental illness (13%), social deviance (12%), and aging (10%).

Throughout the 1960s and 1970s, many remedial attempts were made by researchers studying learning disabilities. The researchers focused on only one aspect of a learning disability at a time. Linguistics, motoric involvement, visual-perceptual approaches, and other problems made it difficult for any one program or research study to treat the LD youngster as a whole person. Though much data was collected on each research approach, learning disabilities continued to be defined and treated in terms of the stress of its own methodology (Hammill & Bartel, 1975). Research focusing on this special population has increased, but its primary focus has been on testing the effects of drugs on the LD individual (Kornetsky, 1975). Safer and Allen (1976) recommended a team approach consisting of parents, teachers, administrative school staff, and health care professionals, with coordination at all levels of service, when working with LD students.

A review of a detailed study of "Resumes of Projects for Handicapped Children Funded under P.L. 89-313 Amendment of Title 1, ESEA," indicated that most school-based recreation projects for disabled students were conducted in special resident or day schools. The study also determined that over 45,000 children were served in all disability classifications; however, the only disability classifications noted were mental retardation, deaf, emotionally disturbed, blind, and crippled (Wilson, 1969). Learning disabilities was not even included as one category of the "all disability classifications."

Another investigator determined the state of recreational programming for children with learning disabilities in Toronto, Canada (Shulman, 1976). Data concerning recreational participation of the children and the activities were collected via questionnaire. Of the original 233 questionnaires, 127 responses (55%) were received regarding the recreational participation of children. Thirty-three percent of the children had previously participated in regular community programs, another 33% were involved in special programs, and 33% did not enroll in any organized recreation program. In terms of integrated recreation programs, interestingly, one of the most frequent reasons stated by both parents and recreational personnel for their hesitancy in integrating LD children was a lack of staff training in how to deal with the children's problems.

Apparently, relatively little emphasis has been placed on an objective analysis of the effects of recreation and play on LD children. One research project that was conducted in this area studied choices of learning disabled children (Cratty, 1970). Approximately 300, 5- to 12-year-old elementary school children were sampled to compare the percentages of children with and without movement problems who indicated a liking for any of 37 games. Among the LD children, clumsy children avoided vigorous active games such as direct contact sports. Unlike their non-LD peers, these children preferred games involving fantasy, such as cowboys and indians.

Trammel (1974) studied play preferences of approximately 200 LD children and compared them with the same number of non-LD peers using a modified Sutton-Smith Play and Game List. The author found that the LD children shared more preferences with their non-LD peers than differences. A chi-square nonparametric statistical technique yielded only 18 games on which both groups differed significantly in preference.

Therapeutic recreational activities were used in one research project to provide the framework for treatment of hyperactive children, one of the most common characteristics of learning disabilities. With the identification of meaningful and measurable goals for each child, Clift, Edwards, Reese, and Vincent (1977) utilized therapeutic recreation to provide children with opportunities to practice new skills, receive feedback regarding progress, and encourage interactions outside the program with others. Five of the six hyperactive children participating in the study achieved significant progress in the attainment of predetermined goals, which included increasing attention span, improved relationships with peers, control of temper, and improvement in personal behavior. Although the study should only be considered pilot work with a small sample, the findings suggested the critical role that therapeutic recreation and leisure education could play in working with these children.

Groups of 20 "normal" and 20 hyperactive LD boys were observed interacting with their mothers in free play and structured-task situations (Cunningham & Barkley, 1979). The interactions and amounts of independent play that occurred during the two experimental situations were compared using a partial interval data collection procedure. The hyperactive subjects were more active, less compliant, and less likely to remain on task than their normal peers. No difference in amounts of time spent in independent play among the two groups was found.

LEISURE EDUCATION AND SOCIALIZATION

In a national survey of families with disabled children, it was found that only a small portion of the subjects (e.g., deaf) had used at least one recreational service (Brewer & Kakalik, 1979). Of the families that did use recreational services, the parents favorably regarded leisure as an end in itself. They were satisfied that their children learned independent living skills and made new friends.

The study cited above is just one example of the interplay between recreation participation and socialization. The fact that social development could be increased through interaction with peers and adults during leisure education was also revealed by Verhoven and Goldstein (1976). Wehman (1979) noted that a major reason disabled children display inappropriate play behavior is that they have limited cooperative play skills and exhibit a lack of social interaction among peers. Paloutzian et al. (1971) noted an inordinate amount of independent or isolated play among severely disabled young children, reinforcing the association between play and social skills.

In fact, children fail to develop higher level social behaviors such as cooperative and competitive play when little peer interaction exists during play (Wehman, 1979). Independent or isolate play is a lower stage of social development than cooperative play. Affective feedback cannot be obtained until social interactions occur between children. As a child becomes more proficient at playing with others, socialization skills will be acquired (Paloutzian et al., 1971). Cooperative play between children leads to learning acceptable modes of socialization, such as sharing, taking turns, and teamwork. Therefore, social play directly influences the development of cooperative play behavior (Knapczyk & Yoppi, 1975; Samaras & Ball, 1975).

In her rationale for leisure education as a process rather than as a specific service in education, Collard (1981) identified the many roles that leisure education can play in assisting in the development of needed social skills. Disabled individuals can learn valuable and critical social skills to facilitate appropriate functioning in the school, on the job, and in the community. Zigmond (1978a) insisted that disabled individuals must be socially competent to attain maximum benefit from classroom instruction in all curriculum areas. Several other authors have cited the importance of proficiency in socialization among disabled individuals to perform successfully on the job (Neal, 1970; President's Committee on Mental Retardation, 1974; Wehman, 1977) and within the community (Collard, 1981; Novak & Heal, 1980; Wehman & Schleien, 1981).

The U.S. Department of Health and Human Services (1979) explained how play teaches children to relate to other people and helps them learn how to live in culturally sanctioned ways. Social rules and mores are learned in this manner. Preparing for adult life through play by practicing principles of give-and-take, sharing similar space, and exchanging information with other playmates was also discussed.

As cited earlier, the inability to cope in social situations and a lack of socialization skills are major characteristics of many disabled children. These limitations significantly affect the development of communication skills, and, inevitably, minimize the effects of play and recreation as a medium of social skills development. The LD child often exhibits extreme difficulty in making and maintaining friends with chronological age peers. Besides language and other communication problems, hyperactivity and distractibility also interfere with interactions and play behavior with peers. Learning disabled children have difficulty functioning adequately in regular community recreation programs because, among other deficiencies (e.g., physical skills), they lack the necessary social skills to participate successfully (Shulman, 1976).

COOPERATIVE LEISURE SKILL ACTIVITIES: AN EXPERIMENTAL ACTIVITY

Most children with learning disabilities are enrolled in special classes in the public schools, to which many of them must be transported by school bus. The relocation to a new environment is often necessary due to the unavailability of appropriate programs close to home, or it may be in the best interest of the child to travel to school (Shulman, 1976). Neighborhood children consider the special child as different, and friendships become difficult to develop or maintain. This problem leads to other problems for LD children, such as a reluctance to participate in neighborhood recreation programs and social withdrawal. LD children do not function adequately in peer group situations, as their social inactivity and deficits in academic areas move them further apart from society.

Further research and investigation into the field of learning disabilities, recreation, and socialization is crucial. As the editor of a symposium concerning learning disability research, Wiederholt (1976) suggested that experimental research designs be used and called for a shift away from ex post facto research in special education to make it possible for other researchers and classroom teachers to replicate studies with equivalent results. Anderson (1976) determined that experimental research designs, in combination with more stringently defined research groups, should provide the necessary answers to questions regarding the efficacy of various instructional methods for LD children. Cohen (1976) called for a shift in balance toward experimental designs when he stated, "It never occurred to me that rigor and scientific excellence are solely the the properties of experimental designs. Or that ex post facto research is illegitimate, or unscientific. My argument is based on need and value. Ex post facto research can be as rigorous as experimental research. The issue is that for replicability and applicability we need more experimental types of designs" (p. 167).

The current investigation, with the understanding of the importance of leisure skills training for the development and maintenance of social skills in LD children and the values of replicability and applicability, attempted to increase cooperative play behavior in this special population within a multiple baseline experimental time series design (Hersen & Barlow, 1976).

This study attempted to answer the question, can an individualized leisure education instructional program produce significant gains in cooperative leisure time use in severely learning disabled subjects? The investigator developed a leisure education instructional program, which was implemented in two special education classrooms. Descriptions of subjects, settings, program description, instrumentation, research design, data collection, and analysis of data follow.

Subjects and Setting

Twenty-three students, diagnosed severely learning disabled and attending a public school in a large metropolitan area, participated in the leisure education program. Subjects, ranging in age from 9 to 13 years, were 21 males and 2 females. All subjects were transferred to segregated classrooms at a special school from the city public school system. A majority of subjects exhibited inappropriate, stereotypic social and play behaviors (e.g., social withdrawal, autistic and aggressive play), limited social skills development, delays in fine and gross motor development, and other learning problems of a neurological origin. Subjects' Wechsler Intelligence Scale for Children—Revised I.Q. scores ranged from 70–123.

The special school that the subjects attended is a public/private school serving disabled individuals between the ages of 3 and 21 years. The students attended the school from 8:45 A.M. to 2:30 P.M., Monday through Friday. The leisure education instructional program was implemented in two preselected classrooms within the school. Classrooms were selected by the school administrator due to an identified need for cooperative play skills for these subjects. High incidents of physically and verbally aggressive behaviors and large amounts of isolate play and social withdrawal were observed daily in the selected classrooms. Two special education classroom teachers were present in each classroom and assisted on a rotating basis with the leisure education program and treatment. There were 11 students in Classroom 1 and 12 students in Classroom 2.

Program Description

The leisure education instructional program of cooperative leisure skill activities, employing a multiple baseline design across classrooms, was composed of the following three components: exposure to games and materials, leisure skills instruction, and positive reinforcement.

Exposure to Games and Materials

New age-appropriate and cooperative leisure-related games and materials were introduced into the two classrooms. Subjects were exposed to games and materials, including *Pokeno, Chinese Checkers, One-on-One*

Basketball, darts (velcro type), *Battleship Toss-a-Cross,* and *Operation* in Classroom 1; and, *Bobby Hull, Hockey, Chinese Checkers, Pokeno, Booby Trap, Carrom Board* set, and *Twister* in Classroom 2. Different board and table games were selected for each classroom since the investigator, school administrative staff, and classroom teachers believed that specific activities were not essential to cooperative play development as long as the activities were age-appropriate, cooperative (i.e., games and activities requiring at least two players for participation), and equal in motor and language response difficulty levels. Also, the investigator attempted to demonstrate the functional control of the independent variable, the leisure education instructional program, over the dependent variable, levels of play, by exposing subjects to games and activities that were classified as cooperative, in order for other educators to be able to select similar, but not necessarily identical, games for the same purpose. Selection of two different groups of leisure skill activities could facilitate program replicability, as teachers and other facilitators of leisure education would not be required to implement a specific set of activities, but, rather, activities having the same characteristics and meeting the same criteria.

Special education teachers and classrooms were surveyed by the investigator prior to games and materials selection and purchasing to determine the average dollar amount spent on leisure-related materials and equipment in each classroom during the previous school year. By determining the dollar amount typically spent on recreation games and materials in a special education classroom ($60 per year) and then purchasing games and materials not to exceed this determined value, the implementation of the current leisure education program would be financially feasible in other school classrooms, thereby facilitating the external validity of the program to other settings.

Leisure Skills Instruction

In addition to exposing subjects to new games and materials, skill instruction was provided. During the initial encounter with subjects, a directed discussion of recreational pursuits and past and present discretionary time use occurred. The investigator (e.g., leisure education instructor) initiated class discussion concerning past recreational experiences, current leisure repertoires, activity preferences, and the purpose for and benefits of cooperative play and recreational participation with peers. Additionally, categories of recreation (e.g., board games, hobbies, sports) and levels of play (e.g., isolate, parallel, cooperative) were compared and contrasted and their individual relevancies discussed. For example, the benefits and feelings derived when playing the card game Solitaire (i.e., isolate play), were compared to playing a group card game, such as I

Doubt It (e.g., cooperative play). Subjects were encouraged to participate cooperatively with their classmates in school and friends at home whenever they had discretionary time. Cooperative activities were consistently, blatantly, and firmly reinforced by the investigator throughout the leisure education instructional program.

Leisure skills instruction relevant to the newly introduced recreational games and materials was provided by the investigator during each instructional session. Before subject participation and immediately following the introduction of a new game to the classroom, playing rules were explained and taught to the subjects within the context of the activities. The instructor would read and review the playing rules to the subjects and then participate with the subjects in the activity for 10 minutes. If a subject did not understand a playing rule, or did not play by the rules or follow appropriate playing procedures, the instructor would model the desired response(s). In this manner, both playing skills and appropriate social interactions were addressed. Subjects were encouraged to select one of four activities that were available in the classroom at any one time during instruction. If a subject wished to participate in an activity where the maximum number of subjects were already playing, the subject was asked to wait until the game terminated or was encouraged to participate in another activity.

Positive Reinforcement

Positive social reinforcement (e.g., pat on back, social praise) was given to the subjects for cooperative play by the leisure education instructor and classroom teacher present during the instructional program. Systematically, and in a rotating fashion, the instructor and classroom teacher would walk in opposite directions from activity to activity and observe the subjects for 30 seconds. Praise and encouragement were immediately offered to any subject who was playing cooperatively with at least one other classmate at the time of observation. If the subject was engaged in inappropriate, isolate, or parallel play during an observation, positive reinforcement was withheld. Classroom teachers responded to verbally and physically aggressive and other inappropriate behaviors in the identical manner in which they had responded prior to the introduction of the leisure education program. This was done in order to discipline the children (e.g., time-out procedure, verbal reprimand) consistently throughout the school year.

Instrumentation

All subjects in the two classrooms were assessed to determine their leisure skill competencies, repertoires, and activity and material preferences. With the use of one-way mirrors (located between classrooms and adjacent observation rooms), a partial interval time sampling data collection method (Bailey & Bostow, 1979; Levy, 1982) was used to assess leisure and social behavior (i.e., social level of play) during subjects' free time over a 1-week period. This baseline assessment of preinstruction competency levels established if and how much each subject was already performing appropriate activities, the amount of peer cooperation during play, and gave some indication of what areas of training were necessary.

Within 15 minutes of free play (12:15–12:30 p.m.) each observer/recorder made 60 recordings (approximately 5 recordings per subject in a 12-subject class). This recording procedure was used twice each week by the classroom teacher throughout the course of the leisure education program (approximately 2-3 months).

The four categories of developmental levels of play (i.e., inappropriate, isolate, parallel, cooperative) were derived from the Social Interaction Rating Scale, an 8-point scale used to measure the level of social behavior of young severely retarded children in a free play setting (Paloutzian et al., 1971). Paloutzian's levels were adapted from those used by Parten and Newhall (1943) for intellectually average children.

The supplement to the Leisure Behavior Data Collection Form, which contained the operational definitions of the modified developmental levels of play (adapted by the investigator) appears below.

- *Inappropriate play:* Percentage of time subject plays or uses free time inappropriately — maniupulates or uses toys, objects, or recreation materials incorrectly; socially inappropriate behavior (e.g., verbal/physical abuse on others); manipulation of chronological age-inappropriate toys, objects, or recreation materials (determined by manufacturer's age level recommendation); nongoal directed, nonfunctional, purposeless behavior; stereotypic behavior (e.g., self-stimulation).
- *Isolate play:* Percentage of time subject plays or manipulates toys, objects, or recreation materials appropriately, but in a solitary manner (not within 5 feet of another peer).
- *Parallel play:* Percentage of time subject plays or manipulates toys, objects, or recreation materials appropriately, in the presence of a peer, but not cooperatively (other peers within 5 feet of subject — does not interact with others).
- *Cooperative play:* Percentage of time subject plays or manipulates toys, objects, or recreation materials in an appropriate and cooperative fashion (i.e., socially interacts with peers, engages in play activity with another peer, displays a cooperative give-and-take manner; no hitting or yelling occurs; shares toys, objects, or game).

Concurrent with baselining, a social validation survey/questionnaire was developed and administered to parents of the subjects participating in the program. Several questions from the Behavioral Characteristics Progression Assessment Chart (Texas Department of Mental Health and Mental Retardation, 1976) and Institute for Career and Leisure Development Indices of Leisure Behavior Form (1979) were used in the survey. A modified Likert procedure was utilized, placing the respondents/parents on an attitude continuum for each statement ranging from "strongly agree" to "strongly disagree." The parent survey was a structured, forced-choice technique. The instrument was also adminstered at the program's termination to the parents, so the parents' responses prior to and following the leisure education instructional program could be statistically compared.

Data Collection

Subjects were instructed for 65 minutes on Mondays, between 1:00 and 2:05 P.M. and for 45 minutes on Wednesdays between 8:45 and 9:30 A.M. Following the leisure education instructional program each Monday, a 15-minute nonreinforced probe was conducted between 2:05 and 2:20 P.M. to acquire data concerning the measurement of the dependent variable (e.g., level of social interactions) for each subject. No data were taken following the program on Wednesdays, since the subjects were involved in other curricular programs. Every Tuesday and Thursday, however, between 12:15 and 12:30 P.M., a classroom teacher in each classroom conducted the partial interval time sampling data collection, resulting in 3 days of observational data per week (Mondays, Tuesdays, and Thursdays). Observations were made in an adjacent room containing a one-way mirror. Leisure education instruction commenced in Classroom 1 and baseline assessment data continued for all subjects in Classroom 2. Following the expiration of a predetermined 4-week time period, treatment began in Classroom 2. During this time (i.e., weeks 5–8), Tuesday and Thursday observations and data recording continued in Classroom 1 for skill maintenance probles. Monday interobserver reliability checks were no longer made in Classroom 1 during leisure education instruction in Classroom 2. However, classroom teachers in Classroom 1 continued to implement the leisure education instructional program on Mondays and Wednesdays, even though the leisure education instructor commenced instruction in Classroom 2 and was no longer available in Classroom 1. Instead of only taking maintenance probes twice weekly, the classroom teachers agreed, with the support of the school principal, to continue the leisure education instructional program on their own.

Data Analysis

Data analysis was divided into two major sections: (a) analysis of levels of play behaviors across classrooms; and (b) analysis of social validation pre-/post-leisure education instruction parent survey. Results of statistical testing of each of the dependent variables mentioned above and results of the hypotheses testing related to each of the null hypotheses of the study follow.

Analysis of Play Behaviors

Figures 4-1 and 4-2 present class averages of all levels of play (i.e., cooperative and inappropriate — Figure 4-1; parallel and isolate —Figure 4-2) for the two classrooms of severely learning disabled subjects. The ordinates show mean percentages of behavior occurrence (as previously defined) at 15-second observation intervals. The abcissas show the number of sessions across baseline treatment, and maintenance phases of the study. In order to analyze the initial dependent variable, levels of play, the study focused on three major questions. First, are the levels of play performed at equal frequencies, or are certain levels consistently exhibited more frequently than others? Second, if the four levels of play are not performed equally, will a treatment procedure designed to increase cooperative play behavior result in a decrease in inappropriate and isolate play

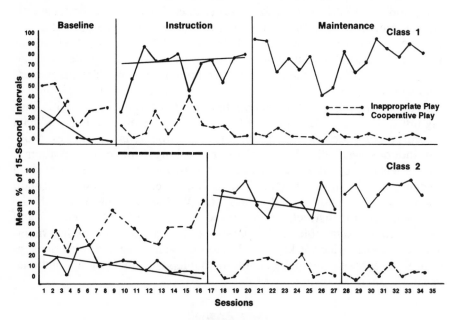

FIGURE 4-1

Mean percent of cooperative and inappropriate play for Class 1 and Class 2 across experimental conditions and split middle analysis of cooperative play across baseline and treatment phases.

and a concomitant increase in cooperative play? Third, will increases in cooperative play and parallel play and decreases in inappropriate and isolate behaviors be maintained after the treatment is discontinued by the experimenter (classroom teacher only instruction)?

Results of the multiple baseline design across classrooms demonstrated that the leisure education intervention produced effects by showing that, at different times, behavior change occurred if, and only if, the intervention was present. The mean percentage for cooperative play remained low and for inappropriate play remained high for each classroom throughout the baseline periods of the study.

An examination of Figure 4–1 reveals that for Classroom 1, the average percentage of 15-second intervals of cooperative play was 11% (range: 0% to 35%), whereas the class exhibited inappropriate play for an average of 34% of the intervals (range: 15% to 52%). The data for Classroom 2 were very similar. The average percentage of cooperative play was 14% (range: 3% to 30%), whereas the average number of intervals in which the class exhibited inappropriate play was 43% (range: 25% to 67%). Thus, the data suggest that if the subjects in the classrooms were left alone, they would not play cooperatively and would exhibit numerous inappropriate social behaviors.

The data concerning the remaining two levels of play (isolate and parallel) in Figure 4–2 present a more confusing picture. For Classroom 1, the average percentage of 15-second intervals of parallel play was 29% (range: 7% to 46%), whereas the same class exhibited isolate play for an average of 44% of the intervals (range: 26% to 58%). Parallel and isolate play for Classroom 2 were almost identical to those found for Classroom 1. The average percentage of parallel play was 38% (range: 15% to 65%), whereas the average number of intervals in which Classroom 2 exhibited isolate play was also 38% (range: 3% to 70%). Thus, the data suggest that if the subjects in the classroom were left alone, they would play in a parallel fashion about one-third of the time and in an isolate manner slightly over one-third of the time.

The effects of the treatment interventions on the classrooms' overall behaviors can be observed in Figure 4–1. The introduction of treatment resulted in an immediate increase (to 28% and 40%) in the percentages of intervals in which the subjects exhibited cooperative play behavior in both classrooms. Cooperative play behavior remained at high levels throughout the instructional phase. In Classroom 1, except for the first session of intervention (session 8), the mean percentage of cooperative play behavior during each treatment session was greater than the largest percentage (35% during session 3) of cooperative play during any baseline session. Similarly, in Classroom 2, all 12 intervention probes resulted in greater mean percentages of cooperative play behavior than the largest percentage (30% during session 5) of cooperative play during the baseline period. Classroom 1

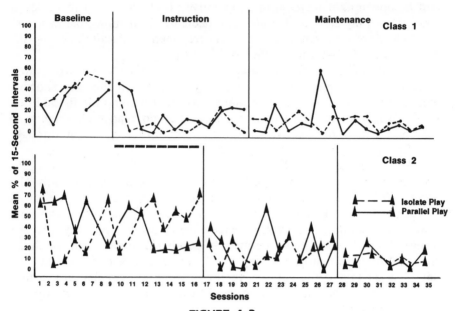

FIGURE 4–2

Mean percent in isolate and parallel play for Class 1
and Class 2 across experimental conditions.

exhibited cooperative play behavior for an average of 67% of the intervals, as
compared to 11% in baseline. Classroom 2 exhibited cooperative play behavior for an average of 66% of the intervals, as compared to 14% in baseline. On
the other hand, the number of inappropriate behaviors decreased substantially in both classrooms, averaging only 14% during intervention, down
from 34% during baseline for Classroom 1, and averaging only 12% during
intervention in Classroom 2, down from 43%. Both parallel and isolate play
decreased in Classroom 1 and Classroom 2 during intervention phases. In
Classroom 1, parallel and isolate play decreased from 29% and 44%, respectively, compared to intervention when these figures were 17% and 3%. Similarly, in Classroom 2, parallel and isolate levels of play decreased from 38%
during baseline to 22% and 15%, respectively, during intervention. For
Classroom 1 and Classroom 2, then, instructional control through the leisure
education instructional program was apparently effective in establishing
cooperative play behaviors and reducing inappropriate social play.

In Classroom 1, the high percentage of cooperative play behavior and
low level of inappropriate social behaviors reached in treatment were
maintained once treatment was no longer implemented by the experimenter but by classroom teacher only instruction (Figure 4–1). In comparison
to the average percentage of cooperative play occurrences made during

baseline (11%), Classroom 1 students played cooperatively an average of 75% after treatment was discontinued by the experimenter. Furthermore, the average number of intervals in which Classroom 1 students exhibited inappropriate social behaviors was consistently less (average 6%) than during baseline (average 34%). Classroom 2 students played cooperatively an average of 78% during classroom teacher only instruction in comparison to the average percentage of cooperative play during baseline (14%). Additionally, the average number of intervals in which Classroom 2 students exhibited inappropriate social behaviors was, once again, less (average 6%) during maintenance than during baseline (average 43%). Not only were mean cooperative play and inappropriate behaviors respectively greater and less than their corresponding baseline rates, but the average performances were also respectively greater and less than cooperative play and inappropriate social behaviors during intervention phases. Mean cooperative play in Classroom 1 and Classroom 2 was 75% and 78%, respectively, during the teacher only instruction maintenance phase as compared to 67% and 66%, respectively, during intervention. Mean inappropriate behavior in Classroom 1 and Classroom 2 was 6% during the teacher only maintenance phase as compared to 14% and 12%, respectively, during intervention.

The data from Figure 4–1 for Classroom 1 and Classroom 2 indicated that (a) cooperative play behavior was not established when the subjects were left to themselves and, as a result, they exhibited a large amount of inappropriate and isolate play; (b) implementing the leisure education instructional program resulted in an immediate increase in cooperative play and a concomitant decrease in inappropriate and isolate play; and (c) the increases in cooperative play and decreases in inappropriate and isolate play reported under the treatment condition were maintained above and below baseline levels, respectively, when treatment by the experimenter was discontinued and classroom teacher only instruction occurred.

On an individual subject basis, without any exceptions in either classroom, all subjects exhibited substantial increases in cooperative play behavior and concomitant decreases in inappropriate behavior from baseline to instruction. The reader is referred to Schleien (1982) for a complete analysis and graphic descriptions of the 23 subjects' individual play behaviors.

The split middle method of trend estimation (White, 1971, 1972, 1974), a technique that provides a method for describing the rate of behavior change over time for a single individual or group, and reveals a linear trend in the data, demonstrated that there was a change in slope from baseline to instruction of 6.74, and a change in level of 24.33 in Classroom 1. These changes summarize the differences in performance across phases. Applying the binomial test (used to determine whether the number of data points that fell above the projected slope of the baseline phase was of a sufficiently low probability to reject the null hypothesis) to the data in which all 12 data points fell above the baseline celeration line, allows for a rejection of the null hypothesis that the data during the instruction phase can be represented by the slope during baseline ($p<.001$). The alternative hypothesis, stating that data during the instruction phase were significantly different from the data during the baseline phase, was accepted.

The statistical test was also applied to the baseline and treatment phases of Classroom 2 to ascertain if any significant differences existed. Figure 4–1 also demonstrates the results for Classroom 2. The change in level was 10.14 and the change in slope was 1.34 from baseline to instructional phases. All of the data points in the instructional phase were above the extrapolation line projected from the baseline phase, suggesting a significant difference between the two phases ($p<.001$).

The split middle procedure results demonstrated the effectiveness of the intervention procedure for both classrooms. In each case, the leisure education intervention resulted in significant increases in cooperative play from one phase to another.

In order to determine reliability for the baseline, instruction, and maintenance records, a reliability check was made by a second trained observer for one session per week. Interobserver reliability averaged .88 with a range of .73 to 1.00 across the two classrooms. Observer agreement was calculated by dividing the number of agreements by the number of agreements plus disagreements (Wehman & Schleien, 1980). An agreement was recorded when a 15-second recording interval for a particular subject was scored by both instructor and observer in an identical manner. That is to say, if both scores recorded a plus for cooperative play in the first 15-second interval for Subject 1, Class 1, an agreement was scored. If the scorers were in disagreement (i.e., one plus for cooperative play and one plus for parallel play) concerning the subject's performance during a particular 15-second interval, a disagreement was recorded. Instructor and observer concurrently were responsible for recording levels of play behaviors of all subjects in the classroom. Those subjects and data were compared.

Analysis of Parent Survey

This section describes the relationship between the pre- and post-program responses of the parents of the 23 subjects who participated in the leisure education instructional program. A telephone interview questionnaire was designed to investigate whether parents of the subjects possessed divergent perceptions concerning their children's use of leisure time and cooperative play skills prior to and following the children's participation in the leisure education instructional program. The telephone survey consisted of a series of 20 questions that were responded to during the baseline phase of the program and repeated within 2 weeks of the completion of the "teacher only instruction" maintenance probe.

Seven questions were responded to in a manner that yielded a mean difference between pre- and postscores of .80 or greater. Question 3, regarding the cooperative play skills of the respondents' children with others, displayed a mean difference of 1.13 (pre — 2.96, post — 1.83) for the 23 respondents signifying a substantial positive change in parental perceptions of children's cooperative play skills. Additionally, approximately 22% of the parents reported a low score for this question during the presurvey. During the postsurvey, however, 80% of the respondents answered with a "most of the time" or "some of the time."

Similar results were found in Question 10, concerning the subjects finding others to play with. A mean difference from pre- to postquestionnaire for this question for the 23 respondents yielded a 1.05 discrepancy score (pre — 2.83, post — 1.78). Again, parental responses moved in a more favorable direction, as only 2 (9%) respondents believed their children found others to play with "most of the time" at the time of the presurvey, but 9 (39%) responded in the fashion following the program.

Concerning the subjects' aggressiveness during play and free time, answers to Question 7, "Does your child fight physically?" and Question 8, "Does your child argue?" lend support to the significance of the leisure education program as more parents responded negatively to both questions during the postsurvey. Mean differences from pre- to postresponses were .83 (pre — 1.78, post — 2.61) and .92 (pre — 1.30, post — 2.22) for Question 7 and Question 8, respectively. Also, 8 (35%) parents and 19 (83%) parents during the prequestionnaire responded "most of the time" to Question 7 and 8, respectively, and 0% of the time following leisure education instruction.

Regarding the acceptance of losing in a game (Question 14) a play-related problem for several of the subjects, parents perceived their children dealing with and accepting losing in a more favorable light following the program. A preinstruction mean for 23 respondents of 3.04 and a post-program mean score of only 2.21 yielded a mean difference of .83. Seven (30%) respondents believed their children accepted losing in a game "most of the time" or "some of the time" prior to the classroom leisure educational program in comparison to as many as 18 (78%) parents responding in this fashion at the program's termination.

Finally, regarding the subjects' verbalizing at home about leisure education instruction and playing with classmates (Question 19), parents perceived the subjects as taking an increased interest in playing with others in school. The difference in means was .62 (pre — 1.74, post — 1.13) from pre- to postinstruction, but more significantly, only 6 (26%) respondents insisted their children enjoyed speaking about playing with classmates "most of the time" prior to program commencement, but 20 (87%) parents during the postsurvey responded in this manner. The most frequent alternative selected during the presurvey for this item was "some of the time" and during postinstruction was "most of the time."

Several methods of analyzing the data exist related to the hypothesis: There will be no significant changes in parental responses regarding subjects' cooperative play skills during leisure activity participation from pre- to postleisure education instruction. The primary analytic method to determine statistical significance for pre- and postquestionnaire items was a series of 20 paired t tests. The hypothesis being tested for each item was the test for zero means ($u_1 - u_2 = 0$). A large discrepancy between pre- and postinstruction mean scores for a given questionnaire item would yield a significant t for that question.

Of the 20 questions analyzed for overall respondent significance at 22 degrees of freedom, 15 (75%) pre-post instruction comparisons were significant at the .05 level. Nine questions were significant at the .001 level; five questions were significant at the .01 level; and one question was significant at the .02 level of significance. Five (25%) pre-post instruction comparisons were not significant at the .05 level.

With the exception of the five questionnaire items that yielded observed values of t less than the critical value at the .05 significance level (i.e., Question 2 — child plays alone; Question 5 — child takes turns; Question 13 — child sticks up for him/herself; Question 15 — child wants to learn new games; Question 20 — age of child's friends), and according to the decision rules, the null hypothesis (i.e., $u_1 - u_2 = 0$) is not rejected, three-fourths of the items yielded observed pre-post mean differences not within the realm of sampling error. That is, parental responses were not identical in their perceptions of their children's play skills prior to and following leisure education instruction.

SUMMARY

The investigation represented an effort to demonstrate and evaluate instructional procedures for teaching cooperative leisure skill activities to 23 school-age children with severe learning disabilities. The purposes of this study were threefold: (a) to develop and implement a program that had instructional elements that were easily replicable by other regular and special educators; (b) to develop a leisure education instructional program that evaluated quality or levels of LD children's play; and (c) to evaluate the program in an experimental design that allowed for verification of the instructional package employed.

The following conclusions were drawn concerning school-based leisure education for children with learning disabilities. First, a traditionally underserved population of severely learning disabled children participated in a leisure instruction program that provided chronologically age-appropriate activities and materials of a cooperative nature. Second, the instructional "package" of modeling, social reinforcement, exposure, and availability of cooperative-type materials was identified as an effective means of facilitating cooperative leisure skills. Third, the intervention program was shown to have a functional relationship with socially appropriate activity; concurrently, inappropriate social behaviors were reduced in all of the subjects. The data support the findings of a previous study (Favell, 1973) demonstrating the deceleration of stereotypic, inappropriate behavior as a direct result of the acquisition of play behaviors. Fourth, children with severe learning disabilities successfully maintained high rates of cooperative play and low levels of inappropriate behavior and isolate play during maintenance probes. The absence of a discriminative stimulus (i.e., experimenter) during the teacher-only instruction maintenance phase did not reduce the frequency of the target behavior, cooperative play. Fifth, following leisure education instruction, parents significantly altered their perceptions of their LD children's play in the home environment. Finally, all subjects generalized appropriate play from the classroom to the home and neighborhood. Results from this study indicated that children with learning disabilities can acquire a more diverse repertoire of social and cooperative leisure skills than has been previously demonstrated in the literature.

This study, as described in this chapter, may be appropriately considered an exploratory instructional program for more in-depth investigations that might include a larger number of subjects who are learning disabled. Several positive implications of this study should be observed. First, successful results were obtained over a relatively short period of time (i.e., one month of instruction). Second, positive results were achieved largely through instruction by special education classroom teachers and teachers' aides who were not previously provided with inservice training to increase their competencies in implementing leisure education. They had no previous exposure to leisure/recreation university courses. Third, the leisure skills acquired by the participants were skills that could be facilitated by family members, teachers, and community recreators following the termination of the study.

The primary implication to be drawn from this study is that LD youngsters need not engage in only solitary leisure activities and competitive sports of a gross motor nature. A major purpose of the investigation was to describe how introduction of leisure options in addition to solitary activity might be facilitated for LD children. Without access to and instruction in the use of different leisure materials and activities, LD youngsters will not be able to enjoy the reinforcing aspects of cooperative play. This study presented a model that regular and special educators can utilize in their respective programs. The instructional components for leisure education intervention have been delineated for the purposes of replication in other school programs. The time of a professional therapeutic recreation specialist in the school would be required weekly.

CHAPTER 5

Service Arrangements

Gary M. Sasso

The assumption that all students do not prosper under the same educational programs is basic to the need for differential programming. Hence, the purpose for assessment and classification procedures has been to match a student's particular characteristics with that of certain intervention programs. In effect, appropriate and effective instruction was viewed as being dependent on the needs of the LD students involved.

Although the focus of this chapter is the LD student, it is difficult to focus exclusively on LD when studying service delivery. Programming alternatives cover all students in the mildly disabled area (mentally retarded and behaviorally disordered). Consequently, information gleaned from all three mildly disabled areas will be presented, although the emphasis will be on LD. According to Madden and Slavin (1983), use of these terms has changed considerably and varies from place to place. In fact, many students identified as educable mentally retarded in 1970 would be labeled as LD today. What is important is to recognize that there are students who are administratively defined as being in need of special services because of learning problems and come under the general mildly disabled designation. When authors cited in this review, however, used such terms as learning disabled, behaviorally disordered, or mentally retarded to describe their samples, these terms are used here.

The logical question to raise is: Do LD students profit from distinctly different educational programs than those offered to behaviorally disordered students? Or it could be asked: Do common components of effective instruction apply across catagories to all students referred to as mildly disabled? Most special education programs operate with specially certified staff (e.g., LD teachers) that reflects the nature of the classification. It would appear that the most important issue here is whether such certification has any functional implications in the classroom and in the development of individualized educational programs.

Although all intervention systems may be effective, it is important to know which types of interventions work with which types of students. It is necessary to ascertain how individual differences in LD students interact with program processes to produce differential outcomes (Burstein & Guiton, 1984). The main issue is whether or not LD students gain more when they receive instruction in regular or mainstreamed settings or when they are placed in resource room or self-contained settings.

MAINSTREAMING

In accordance with PL 94-142, providing equal educational opportunities for LD students requires designing and implementing high quality, comprehensive, yet least restrictive educational services. It was in response to this law that the concept of mainstreaming gained prominence. Mainstreaming refers to multiple service levels in which a range of administrative and instructional options are available. It is these multiple service options that stand out in contrast to the initial conceptualization and organization of special education as a system from general education (Kaufman, Gottlieb, Agard, & Kukic, 1975). Even though the term *mainstreaming* has been used frequently, it is not possible to find consistent agreement regarding the specific features that depict a mainstreaming program (Adelman & Taylor, 1985; Kaufman et al., 1975; MacMillan & Semmel, 1977; Palmer, 1980).

Unfortunately, discussions of mainstreaming have concentrated on administrative arrangements (for example, the amount of time students spend in general education settings) rather than on instructional variables in the regular classroom. Consequently, temporal integration is one of the most frequently used characteristics of mainstreaming in efficacy studies. Hence, the amount of time an LD student spends in the regular classroom with nondisabled peers might be considered a criterion for a mainstreaming program (Algozzine & Korinek, 1985; Carlberg & Kavale, 1980; Salend & Lutz, 1984; Semmel, Gottlieb, & Robinson, 1979; Smith & Smith, 1985; Vaughn & Bos, 1987; Wang & Baker, 1985–86; Ysseldyke & Algozzine, 1982).

CASCADE MODEL

The most common scheme for organizing special education programs along a continuum of instructional arrangements is illustrated by Deno's

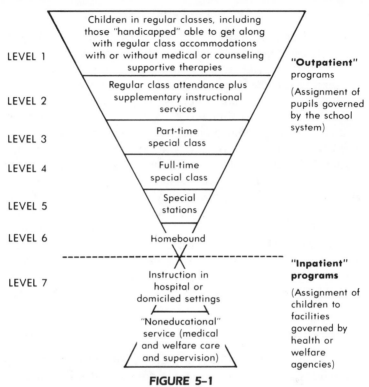

FIGURE 5-1

Deno's Cascade System of special education service. From "Special Education as Developmental Capital" by E. Deno in *Expectional Children, 37,* 1970, p. 235. Copyright 1970 by The Council for Exceptional Children. Reprinted with permission.

cascade (Figure 5-1). Basically, Deno's model (Deno, 1970) for special education services proposes a continuum of settings within which specific instructional programming is emphasized at each level. Supposedly, there is more commonality within each level of this continuum than among the levels. The degree to which the environment is structured differs among the levels, with the greatest degree of special education at Level 7. Levels 5, 6, and 7 would not typically be considered for LD students.

Deno's model emphasizes several points: (1) relatively fewer students will be found at each succeeding level from Level 1 to Level 7; (2) students should not be moved downward in the system (toward Level 7) unless it is absolutely necessary and clear documentation is available to warrant such a move; and (3) each student should be moved upward in the system (toward Level 1) as far and as quickly as possible.

Level 1 — Regular Class

This is the most integrated level, with LD students attending class with other students their age. Because of functional disorders of various types and degrees, however, LD students may require adjustments in their environment that exceed the usual demands of their peers. The kinds of supportive services that will most often be found in Level 1 classes for LD students vary from slightly altered regular instructional methods and materials to unique instructional materials and audiovisual aids. The regular class teacher will usually consult with someone within or outside the school about a special problem pertaining to a given LD student. Consultation with a special resource teacher, reading consultant, school psychologist, or educational diagnostician should take place as frequently as necessary to obtain information that will lead to the best instructional atmosphere. The key to success for an LD student located in a regular classroom is the teacher, because whatever adjustments are needed to accommodate a particular LD pupil will have to be initiated and followed up by the classroom teacher (Bruininks, 1978a; Olson & Midgett, 1984; Roddy, 1984; Rose, Lessen, & Gottlieb, 1982; Smith, Flexter, & Sigelman, 1980).

Level 2 — Regular Class with Instructional Support

For a majority of LD students, this is the most popular program option. Students are assigned to a homeroom in a regular class and spend most of the school day there, but part of their instruction is provided in a resource room. The resource room teacher carries out an individually prescribed instructional program for each student or for small groups. Upon completion of the lesson, a student returns to the regular classroom. Although resource room teachers may have different specialties, they are highly skilled in meeting most of the instructional needs of LD students. Reading specialists, speech therapists, and counselors may be viewed as itinerant resource room consultants, usually available if needed.

Regardless of the programming configuration, the main purpose is to allow LD children to receive as much instruction in the regular program as possible and to provide effectively for their individual educational needs without calling undue attention to their learning deficits. Students with a wide range of disabilities may receive instruction at the same time if their functional level and instructional needs are similar (Polloway, 1984; Sindelar & Deno, 1978; Tindal, 1985).

Level 3 — Part-Time Special Class

Every school system has LD children with educational problems that require an instructional setting or educational delivery system that is highly specialized or unique. Such a learning environment is necessitated when (1) a student has deficits in several subject areas, (2) the complexity of the problem exceeds the expertise of the regular instructional staff, and (3) the magnitude of instructional needs exceeds the normal capabilities of the resource room. When all three of these circumstances exist, the LD student may be a likely candidate for a part-time special class, with the remaining portion of the school day in either the resource room or the regular class.

It is important to note that the characteristics of a part-time special class will differ dramatically among school districts because of the differences that exist among teachers in their philosophy, orientation, attitudes, and talents. The character of the part-time special class will change according to the children's needs and the teacher's skills.

Level 4 — Full-Time Special Class

Some LD students profit from placement in an educational setting on a full-time basis. An arrangement of this type affords the teacher more contact on a continuous basis and in all instructional areas of the curriculum. It is easier to engineer the educational program so that instructional work accomplished in one subject or area of the curriculum can be more carefully and appropriately integrated into all aspects of the instructional program. Furthermore, it should be noted that although some studies have shown that special class placement may stigmatize students, who may then reject the special class, these outcomes are by no means necessary. In fact, both positive and negative attitudes regarding special classes were expressed by disabled and nondisabled students (Jones, 1974; Warner, Thrapp, & Walsh, 1973).

COMPARISON OF SPECIAL CLASS AND RESOURCE ROOM

It should be readily apparent that all educational delivery systems have both positive and negative characteristics. A closer look at two of these educational delivery systems — the resource room (in vogue today) and the special class (in vogue 20 years ago) — will illustrate this point.

What are the advantages and disadvantages of using the resource room in teaching the LD student (Glavin, 1974; Sabatino, 1971; Salend, 1984; Thurlow, Graden, Greener, & Ysseldyke, 1982; Wang & Baker, 1985–86)? The advantages of the resource room as an instructional delivery system are numerous. Students can be left with "normal" peers for the majority of the school day, but specific problems can be attacked by a specially trained teacher. A large number of students can be worked with over the course of a school year and it is easier to phase students in or out of the resource room program any time they appear ready for such changes. Currently, there is little or no stigma attached to this particular educational delivery system and teachers, parents, and students seem to accept this arrangement more readily than other arrangements.

This is not to say that the resource room does not have its liabilities (Heller, Holtzman, & Messick, 1982; Stainback, Stainback, Courtnage, & Jaben, 1985). For example, the role and function of resource teachers are still not clear. Should their roles be primarily remedial or tutorial, or should they work as much with regular classroom teachers via inservice programs as they do with students? Determining which children would benefit most from this instructional system is still difficult. Is it the child with minimal problems or difficulties, or the one with severe involvement? Efficient and effective scheduling is a Herculean problem. Can the resource teacher do the most effective job of teaching by seeing a child daily for short periods of time, or two or three times a week for longer blocks of time? How can the resource teacher remain in touch with the regular classroom teacher? What is the best communication system to keep these lines open?

What are the advantages and disadvantages of using the self-contained special class in teaching the LD child? The most obvious advantages of the self-contained classroom include a low teacher-pupil ratio, which affords the maximum opportunity for individualizing instruction. Teachers who work with LD children exclusively have special training, and continuous contact with the same teacher over a long period of time affords efficient, systematic instruction for each student. A well-defined, organized curriculum content in terms of sequence, scope, continuity, and balance of program is available in special classes and a high degree of homogeneity among pupils makes it easier to differentiate instruction. Reduced competition among students reduces the need to outperform other students and reduces the probability that students will develop negative self-images. However, just because these positive possibilities exist does not mean that they will necessarily be taken advantage of by the special education teacher (Blatt, 1958; Denham & Lieberman, 1980; Elenbogen, 1957; Fisher & Berliner, 1985; Guskin & Spicker, 1968; Leinhardt & Pallay, 1982; Mullen & Itkin, 1961; Myers, 1976).

The disadvantages of the self-contained special education classroom have been delineated (Caroll, 1967; Cegelka & Tyler, 1970; Elenbogen, 1957; Goldstein, Moss, & Jordan, 1965; Kaufman & Alberto, 1976; Mullen & Itkin, 1961; Stanton & Cassidy, 1964; Tucker, 1980; Vacc, 1968). They include the tendency for students in special education classes to be segregated from other students, not only academically but at other times as well (e.g., arriving at different times, eating at different times, having recess at different times). Once placed in a special class, there is a tendency for individuals to be kept in the program, whether they are still benefiting from it or not. Having the same teacher year after year is a liability if the teacher is not competent, or if a personality conflict develops between the student and teacher. Lack of a well-defined, organized curriculum can also be a problem. Finally, homogeneity on one dimension (e.g., cognitive level) does not mean homogeneity among the children on other aspects of their development.

Reynolds and Birch (1982) pointed out several positive features of the cascade model. One, such a model amplifies the point that one means of meeting the needs of LD students is to provide support in regular classrooms. Second, although it provides a framework for placing students in more restrictive settings when necessary, it also implies that they should be moved to less restrictive settings as soon as feasible. Third, the need for a closer working relationship between regular and special education is conveyed so that adjustments in level can be easily accomplished in terms of the students' educational needs. Fourth, a sharing of responsibilities for students between special and general educators is clearly indicated. Fifth, this model implies that overwhelming evidence should be required to remove a student from a regular class.

It should be noted that within the cascade model, attention is focused on the setting in which special education is provided. The setting is a macrovariable that has recieved considerable attention with respect to policy decisions (Leinhardt & Pallay, 1982). The setting has been viewed as a form of treatment for students who have had difficulty in the regular class, and hence, it has been examined as an independent variable that directly influences student achievement.

EFFICACY RESEARCH

In the past, special education was generally viewed as a positive event because the intent was to provide services for students experiencing difficulty in general education. An accepting environment, modified instructional goals and techniques, and teachers with special training in areas of exceptionality were presumed to lead to more effective educational programs for LD students. Special programs usually received little systematic scrutiny since the assumption was that they were beneficial, although data regarding the efficacy of LD programs typically were unavailable. It was not possible, therefore, to determine the relative effectiveness of various instructional programs with LD students (Sheehan & Keogh, 1984).

Recently, however, economic and professional pressures have made evaluating and demonstrating program impact a high priority for LD personnel. Since evaluation data are needed to improve educational practice, this emphasis is fortunate. It appears that data on program evaluaton will continue to be of great importance as LD programs compete for tighter funds. To evaluate program effectiveness, systematic collection of data is needed (Sheehan & Keogh, 1984).

Two questions need to be addressed when assessing the efficacy of special versus general education placement for LD students. First, do students experiencing difficulty in school fare better when placed in special education settings, such as resource rooms and self-contained classes, or when allowed to remain in regular classrooms? Second, what is the content of special education instruction and how is it different from the content offered in the regular classroom?

In reviewing "efficacy" studies, it is important to note that the literature has been criticized for possessing serious methodological flaws (MacMillan, 1971). Interpreting the results of efficacy studies must be viewed cautiously for two reasons: (1) attention has focused mainly on the setting in which special instruction is provided rather than on the components of instruction; and (2) the assumption that instructional programs are similar characterizes much of the evaluation literature.

Special programs for LD students may be of questionable value if they show no advantage over regular class placement. In fact, in some instances special education placements may have a detrimental effect on LD student progress (Glavin, 1974; Glavin, Quay, Annesley, & Werry, 1971; Sabatino, 1971; Sheehan & Keogh, 1984; Tindal, 1985; Walker, 1974). This disappointing finding may have two possible explanations: (1) special education intervention may be ineffective, or (2) the methodology for measuring treatment and program outcome may be questionable.

There are at least five methodological concerns that must be examined when evaluating data regarding the effectiveness of special education services. They are (1) population served, (2) variability among definitions, (3) historical changes in classifications, (4) placement histories, and (5) assignment to treatment. The extent to which studies have considered each of these methodological concerns and their control determines the validity of the results (Tindal, 1985).

Classification

Each particular category of exceptional students represents a heterogeneous group of individuals who have been classified according to diverse, and often ambiguous, criteria that may vary from district to district and from state to state. Students classified into the LD category in one setting are very likely to be different from those similarly identified in another setting. Even assuming that assessment personnel were able to reach consensus on a definition, differences are almost sure to remain in the way that definition is operationalized (Landers, 1987). Identification of the same students (Epps, Ysseldyke, & Algozzine, 1985), or even the same number of students (Epps, Ysseldyke, & Algozzine, 1983), does not necessarily result from the selection of one operational definition over another. Classification in a certain area of exceptionality depends not only on pupil characteristic but also on the classification formula and the specific tests used to derive scores that are entered into the formula (Olson & Midgett, 1984). Therefore, a classification made when using one group of tests is not always generalizable to other instruments.

Additional complications arise when attempts are made to operationalize the definition of LD. Not only are there differences among operational definitions because of the use of different tests, but results may be differentially biased depending on the match between curriculum and test (Epps, Ysseldyke, & Algozzine, 1983, 1985; Jenkins & Pany, 1978). Then, too, operational definitions are influenced by the amount of decision making required of diagnostic personnel, especially when tests having low reliability are used (Salvia & Ysseldyke, 1985). Effective instruction is more likely to depend on a student's characteristics as a learner than on a particular special education classification. Therefore, the variation in the definition of LD and the subsequent heterogeneity obviously limit the conclusions that can be drawn from most of the efficacy research (Heller, Holtzman, & Messick, 1982).

Algozzine and Korinek (1985) raised the question, "What if the programs these students are in (resource rooms, etc.) are not effective?" In addressing this point, Gerber (1984) noted, "Over 1.6 million American school children are being treated as LD and their school experiences are often drastically changed without unequivocal demonstration that such changes benefit them over the course of their public school education or produce desirable, long-term life outcomes" (p. 222).

Historical changes in classification practices present an additional difficulty in interpreting efficacy research. For example, in the past decade there has been a rapid increase in the number of students identified as learning disabled, but a sharp decrease in the number of students identified as educable mentally retarded (EMR) (Tucker, 1980; U. S. Department of Education, 1987). As a result, students currently classified as EMR who are placed in self-contained settings may be more disabled than their counterparts who were classified as EMR in previous years. Therefore, the results of efficacy studies done some years ago may not be generalizable to the current group of educable mentally retarded students (Heller et al., 1982).

Placement Histories

The potential of different placement histories to affect students' progress in educational programs must be considered. This suggests that the apparent effect of each successive intervention may be confounded by its order in the placement sequence. Consequently, the effects of multiple treatments seriously limit the applicability of experimental findings (Campbell, 1969). Some authorities feel that long-term studies are less likely to be subjected to this threat to internal validity introduced by different placement histories (Sindelar & Deno, 1978).

It is evident that the characteristics of LD students are more diverse than the single label given to them suggests. It is possible that some students may profit more from instruction in the regular classroom whereas others may profit more from special class instruction. Goldstein, Moss, and Jordan (1965) studied EMR student placement and found such a result. Students with IQs in the range of 81-85 who were instructed in regular classrooms had slightly, although not significantly, higher achievement test scores than did students within the same IQ range in self-contained classes. The opposite pattern was found for students with IQs less than 80; students in special classes had higher math achievement test scores than did those in regular classes.

Assignment to Treatment

The means by which subjects are assigned to treatment is important for controlling threats to internal validity, such as history, maturation, testing, instrumentation, regression, selection, mortality, and the interaction of selection and maturation (Campbell & Stanley, 1979). These factors can invalidate test results; outcome data may be unrelated to treatment.

"Comparison" groups are not likely to be comparable without random sampling. Randomness was not achieved in many of the early efficacy studies. Subject selection included the use of preexisting groups, which were not placed into alternate forms of educational intervention on a random basis. Some schools transfer students with the most severe problems into segregated classes and retain other students who are less of a problem in regular classes. This results in the students most repugnant to the general educators being disproportionately represented in special classes. The complex referral and identification process contains considerable potential for bias (Ysseldyke & Algozzine, 1982; Ysseldyke & Thurlow, 1983). In addition, the school and adjustment histories of students in special education may not be similar to those who remain in regular classes. Therefore, it may be that any differences between groups are due to antecedent conditions rather than to the effects of educational intervention (Kaufman & Alberto, 1976). Such biases in sample selection are serious enough to make the results suspect.

A more frequently used procedure, given the difficulty of randomization, is to match students on various characteristics such as IQ, sex, and age. However, matching background characteristics other than the outcome measure is usually ineffective and can be misleading. It appears that there have been few studies in which students were matched on the outcome measure (e.g., Franklin & Sparkman, 1978; Vacc, 1968; Walker, 1974).

Efficacy research has generally focused on determining the type of administrative setting associated with the greatest treatment gains. The performance of LD students in special classes and that of LD students placed in a variety of integrated settings are compared to determine the effects of mainstreaming. The service options in these settings range from treatment in full-time special education to regular class placement with resource room support and regular class placement with supportive services offered within the regular classroom.

COMPARISON OF REGULAR AND SELF-CONTAINED SETTINGS

Only a few of the earlier efficacy studies (pre-1970) are reviewed in the following section because significant methodological problems make it unwise to place much emphasis on their results. The populations studied were mainly EMR, but results can be generalized to illustrate the problems in educating LD students.

Elenbogen (1957) compared the academic and social adjustment of two groups of EMR students. One group had been placed in special classes while the other remained in regular class during the 2 years prior to the study. The two groups were matched by chronological age, sex, IQ, and school district. As measured by the Stanford Achievement Test, the results in reading and arithmetic revealed significantly higher mean scores for students in regular classes. It might be concluded that general education placement was superior to special education since achievement was higher for students who remained in the regular classrooms. However, this interpretation is not warranted in light of several significant methodological shortcomings. Random selection of the students placed in special classes with the remaining students serving as controls did not occur. Students were matched on several characteristics, but not on achievement level. Because the subject selection bias gave the regular class group an advantage, the two groups were not equivalent. It is quite likely that students not placed in special classes probably were superior on other school-related characteristics. In addition, the study provided no information about the curriculum used in each setting.

In a study by Mullen and Itkin (1961), conducted over a 2-year period, 140 pairs of EMR students in special and regular classes were matched for age, IQ, sex, socioeconomic status, foreign language spoken at home, and reading achievement. The students in regular classes showed significantly greater gains in arithmetic, but in no other area, at the end of the first year. There was no maintenance of this effect, however, after two years.

Blatt (1958) and Stanton and Cassidy (1964) also found that regular class students who received no special help, performed as well as or better than special class students. Others (Leinhardt & Pallay, 1982) who reviewed studies conducted during this period found similar results. There was a problem, however, in concluding that the special class setting itself had a negative impact. Students in the more segregated environments often received only a watered-down curriculum, leading to a general reduction in the intensity of instruction as well as little systematic alteration of instructional techniques (Guskin & Spicker, 1968).

One earlier study can be singled out as an attempt to cope with the problem of subject selection bias by randomly assigning students to classrooms. Goldstein et al. (1965) used the Primary Abilities Test to screen 2,000 students entering first grade in 20 Illinois school districts. The Stanford-Binet was administered to those who scored below 85. The students who scored between 56 and 85 on both measures were assigned randomly to either self-contained classes or regular classes. At the end of each of the 4 years of the project, achievement measures were given to the students. After the first 2 years, there were significant differences between the experimental and control groups for the total sample, with the control group obtaining 0.5 and 0.3 grade-equivalent scores higher. There was a significant difference in math between groups, but only after the first year, with the control group scoring 0.3 grade equivalents higher. Students in regular classes outscored those in special classes in both reading and math for the total sample, but this advantage did not maintain itself.

The Goldstein et al. (1965) study represented a significant contribution to the literature because it controlled for some of the methodological weaknesses of previous investigations, such as (1) random assignment of subjects to treatment; (2) differences in school experiences prior to special class placement; and (3) specification of the special class educational program. The data, however, did not provide unequivocal support for the superiority of special class placement. The fact that the special class curriculum placed a greater emphasis on practical knowledge, social skills, and emotional development than the regular class curriculum might be one reason for the lack of greater academic gains. Hence, curriculum test overlap was significantly reduced (Jenkins & Pany, 1978).

Any conclusions drawn from this study (Goldstein et al., 1965) must take into account several weaknesses. First, children were placed in self-contained or regular classrooms on the sole basis of an IQ score, and a considerable number had scores above 85. Goldstein's experimental group may not be comparable to students typically served in special classes. Second, the standardized achievement tests used to document student progress may not have been sensitive in detecting changes. Third, the significance of small differences tend to be exaggerated when grade equivalent scores are used.

In the early 1970s, a trend toward less segregation of the disabled began. This may have been due, in part, to the unimpressive results of earlier efficacy studies. Increased interest in the mainstreaming philosophy brought about a new series of studies designed to test the hypothesis that disabled students would profit if they spent at least part of their school year with their nondisabled peers (Heller et al.,1982).

The results of studies concerning the academic benefits of self-contained and regular classes have been inconsistent. The efficacy of a special day school, self-contained class, and regular class for the EMR students was examined by Myers (1976). There were no significant differences in grade level gain scores among the three settings based on the Wide Range Achievement Test (WRAT) as a measure of academic achievement. There were significant differences in grade level gain scores, however, when the three groups of students were divided into low IQ (Slosson IQ of 49–70) and high IQ groups (Slosson IQ of 71–85). For example, in both reading and spelling, low IQ students in the special school demonstrated significantly greater gains than either the special class or regular class group. Students remaining in regular classes made significantly greater gains in reading than students in self-contained classes for the high IQ groups. Low IQ students made more academic gains in a segragated setting whereas high IQ students made more gains in the regular class. In arithmetic, however, there were no significant differences among the three treatment conditions for either the low IQ or high IQ students.

Myers' (1976) study and a study by Sabatino (1971) both produced favorable results regarding self-contained classes, although regular class placement tended to be favored when Myers' high IQ group was considered. The effectiveness of a self-contained classroom, regular class placement with tutoring 2 to 5 hours per week from certified teachers, and regular class placement with no additional help for children who had been identified as neurologically disabled, was examined by Bersoff, Kabler, Fiscus, and Ankney (1972). No significant differences were found among the three treatment groups in WRAT reading or arithmetic scores. Academic performance beyond what was obtained in regular classrooms did not result from either special class placement or individual tutoring.

Special class placement is affected by the negative attitudes of students who have been placed there. Although student rejection of special class placement is clear, great caution needs to be taken before generalizing about reactions of disabled students to their special classrooms and overall school experiences. For example, the results of a study by Jones (1974) revealed clearly that neither exceptional nor nondisabled students held homogeneous school attitudes. Members of both groups expressed positive and negative attitudes toward instruction and school relationships. In many instances, attitudes toward classroom and school held by disabled students were no different than those held by nondisabled students.

It seems clear that the wholesale attribution of negative school attitudes to LD students is incorrect. This does not mean, however, that data on stigma associated with the LD label and special class placement are any less real. It should be realized that although it is important to reduce negative school attitudes associated with special classes, it does not follow that all the LD student's problems will be eliminated when this objective is obtained. That is to say, placement of the LD student in a regular class-room, without the provision of supportive services for the remediation of deficiencies in academic skills and interpersonal relationships, might well lead to the creation of problems as serious as those that are believed to result from placement in the special class.

A meta-analysis by Carlberg and Kavale (1980) studied the efficacy of special versus regular class placement for exceptional children. Fifty primary research studies of special education versus regular class place-ment were selected. Each study provided a measure of effect size (ES), defined as the posttreatment differences between special and regular place-ment means, expressed in standard deviation units. Effect size was used as a dependent variable to assess the effects of independent variables such as placement, type of outcome measure, and internal validity. Special classes were found to be significantly inferior to regular class placement for students with below average IQs, and significantly superior to regular classes for students with behavioral or emotional disorders and for LD stu-dents. It was reported that traditional reviews of the literature generally fail to reveal unilateral evidence that establishes the superiority of one educa-tional delivery system over another on academic or social criteria. Further-more, equivocal results were found in most studies comparing integrated versus segregated placement for LD children.

Carlberg and Kavale (1980) summarized their results by stating that no conclusion about the relative superiority of special versus regular class placement can be drawn from simple inspection of empirical findings. No significant differences in either academic achievement or perceptual motor functioning among LD children in integrated and segregated settings were reported in several other studies (Bersoff, Kabler, Fiscus, & Ankney, 1972; Sabatino, 1971; Spollen & Ballif, 1971).

It is often assumed that the skills and behavior learned in a special class or resource room will be transferred to the regular class, although it is well known that the two settings (special class and regular class) are quite different in terms of instructional materials, rules, directions, reinforce-ment, and individualized instruction. For example, Rose, Lessen, and Gott-lieb, (1982) reported that 82% of the special education teachers surveyed in their study employed a 1:1 instructional ratio more than one-third of the day per student. It is clear that merely shifting students from one setting to another will not result in improved performance regardless of how effec-tive the student performed in a special class setting. Transfer of training is not likely to be spontaneous.

Olson and Midgett (1984) examined the similarities and differences in characteristics of 35 LD students in resource programs and 50 LD students in self-contained programs. Performance was compared on the Wechsler Intelligence Scale for Children, the Picture Story Language Test, the Peabody Individual Achievement Test, and selected subtests of the Detroit Test of Learning Aptitude. The subjects were also compared on the factors of retention, age, and subjective indices of behavior. The results of a discriminant function indicated a difference only in the intelligence factor between the two groups, favoring those LD students placed in the resource room. The overall results, however, showed that the basic test battery criteria used for LD placement did not differentiate between those subjects in self-contained classrooms and those in resource classrooms.

RESOURCE ROOMS

Results are not definitive when self-contained and regular classroom settings are compared with resource room placements. The small body of research has offered conflicting findings, for example, with the EMR population. In a study by Carroll (1967), a resource program was compared with a full-time special class. After 8 months, a statistically significant but only moderate increase in students' performance on the WRAT for both groups was obtained. The integrated group, however, made significantly greater gains on the reading subtest. There was some question about the relative equivalence of these two groups. More specifically, the resource room students had higher initial scores on all three subtests and may have been better students. Other significant differences between the groups may also have been in effect.

Walker (1974) reported that students in a resource program outperformed students in a special class on both word reading and vocabulary subtests of the Stanford Achievement Test. There were no significant differences in achievement when a resource program was compared with regular class placement (Smith & Kennedy, 1967) or a resource program with special class placement (Budoff & Gottlieb, 1976). Leinhardt and Pallay (1982) reported inconclusive findings in a comparison of resource room and self-contained class with nonretarded populations.

Several studies contrasting resource rooms with regular programs suggest resource rooms may be superior (Glavin, Quay, Annesley, & Werry, 1971; Sabatino, 1971). In the Sabatino (1971) study, students in self-contained and resource room classes performed better academically than the regular class controls. This study tended to support the resource room over the special class, but that depends on which outcome measure was used. Highly significant differences in academic gains occurred on the reading subtest of the WRAT. Students in the resource room for 1 hour each day gained 1.9 age equivalents compared to 1.4 for self-contained and 1.2 for students in the resource program 1/2 hour a day. The control pupils gained approximately 0.1 age equivalent. The use of the Gilmore Oral Reading Comprehensive Subtest brought about a different pattern of results: students in the self-contained class gained 2.0 age equivalents, those in the resource room 1 hour each day gained 1.5 age equivlents, and those in the resource room for 1/2 hour each week gained 1.0 age equivalents.

The Glavin, Quay, Annesley, and Werry (1971) study viewed the performance of children with behavioral disorders in resource and regular classes. The subjects were then randomly selected for part-time participation in a resource room or a regular class. In the experimental group (part-time resource room participants), some of the students attended the resource room for two periods a day receiving instruction in reading and arithmetic; others attended for one period a day and were instructed in arithmetic or reading only. It was concluded that both groups significantly reduced deviant behavior and increased on-task behavior during the program. There were significant differences in all three classes of behavior when the experimental group's behavior in the resource room was compared with the control group's behavior in the regular classroom. Academic achievement for the experimental group had significantly higher gain scores in reading comprehension and arithmetic fundamentals. There were, however, no significant differences in reading vocabulary and arithmetic reasoning. Furthermore, Quay, Glavin, Annesley, and Werry (1972), in a study of the second year of the program described in Glavin et al. (1971), reported the resource program group scoring significantly higher than the regular class group on the California Achievement Test in reading vocabulary, total reading, arithmetic fundamentals, and total arithmetic. This was not true for reading comprehension, however. Following termination of this 2-year program, a first year postcheck revealed a continued significant difference in arithmetic fundamentals only. Unfortunately, the second year postcheck did not show any significant differences between the two groups (Glavin, 1974).

It appears that resource programs, in general, are effective in improving the academic performance of all populations, although this has not been clearly established. Some studies have found resource room placement to be superior to full-time placement in the regular class. However, an additional issue may need to be addressed: Does the effectiveness of resource rooms vary depending on whether students have motivational problems?

SUMMARY

Although earlier efficacy studies (pre-1970) had major methodological problems, some general conclusions may be drawn. Mildly disabled students in general, and LD students in particular, fared at least as well as or better in the regular class than in the self-contained class with reference to academic measures (Elenbogen, 1957; Leinhardt & Pallay, 1982; Mullen & Itkin, 1961; Stanton & Cassidy, 1964). After a meta-analytic review of studies of special class versus regular class placement, Carlberg and Kavale (1980) concluded that the literature failed to reveal unilateral evidence that establishes the superiority of one educational delivery system over another in terms of academic or social criteria. Equivocal results were found in most studies comparing integrated versus segregated placement for LD children. Several additional studies (Bersoff, Kabler, Fiscus, & Ankney, 1972; Sabatino, 1971; Spollen & Ballif, 1971) reported no significant differences in academic achievement or perceptual motor functioning among LD children in integrated and segregated settings. Hence, no confident conclusion regarding the relative superiority of special versus regular class placement can be deduced from simple inspection of the empirical findings.

It appears, however, that resource rooms in general are more effective in improving the academic performance of all disabled populations, especially LD, than other special education delivery systems. Resource rooms also appear to be superior to full-time placement in the regular class (Caroll, 1967; Glavin, Quay, Annesley, & Werry, 1971; Sabatino, 1971; Walker, 1974). In fact, resource rooms were better than regular class placement with no support and seem to hold their own against self-contained placement (Leinhardt & Pallay, 1982; Sabatino, 1971).

Some special educators state that the issue of efficacy of special classes is a dead one (Milazzo, 1970) and that future research should be directed toward variables that are functionally important in changing student behavior. More specifically, it is felt that the focus of research should be directed at developing systems for measuring the implementation of instruction as well as the consequence of its effects (Millazzo, 1970). These issues must be investigated as covariates. Each variable should be considered in relation to, not independent of, the other variable.

In conclusion, it would seem prudent to ponder the following points made by Leinhardt and Pallay (1982). They suggested that setting does not operate directly on student academic and social growth, but rather indirectly through instructional and affective processes. Achievement is the result of the actual teaching processes that may be influenced by the manner in which children are grouped, but achievement is never the direct outcome of a particular grouping arrangement. Furthermore, Leinhardt and Pallay suggested that setting is a macrovariable that masks more significant and fine-grained microvariables. The point is that a service delivery arrangement is important, but not of ultimate importance because, "Its visibility and alterability make it worth studying, *not* the magnitude of its influence on achievement" (Leinhardt & Pallay, 1982, p. 560).

Computer Technology

The three chapters in this section deal with the use of computers. With the increased use of computers in schools, it is important to understand their role and potential usefulness. Chapter 6 describes how computers may be used for the purpose of instructional management of LD students. A systems approach is described for organizing and managing instructional information along with evaluative comments about available systems and software. Chapter 7 provides an evaluative framework for software and demonstrates its use with available software in language arts and math.

The final chapter in Part III deals with computer applications for LD students and their teachers. Specifically, information is presented in the development of a systematized computer training program for LD professionals and integrated classroom applications for LD students, particularly with regard to computer literacy and language processing. These applications hold great promise for the LD field, but require careful thought and planning.

CHAPTER 6

Computer Management

David L. Hayden
Lois T. Pommer
David S. Mark

T his chapter examines the use of personal computers to manage instructional materials for the learning disabled and provides a rationale for collecting and processing data. It begins with a review of a system approach to general education and then reviews special education materials systems and information for teachers. It presents a model for organizing information and, in the last section, describes various software programs that are available for personal computers and suggests some innovations in instructional-material management for teachers.

DEVELOPMENT OF EDUCATION SYSTEMS APPROACHES

The need to apply systems approaches to educational processes has led educational psychologists such as Gagne (1968) to concern themselves with objectively describing conditions of learning based on psychological principles. These descriptions and principles are embodied in design criteria during systems development. Other writers, such as Mager (1962) and

This chapter originally appeared as an article by **David L. Hayden, Lois T. Pommer,** and **David S. Mark** in *Learning Disabilities: An Interdisciplinary Journal* (Vol II (7), 83–97, 1983) and was adapted by permission of Grune & Stratton for inclusion in this *Handbook.*

Popham, Eisner, Sullivan and Tyler (1969), have taken the position that an operational definition of teaching and learning objectives is necessary for the systematic management of learning. Bose (1970) was concerned with the application of Program Evaluation Review Techniques (PERT) to educational systems. McIntyre and Nelson (1969) were concerned with the development of techniques for empirically testing the effectiveness of instructional materials (a necessary prerequisite for effective instructional-systems development). A personal-computer-based management system is proposed to facilitate the engineering job of translating these components into an operational instructional system for teachers. As noted by Hannaford and Sloane (1981), personal computers are of little use unless they are accompanied by good educational software programs.

DEVELOPMENT OF SPECIAL EDUCATION SYSTEMS APPROACHES

In 1966, the federal government recognized the need for coordinating instructional-materials information for teachers of the handicapped. In the years that followed, the federal Office of Special Education established a network of Special Education Instructional Materials Centers (SEIMCs) in various regions across the country to serve the purpose. The need to use standard terminology for describing instructional materials and strategies for handicapped students became a national problem in the attempt to evaluate and coordinate information among the SEIMCs. This problem was addressed by Armstrong (1973) and Oldesen (1974).

In 1974, the six experimental resource centers dealing with diagnostic-prescriptive services were replaced with a national network of thirteen regional resource centers and the SEIMC network was realigned to cover the same regions as the regional resource centers. There was a title change to Area Learning Resource Centers (ALRCs), though the functions remained primarily the same. The need for standard terminology for describing diagnostic tests and learner characteristics of disabled students that provide specifications for selecting instructional materials and strategies could be addressed. Close cooperation among the 13 regions made possible a national network, and sharing resources gave a wider base of experiences to draw from than any single center or teacher could achieve.

The creation of special centers for analyzing and indexing recommended instructional materials for various types of disabling conditions and the creation of one national center for dissemination of special education media and material information enhanced the coordination of information and services. Through these national efforts, a series of models for organizing diagnostic and prescriptive information were developed and field tested. These models now have practical applications in organizing information using personal computers to assist in managing instructional strategies for LD students. For example, the National Information Center for Special Education Materials (NICSEM) system was designed by Risner (1979) to assist special educators in meeting the requirement of Public Law 94-142 that an individualized educational program (IEP) be developed for each handicapped child receiving special education services.

The five-level NICSEM Special Education Thesaurus, which encompasses the full range of learning characteristics, learner skills, curriculum content areas and parent/professional topics, serves as the controlled indexing vocabulary for instructional and professional materials in the NICSEM data base. The structure of the learner segment of the thesaurus allows for the retrieval of materials based on the specificity or generality of a particular instructional goal and the discrete learner skill or content area that has been targeted. The thesaurus thus facilitates the ability of special educators to use the retrieval system to select materials in accordance with a child's IEP. The five levels are used to describe and retrieve materials. The levels of the hierarchy are illustrated in Table 6-1.

SYSTEM COMPONENTS

Learning Objectives

In order to coordinate and evaluate the usefulness of resources for teachers of LD students, it is necessary to have objectives around which resources can be coordinated and evaluated. Learning objectives are generated from the school curriculum, teacher guides, and course outlines, or are implied from the instructional materials and methods selected by the teacher for LD children. By beginning with learning objectives, it is possible to develop a cross-indexing system that will serve to (a) identify

TABLE 6-1
The Five Levels of the NICSEM Special Education Thesaurus

Level	Code	Target Area
Level 1	H	Communication skills
Level 2	HF	Reading skills
Level 3	HF-06	Visual skills
Level 4	HF-0603	Visual discrimination
Level 5	HF-0603.03	Color discrimination

materials that are purported to be suitable for achieving specific objectives; (b) identify standard criterion tests for measuring each learning objective; (c) identify methods of using the materials to achieve these specific objectives; (d) identify disabled children which certain identifiable learning characteristics for whom specific learning objectives have been achieved in the past; (e) define learning environments in which materials and methods have been used successfully in the past to achieve stated objectives; (f) cross-reference critical skills required of implementors (such as teachers, aides, and parents) to use materials related to specific learning objectives with a child who has certain identifiable learning characteristics; and (g) specify average time required to obtain specific objectives with LD children who have certain identifiable learning characteristics, using the specified materials, methods, and learning environments.

Such a cross-indexing system using a personal computer provides a mechanism for identifying and managing the resources needed to achieve specific objectives with LD children who have certain identifiable learning characteristics. Therefore, by building on learning objectives, it is possible to develop an instructional management system for teachers of LD students.

Standardized criterion test must be developed to measure specific short-term instructional objectives to meet the PL 94-142 requirements. The word *standardized* applies to methods of administering the test, to the materials used, and to methods of scoring. After learning objectives have been specified, the teacher will be able to select from a pool of test items those that have been developed as appropriate measures of each objective. Through the use of standardized criterion tests, it will be possible to obtain data across various curricula as children enter into the individualized educational programs, and to obtain posttest results after the children have been exposed to instruction based on that IEP.

There is also a need for a personal computer instructional management system that has the capacity for storing a bank of criterion-referenced test items indexed to specific objectives.

Comprehensive Achievement Monitoring System

It would be useful to develop a comprehensive achievement monitoring system for the teacher that makes it possible to evaluate and manage individualized educational programs for LD students. Such a system would provide the teacher with information concerning mastery of each learning objective in the IEP and for grouping students based on IEP objectives. Criterion tests are the critical components for the achievement monitoring system to evaluate student progress on specific objectives.

The personal computer instructional management system should be able to store user-history data and generate status reports on specific objectives for each student.

Learner Characteristics

To select appropriate instructional strategies, the management system needs to identify critical learner characteristics that coordinate with learning objectives in the IEP. The teacher needs learner-characteristic information to make a professional judgment regarding the probability of achieving a specific objective with a learning-disabled child who has certain indentifiable learning characteristics. It is not enough to say that a child is learning disabled; one must look at the child's learning characteristics. These serve as prerequisites for the child to master specific enabling tasks related to objectives. It will be possible to analyze diagnostic tests and match (index) objectives.

By specifying learning objectives and by using computer-based instructional management systems that keep records of materials, methods, and learning environments, it will be possible for special education teachers and administrators to build a sequential curriculum of learning objectives that have been evaluated (having a user-history of being successful) for disabled children with certain identifiable learning characteristics.

Instructional Materials

Three major efforts are required to organize information for a computer-assisted management system for teachers. First, instructional materials and equipment that is suitable for LD children must be identified. There is a need for bibliographic (media-graphic) processing of instructional materials and equipment at the level of specificity that would indicate pieces of materials or equipment that can be used independently. This information is needed to reduce instructional materials by content and context analysis into single concept materials to be coordinated with learning objectives in the instructional strategies system.

Next instructional materials that are part of a backup system the teacher has available to use in teaching LD students must be located. These materials may be located in the teacher's own classroom, in the school library, or in the instructional-materials center in the local education agency. At present, a major problem for the teacher of the disabled child has been the delay in obtaining materials after the child's needs have been identified, especially in such cases where these needs were not identified at the beginning of the year and consequently could not be considered in initial planning and budgeting.

Finally, instructional materials must be analyzed by content and context analysis of the learning objectives and learning methods inherent in the materials. Identification of the sequence of enabling steps relating to the learning objectives is also important. Once content analysis has been completed and the learning objectives have been identified, it will be possible to develop a cross-index system. Also, it will be possible to evaluate and compare instructional materials according to their usefulness with specific learning objectives. Content and context analysis will provide a tool for teachers to select appropriate instructional materials for children, based on objectives outlined in their special curriculum as suitable for LD students with a certain developmental age and certain identifiable learning characteristics.

Methods and Procedures

There is a need to develop a system to identify and describe methods for using materials to achieve specified learning objectives. The importance of examining author-intended methods for using materials to achieve specified learning objectives is that it provides a more efficient way of classifying methods according to given recommendations. All materials, such as teacher guides and manuals, recommend certain methods. In the past, adjusting the method to meet the need of the child was a major area of work and concern for the teacher. By beginning with the method recommended by the author, and classifying it using the NICSEM Special Education Thesaurus, it will be possible to field test the appropriateness of a method for using materials to achieve specific objectives. The use of a computer-based instructional management system that keeps records on how materials were used with LD children can help teachers devise more appropriate methods for using these materials and strategies to achieve specific learning objectives.

Personnel

Three major efforts are required in the area of support personnel for special education teachers. The first task is to identify special education technical support personnel with competencies in each of the diagnostic-prescriptive educational programming components discussed previously. It is necessary to identify the skill competency of special education support personnel and the teacher who has the responsibility for implementing prescriptive educational programming to achieve specific learning objectives with LD children in various learning environments. Such information is also needed by special education administrators to determine the appropriate support personnel needed by the teacher.

The second effort involves the location of special education technical support personnel to assist teachers. Such personnel may be located in the teacher's own classroom (aides), the school building (counselor, nurse, other resource room teachers), or in the local education agency (curriculum specialist, school psychologists, pupil personnel, staff, community support agencies).

Third, competency-based skill analyses should be performed on a schema of competency skills required for using various methods suitable for working with LD children. This competency skill analysis should be completed at the level at which the teacher needs the information.

Learning Environment

It is also important to identify learning environments in which various tests, materials, methods, and staff have been used successfully with LD students with certain learner characteristics in achieving specific sets of objectives.

The use of an instructional classification system for coding materials addressing the *how* as well as the *what* of instruction by Tannenbaum (1970) takes into account the teacher's function in (a) organizing instructional content logically and sequentially; (b) transmitting instructional stimuli through any of the pupil's receptive sensory modalities; (c) eliciting responsiveness through any of the pupil's expressive channels of communication; and (d) mastering the total range of instructional modes (or styles) and settings (pupil grouping arrangements) available for utilization. The *how* of instruction refers to the teaching strategy used in presenting content. There are four basic components of this aspect of the taxonomy: instructional setting, instructional mode, sensory modality input, and sensory modality output. This aspect of the taxonomy is shown in Table 6–2.

TABLE 6–2
The Four Components of theTaxonomy

Sensory Modality Input	Sensory Modality Output
Kinesthetic	No response
Auditory	Motoric response (gestures & movement)
Auditory kinesthetic	Vocal response
Visual	Motoric response
Visual kinesthetic	Vocal-motoric response
Auditory visual kinesthetic	

Instructional Setting	Instructional Mode
Teacher–student	Play puzzle
Student self–instruction	Play chance
Student-student (parallel)	Play competition
Student-student (interactive)	Test response
Teacher-small group	Role play
Student-small group	Exploration
Teacher-total group	Programmed response
Student-total group	Problem solving
	Exposition

By using these four components, the strategy aspects of instruction can be categorized. For example, a student may be working with the following content: basic skill, basic subskill, sequential level, interest level/language analysis, consonants, grades 2 and below, middle school age. Further, the student may be using the following strategy: instructional setting, instructional mode, sensory modality input, sensory modality output/teacher-student, test response, auditory/visual, vocal. By referring to the taxonomy, the teacher may find activities for individual students in various learning environments.

IEP Evaluation

By examining component interrelationships, it will be possible to ascertain the effectiveness and cost of IEPs for LD students with certain identifiable learning characteristics.

Since the implementation of PL 94-142, over 4 million individualized educational programs are prepared each year by teachers and administrators. Along with increased services and emphasis on mainstreaming, special education teachers often assume the roles of team teachers and educational consultants to regular teachers. To function effectively, special education teachers now require more detailed curriculum analyses and planning tools to manage special education services for individual students and to report information. In all of these areas, computer support systems could reduce paper work and improve instructional management for teachers and speed up generating reports for administrators.

ORGANIZING INFORMATION

To evaluate the usefulness of existing computer-assisted instructional management systems for teachers, a specific model has to be established to serve as the basis for decision making. Although it is well known that models are not always accurate descriptions of what procedures are actually needed (Goodlad & Klein, 1979; Lindvall & Cox, 1970), they can serve to identify necessary system components that might otherwise by overlooked.

A review of a broad range of diagnostic-prescriptive (DP) models shows that the models are not comprehensive but rather reflect various emphasis and philosophies (Dobbert, 1973; Flack, 1973; Glaser, 1972; Tannenbaum, 1970; Shram, 1973). Each focuses on instructional material selection, instructional methodology, or assessment, but not on all at once. A comprehensive information system must be capable of delivering information to anyone who has an information need. This can only be accomplished with a broad-based model that includes all components of other DP models, not with a model restricted to the needs of persons with a particular philosophy.

The DP model by Olsen (1973) is based on the system-design concept paper by Hayden (1972), and on a series of applied-research studies dealing with various components of a state-wide, computer data-based operating system in Pennsylvania known as "Special Education Resource Location Analysis and Retrieval" (SER-LAR) and the Maryland Statewide Special Services Information System. The DP models (Table 6–3) define four levels of diagnostic assessment, a diagnostic prescriptive link through learning objectives, and a broad interpretation of prescriptions. This DP model is being used in Maryland to design the Special Education Manage ment System.

A number of writers have addressed the issue of norm-referenced versus criterion- or domain-referenced measurement; most take an either/or position (Glaser, 1972; Hambleton, 1973; Millman, 1973). In Olsen's (1973) model, the test-teach-test sequence occurs for norm-referenced measurement on specific aspects of that curriculum (levels 5 and 7). This approach provides a compromise and defines the place of both types of measurement within the model. It should be noted that in the diagnostic assessment levels of the model, formal testing may not have occurred. The decision making at these levels may involve a review of available data, interviews, observations, and informal tests and checklists.

This assessment process focuses on defining a specific target-behavioral learning objective, the optimal characteristics of the prescription to be used during the instruction, and how the instruction should be provided.

After the objective has been identified and verified through an objective-referenced measure, an IEP is written that takes into account the parameters of an optimal prescription. Monitoring student progress takes place during implementation.

After an agreed upon time, the objective-referenced measure is readministered and the results are interpreted in one of three ways: as showing a need for modification of the prescription components, as showing a need for a new objective, or as showing that monitoring is no longer needed.

When monitoring is no longer necessary, the student is placed back into regular curricula and at the end of the school year is posttested in the curricular area of concern with the same norm-referenced instrument that was used as a pretest.

The SER-LAR system, using a minicomputer, was successfully field tested and implemented in Pennsylvania over a 4-year period. The model served in programs for the severely and profoundly retarded as well as for learning disabled and emotionally disturbed children. It was implemented in self-contained classes, in resource rooms, and through itinerant services. It was used for early childhood programs and for junior and senior high school and vocational programs. This model was general enough to meet the needs of a broad range of students, but was specific enough to allow for the monitoring of its use.

TABLE 6-3

Diagnostic-Prescriptive Model

Objective	Prescription
Identify student	Level 1. Obtain identifying data and verify student's eligibility for service according to state standards.
Pretest level of skill	Level 2. Determine the student's functional level in curricular area(s) of concern prior to intervention.
Diagnose for content	Level 3. Determine student's strengths and weaknesses within curricular area(s) of concern.
Diagnose for process	Level 4. Determine, if necessary, student's process characteristics, e.g., modality and reinforcement preferences, learning style and level of interaction needed.
Identify learning objectives and administer ORM	Level 5. a. Identify or create learning objective(s). b. Identify or create test/task to measure objective(s). c. Administer objective-referenced measure (ORM). d. Make decision on whether to initiate instruction or to identify new objective.
Identify prescription: implementer, environment, material, method	Level 6. a. Choose implementer and student-implementer interaction (WHO). b. Choose learning environment (WHERE). c. Identify instructional materials/methods appropriate to student/objective/implementer/ environment (WHAT/HOW). d. Document prescription.
Coordinate and monitor prescription implementation	Level 7. a. Deliver/demonstrate prescription components. b. Monitor implementation of prescription. c. Readminister objective-referenced measure. d. If criteria are not met, return to alter prescription. e. If criteria are met and further monitoring is desired, return to identify new objective. f. If monitoring is no longer necessary, terminate program.
Posttest level of skill	Level 8. Determine student's functional level in curricular area(s) of concern after intervention.

Identifying Information Needs

Once the DP model was agreed upon, the next step in system development was to identify the information needs inherent in the SER-LAR model. The needs of teachers were categorized as informational needs relating to students, test information, learning objectives, objective-referenced measures, instructional materials, instructional methods, human resources, and learning environments.

The SER-LAR model defines the input and output of the special education information management system. As persons who are implementing the model work with students and use tests, objectives, materials, and methods, they document the use of these resources on initial referral forms, test score records, and prescription records. These forms serve a twofold purpose: (a) they provide a structure for the users to maintain diagnostic prescriptive records for each student, and (b) they allow for processing diagnostic prescriptive data. Staff members have access to computer-generated reports to assist them in two ways: (a) to help them find appropriate resources for their particular students and (b) to help them document diagnostic prescriptive interventions. Supervisors and curriculum experts analyze the reports and can revise them and develop new information for future system users.

Information Matrix

To relate the incoming user documentation to existing information in the various information areas, it was necessary to develop an information matrix that would accommodate input and output. One dimension of that martix was outlined as the seven areas defined as information needs in the DP model. The other dimension of the matrix was developed according to types of information. There were four types of information defined: (a) identification information that answers the question: What is the item? (e.g., accession number, title, author, publisher); (b) historical/usage information that answers the question: How was this item used? What is its history? How effective was it in that case? (e.g., all of the materials, methods, and personnel used for various students to reach learning objectives form the history of that objective); (c) analytical information that answers the questions: What can this item be used for? What are its characteristics? (e.g., a description of an instructional material indicating its potential, usually which is someone's judgment of content applicability, input and output modes, and appropriate handicaps); and (d) evaluation information that answers the question: How good is it in contrast to comparable items? (e.g., comparative items or scholar judgments of instructional materials).

MANAGING INSTRUCTION WITH PERSONAL COMPUTERS

Personal computers are gaining widespread acceptance as important tools for teachers in special education planning, monitoring, and evaluation. Although much has been written about computers as tutorial aids, very little has been written about computers as special education instructional management tools for teachers. Computers not only enable better planning and more accurate reporting, but they also offer the availability of advanced management techniques considerably more powerful than traditional special education planning and management practices (Friars & Gelmann, 1981; Parker, Friars, Gelman, & Kowacki, 1980; Wilson, 1981; Hayden, Vance, & Irwin, 1982).

There are two major ways to interact with a computer: one is "on line" for each response and the other is "batch mode" for a series of responses. The batch mode approach typically uses a large centralized computer in an administrative data-processing center and is staffed with computer specialists who can provide efficient services to both teachers and administrators (Spuck, Junter, Owen, & Belt, 1975; Clark, 1980; Holt, Kocsis, & Reisman, 1980). The batch mode approach is usually simple and straightforward, requiring no more than reference to a manual or catalog of procedures. Typical procedures include generation of IEP objectives and standard reports and scoring tests. IEPs are created by selecting numbered goals and objectives and writing their numbers on a preprinted form or optical scan sheet. Generating standard reports follows a similar request procedure. Testing scoring utilizes an optical scan sheet. Of course, some batch mode data-collection forms are better organized and easier to use than others. To the extent that users plan their work in advance, reports and information can be computer-generated and delivered with considerable savings in time and energy. This type of system allows teachers to make lesson plans away from the computer, input information into the computer quickly, and then request different types of reports.

The alternative to the batch mode is the "on line" or direct-access approach in which the teacher in a classroom or the administrator in an office can interact directly with the computer by typing on a computer terminal keyboard (Snodgrass, 1980). The computer answers requests immediately by printing information on the terminal display screen. Talking directly to a computer requires training. Some direct-access computer systems are hard to talk to (that is, they require error-free typing of technical commands) whereas others are more flexible and "friendly" (that is, they offer various kinds of help to the person typing at the terminal keyboard and are designed to reduce the chance of making an error).

The best decision for designing a software program for teachers is to have a combination of "on line" and "batch mode" information entry. Computers can provide the following kinds of support to special education classroom teachers: print IEP objectives by selecting from a curriculum bank, group students based on their status on IEP objectives, score tests and update student's status on IEP objectives, generate progress reports based on IEP objectives, recommend instructional strategies for students based on a set of descriptors, group students based on specific instructional strategies, describe diagnostic tests by descriptors and indexes to materials, report on student due-process status, generate class lesson plans, generate report cards and personalized mail to parents, assist in writing assessment reports, log evaluation status of students, maintain an instructional materials index to curriculum objectives and to instructional strategies, locate instructional materials and list them by content descriptors, report student achievements in content areas or on specific objectives, generate state and federal compliance reports, report staff caseload by handicapping conditions and services provided, maintain data needed by administrators, aid in keeping an inventory of materials, and assist in curriculum management. Taber (1983) listed additional administrative uses for personal computers.

Problems Affecting School Computer Use

The potential for computer-based education management will be reached when computers are as handy and usable as typewriters, and when they are received by teachers and administrators as routine tools. To achieve their potential, systems can no longer be limited to one or two planning or reporting functions. There have been two major problems in advancing the use of computers in schools: (a) teachers feel uncomfortable with computers and fear losing control over classrooms and (b) there are no trained computer personnel for the schools. However, these problems and fears need not diminish the use of computers as a means of meeting enormous management and instructional needs.

Problems Affecting School-Based Education Management Systems

The implementation of PL 94-142. *The Education for All Handicapped Children Act,* has resulted in impressive gains in programs and services for handicapped children. However, as state and local education agencies attempt to establish effective practices in educational programming using a management-by-objective format for children with special education needs, they encounter great developmental difficulties and complex problems associated with changing roles, new procedural requirements, and expanding services. Among the most difficult challenges have been resource allocation and instructional management, tasks that demand that special education administrators organize data effectively and without duplication in data collection by school-level staff.

There is a need for a school-based information management system that interfaces with the district-operated system and the state system so that duplication in data collection can be minimized.

It is also necessary to develop software programs for personal computers that interfaces with school-based systems so that teachers will have access to curricula information. The special education teacher will then have more time for planning and instruction of students. For example, there are currently several educational management systems operating at the school level within Maryland for implementing individualized educational programs: Special Education IEP for handicapped students, Early Identification programming for Learning Problems (House Bill 234), Educational Management Plan (EMP) for high risk students, the Chapter I project for disadvantaged schools with high risk students, and Project Basic appropriate assistant plan for students who fail to make adequate progress. In some cases, teachers are asked to operate or maintain two or more systems for the same students. There are, however, at least four "main" faults with operating multisystems. First, they are redundant. The same tasks are carried out by each staff member with minimal cumulative learning or benefit. Second, they are expensive. Creating educational plans is labor-intensive, requiring not only writing skills, but also organization and access to resources used in creating the IEP, and for typing draft and final copies. Third, there are inconsistencies. The language and conceptual framework of each IEP is dependent on one or more individual staff contributions. Goals and objectives are not stated in a common vocabulary or format. The fourth problem is distribution. IEP data cannot be aggregated for administrative decisions regarding personnel, equipment, transportation, or budget planning.

Educational management systems must effectively implement the requirements of PL 94-142 and other related education laws and regulations. Ideally, such systems should support long-range special education programs so that common problems and effective solutions can be identified and shared.

There are four levels of management in which a computer may be of assistance: (a) administrators — assisting in local planning and evaluation and responding to federal and state reports (e.g., number of students served, number of facilities available for serving handicapped children); (b) supervisors — managing special education curriculum (e.g., suitability of curriculum for specific content areas for various types of handicapped children; coordinating the suitability of curriculum objectives, materials, strategies, and evaluation criteria); (c) special education teachers and related services staff — managing IEP development and implementation (e.g., writing IEPs, grouping children with common needs and objectives, progress reports); and (d) students — using computers in instructional programs and monitoring student progress.

MANAGING INSTRUCTIONAL MATERIALS
WITH PERSONAL COMPUTERS

A school-based curriculum management system provides for continuous monitoring of the progress of all students in the school curriculum. This system provides an inventory of the available instructional materials designed to meet unique needs of students in learning specific objectives.

School districts in Maryland have begun to use computers to assist in the management of curriculum development and utilization. The computer provides a flexible structure for indexing materials and strategies to curriculum objectives and for monitoring the selection of objectives by staff for various types of handicapped students. Special education curriculum and instructional objectives are stored on disks. For example, Worcester County, Maryland has its total early childhood through high school special education curriculum objectives (2,500) stored on computer disks. The computer counts the frequency of use of each objective, and distributes the results annually to special education teachers and related services staff to assist in updating curriculum objectives.

These computer-assisted IEP management systems are designed to aid the special education teacher and related services staff in writing IEP objectives selected by the teacher, parent, and staff and to track individual students on a set of procedural safeguard issues.

The procedural safeguard report indicates the action taken at each step from initial referral through permissions, assessments, meetings, IEP development, placement, and reviews. It enables staff to know exactly what procedural safeguard activity has been met and when the next action is required.

Operational Systems

Although the programs that integrate these educational support functions are highly complex to build and maintain, they have to be easy to use. Programs, many recently updated, with multiple capabilities that have attempted to encourage instructional material management follow.

The MicroPlanner Curriculum Management and Teacher Planning System, developed by Learning Tools, Inc., Brookline, Massachusetts, can be used on the Apple II and other personal computers. Teachers can use the curriculum management system to organize goals and related objectives, methodology, materials, test items, assessment, and user-defined categories. The system can print eight different reports, including the IEP, Summary of Instructional Plan, IEP Due Process Report, Diagnostic Report, Health Report, Speech and Language Report, Contracted Services, and Missing Information Report.

Modularized Student Managment System (MSMS), Education TURNKEY Systems, Inc., Falls Church, Virginia, has a modularized student management system that meets most of the requirements in the administration of the special education process. It can assist in the development and maintenance of pupil records, print the instructional portion of an IEP package, sort through all records for numerous characteristics, and perform descriptive statistics on selected pupil data. The complete program has several modules that perform various tasks, including the preparation of summary data for state and federal reporting requirements.

D.I.M.E. System: Desktop Information Management for Education, is a multiuser 40M BYTE hard disk, personal computer, school-based management system. The Maryland State Department of Education (MSDE), in conjunction with the Frederick County public schools, is developing and field testing the system. The first years' objectives are to make available for teachers an automated IEP program for up to 2,500 students, a financial aid/scholarship search program, a vocational placement program, and a career information program. The multiuser system will utilize existing personal computers, regardless of make, as terminals to download information on floppy disks. The software program is CPM. Documentation and evaluation data can be obtained by contacting MSDE. Staff training requires two days.

SEMES — CAM/IEP Maryland Special Education Management System provides computer-assisted management of IEPs for teachers. This personal computer software program is designed to print IEPs, to group students based IEP objectives, to generate IEP progress reports, to generate procedural safeguard status reports, and to generate and score criterion-referenced tests. It will assist in curriculum management by allowing development, assessing, editing, and printing of curriculum in any subject area. Objectives are indexed to instructional materials and criterion-referenced tests. The CAM/IEP is a school-based system operated and field tested in about 100 Maryland schools. The software operates on a TRS 80 Model III, 48K two-disk-drive computer. The system has a teacher user manual and a three-day training program for installing the system at the school level.

PIE — Programming Individual Education was developed by Educational Growth Strategies Inc., Delaware. Target schools in Delaware are using the software. PIE can be used on the Apple II, 64K two-disk-drive computer and on others. The teacher can use the system for IEP development and instructional management along with IEP due-process tracking and curriculum management of objectives and instructional materials. The software program can interface with a mainframe computer to automatically sent data to the state department to meet federal and state reporting requirements.

APPLE PIE, Inc. (Lawrence, Kansas) was designed for teachers to assist in developing IEPs for handicapped students. The software operates on the Apple II personal computer.

Prescriptive Material Retrieval System (PMRS) was commerically developed to adapt an instructional materials retrieval system (SEIMC) on a personal computer. The system provides for the indexing and classifying of instructional materials. It is sold by B. L. Winch and Associates of Rolling Hills Estates, California. The manual system design was developed to assist teachers in selecting materials to fit students' needs. The system has 418 descriptors across eight major areas for about 10,000 instructional materials. The computer system now operates on an IBM mainframe. The company is in the process of making the system available on a personal computer.

Mainframe Systems

The following mainframe IEP systems, which could be adapted to operate on personal computers, also attempt to organize instructional materials around curriculum objectives to assist the teacher with management of instructional materials.

Organized Resource Bank for IEP Text (ORBIT), was developed by Montgomery County Public Schools, Maryland, and has a system that operates on an IBM 370 mainframe computer. Teachers access the system by terminal or through batch mode order forms. The system generates IEP objectives based on teacher selection from special education guides. Special education curriculum objectives are indexed (matched) to criterion test items, instructional materials, and instructional strategies. Diagnostic test skills are cross-referenced to curriculum objectives to assist teachers in selecting appropriate IEP objectives based on test results and in selecting appropriate assessment instruments to measure mastery of IEP objectives. Materials descriptors are used to assist in selecting appropriate materials based on students' learner characteristics.

The Gacka Computer Aided IEP is offered by Curriculum Associates, Inc., North Billerica, Massachusetts, for school systems that want a quick and efficient service bureau support system. The system generates IEP objectives based on teacher selection. Curriculum Associates also markets a variety of educational and diagnostic materials for special educators.

The Child-Based Information System, provided by the Central Susquehanna Intermediate Unit, Lewisburg, Pennsylvania, is a multidistrict special education, batch-processing management service system. Teachers use a manual of goals and objectives to specify on optical scan sheets what they want to include in computer-generated IEPs. The system also monitors student progress and generates report cards, teacher attendance, grading, and class lists.

Modular Educational Achievement Descriptor (MEAD) was developed in 1974 by Oakland School, Michigan. This is an IEP and curriculum management system that special education teachers can access by terminal or batch process through forms. The system now has a data base and user history on about 20,000 students in Michigan and Iowa. Curriculum objectives are indexed to instructional strategies, criterion-referenced tests, and norm-referenced tests. They are also cross-referenced to diagnostic test skills to assist teachers in selecting appropriate IEP objectives and appropriate test instruments to measure most of the objectives. Students are grouped by objectives for individual teachers. Curriculum objectives are reviewed and revised by specialists based on user history with various types of handicapped students.

EX-ED, sponsored by Computer Systems, Inc., offers a comprehensive information management system for special education. Offered in the system are federal and state compliance programs, individual educational programs, instructional management services, and office automation. Initially, EX-ED constructs a framework for the development of an individual student information record and a behavioral objective (based upon the student information record). This section can be used directly by teachers. A database is also offered. IBAS (Instructional Based Appraisal System) was developed by Dr. Edward Meyer of the University of Kansas, and provides a structured format for managing a teacher-developed curriculum which considers materials and activities appropriate to individual students. Reports can be generated through the EX-ED Service Bureau but require the purchase of additional hardware.

The Insight System, developed by Insight Unlimited, Inc., Muncie, Indiana, is an integrated system running on a large computer providing testing/screening and IEP development for LD students. A variety of prescriptive activities and resources are provided for teachers and parents.

Project Recipe, developed by Sarasota County Schools, Florida, is intended to provide computer-based instructional management for exceptional student programs. It matches test results with goals and objectives and provides a variety of IEP and related progress reports. It is accessed by terminals in schools connected to a large computer. The primary users are resource teachers working with students.

Worchester County, Maryland, Computer Assisted IEP System for Teachers and Administrators has software that operates on IBM 34 Mini Computers. Teachers access the system through review of curriculum objectives that are matched (indexed) according to instructional strategies, criterion-referenced test items, etc. The system also generates a series of administrative reports such as staff caseload, child count by handicapping condition, and child find reports.

Data-Based Management Systems

Special education teachers should look for commercially available data-based management systems that operate on personal computers. *Pro-*

file III Plus is a data-based management system designed by Radio Shack for use with the TRS 80 personal computer. Although not specifically designed for educational purposes, this system is easily adapted to the needs of school administrators. The user can design a management format for a variety of school-related areas such as student classification, student demographic data, and managing by objectives. Additionally, this program has the capability of operating interactively with Visicalc and Super SCRIPSIT for such purposes as generating student progress reports and developing and managing IEPs for students with a variety of handicapping conditions. *Data Factory,* which was designed for use with APPLE personal computers, also offers a versatile data-based management system. The clarity of the operator's manual and the appropriateness of the computer prompts allow for easy integration in an academic framework. This system allows the user to design, append, transfer, and/or update files based on the needs of school administrators and classroom teachers. Data Factory permits the user to conduct a variety of searches. With the addition of a printer (any variety that is compatible with the APPLE), it is possible to generate complete file reports or partial summaries resulting from user searches. Upgraded and new versions of these systems are now available as are new data-based system programs.

Criteria for Evaluating Software

Holznagel (1981) noted that software evaluation should follow a consistent procedure and set of criteria. The Maryland State Department of Education developed the criteria shown in Table 4–4 to help special educators evaluate available software and to design software for use as an instructional management system.

SUMMARY

Systems for using personal computers to manage instructional materials for LD students are just beginning to be developed. Resources that may be helpful in evaluating software include the *Evaluator's Guide,* developed by the Northwest Regional Educational Laboratories' Computer Technology Program at the University of Oregon. The Maryland State Department of Education, Division of Libraries, has developed *Criteria for Evaluating and Selecting Computer Courseware.* The Maryland State Department of Education, Division of Special Education, has composed *Criteria for Evaluation Microcomputer Software for IEP Management Systems,* which was partially delineated in Table 4–4. All of these guides provide information that enables the reviewer to look objectively at instructional management software for the learning disabled.

TABLE 6-4
Criteria for Software Evaluation

Ease of Use and Wide Applicability

Initial training required to use software
Start up delay (request to implementation)
Availability of technical support
Adaptability to procedures/needs
Compatability with curriculum
Ease of changes to entries
Editing facilities for text input
Useful for range of school staff members
Parent and community understanding/acceptance
Compatible with present school district and state objectives
Usable for different populations of students
Modifications ease
Modular, flexible, or fixed programming
Variable information allowed in data base
Output flexibility

Specific Features

Normative provision
Criterion provision
Aptitude indicators
File security system
Accountability aspects
PL 94-142 compliance aide
Annual goals output
Short-term objective output
Complete file output
Student groupings by objective
Student scheduling
Student interaction/assistance directly
Standardized test file provision
Team concept vs. individual school staff aide
IEP aide
Individualized student files vs. fixed data
Computer assisted test generation (CATG)
Interactive vs. batch capability
Automatic file scan provision for
   (a) research/statistics
   (b) summary administrative reports
   (c) listings of children by commonalities

Technical and Other Considerations

Characteristics of objectives considered
Validated in pilot project
Ongoing present use in school district
Documentation completeness

Technical and Other Considerations *(continued)*
Manual flexibility
Compatibility with other peripherals
Multiple domains/curriculums provision
Software and hardware availability and cost
Limit to number of objectives, domains, etc.
Length limit for objectives, headings, etc.
School based versus central office based
Copyright limits/method of purchase

APPENDIX 6–1: GLOSSARY

AUTOMATIC FILE SCAN PROVISION: accessing the same type of data across many records by using software commands; scanning for common characteristics

BASIC: (Beginner's All-purpose Symbolic Instructional Code) one of the simplest computer languages used on personal computers

BYTE: a unit of memory; with personal computers, a byte is 8 bits

BIT: the smallest unit of information that can be known; a binary number that can be a 1 or 0

BUG: an error

CPU: (Central Processing Unit) the brain of the computer; in personal computers, the CPU is a single component called a microprocessor

DATA: information of any kind that can be processed or used by a computer

DISK: a circular, vinyl material coated with a magnetic substance on which programs are written and saved

DISK DRIVE: a peripheral that can store and retrieve information from a disk

DOS: (Disk Operating System) a compilation of programs that facilitates the use of a disk drive

EDIT: making changes or corrections in a program

FILE SECURITY SYSTEM: keeping entry and retrieval of confidential information on computer files restricted to authorized personnel

FIXED PROGRAMMING: a program without provisions for change (see flexible programming and modular programming)

FLEXIBLE PROGRAMMING: a program with provisions for change (see modular programming and fixed programming)

FLOPPY DISK: a 5¼ × 8 inch circular, vinyl disk that is flexible and coated with a magnetic substance on which programs are written and saved

FLOW CHART: a number of simple symbols that depict typical computer operations

HARDWARE: the physical components of a computer

HARD DISK: a circular, vinyl disk that is rigid and coated with a magnetic substance on which programs can be written and saved

IC: (Integrated Circuit) a solid state device containing hundreds of electrical circuits on a single chip of silicon

INTERACTIVE CAPABILITY: a computer system that responds within a second for typical information

MICRO: very small in size

MICROPROCESSOR: an integrated circuit that contains a computer's central processing unit

MODULAR PROGRAMMING: a set of programs with clearly defined functions that communicate with each other and use the same data base of information (see flexible programming and fixed programming)

PERIPHERAL: a contrivance that can transmit information from the user to the computer and vice versa; examples include disk drive, printers, and television sets

RAM: (Random Access Memory) main memory of the computer where information and programs are stored during use

SOFTWARE: instructions used by the computer to perform any function; examples include languages and programs

TERMINAL: the keyboard the user employs to send information to the computer

VIDEO MONITOR: a specialized television set that can be connected to a computer

CHAPTER 7

Computer Software

Lois T. Pommer
David S. Mark
David L. Hayden

According to a recent survey by Connecticut-based Market Data Retrieval (1982), the percentage of school districts using computers as part of their instructional program increased from 39% during the 1981 to 1982 school year to 58% by fall, 1982. Computer use provides many advantages for the general school population and specific benefits for LD students (Bork & Franklin, 1979). Public Law 94-142 mandates that special education teachers individualize instruction. With carefully designed software, a personal computer can be a tremendous aid in this regard (Palmer, 1985). Software can be developed that enables students to work at their own pace, according to their strengths and weaknesses, with tasks broken into appropriate steps, thus individualizing instruction according to specific needs (Lieber & Semmel, 1985).

Taber (1983) noted that "individualization is especially important because branching to appropriate conceptual and reading levels can occur with presentations that remain at the same interest level" (p. 67). Varnen (March, 1983) described the enthusiasm students display when working

The chapter originally appeared as an article by **Lois T. Pommer, David S. Mark,** and **David L. Hayden** in *Learning Disabilities: An Interdisciplinary Journal* (Vol. II (8), 99–110, 1983) and was adapted by permission of Grune & Stratton for inclusion in this *Handbook*.

with computers. This is largely due to appropriate instructional content and to student-computer exchanges. The personal computer and the student interact closely, offering the student some control over the immediate environment. The way in which the student responds to prompts from the computer causes the computer to output additional information. This information takes the form of either continuation of the prescribed lesson or feedback specific to the student's interactive responses. Most feedback is characterized by "user-friendly" language of a positive and/or nonpunitive nature. The combination of user-friendly language and immediate feedback facilitates active participation in learning and lends itself to continued interactions between the student and the computer (Kolich, 1985).

The personal computer can assist LD students with memory deficits by providing prompts on the screen or utilizing multisensory approaches to learning (Weir & Watt, 1981). Students who react quickly and impulsively can be taught to slow down. The program can be designed so that keys can not be depressed until a specific time period has elapsed from problem presentation or reminders to slow down can appear on the screen.

Of great importance to the LD student is the emergence of "talking programs" using voice synthesizers. These programs can be extremely beneficial to nonreaders or very poor readers. Varnen (April, 1983) noted that "talking programs can open up the world of computers to (students) who have trouble reading the traditional keyboard . . . and (students) who have auditory or other learning difficulties that affect their ability to read" (p. 195).

Some research (Gleason, 1981) has indicated that retention of material taught by the computer may be equal to or better than that of traditional instruction. More research needs to be done on specific aspects of computer instruction to determine what has a positive influence and how it does so (Mineo & Cavalier, 1985).

Teacher-developed software (Weisgerber & Rubin, 1985) has been excluded from this chapter. Generally, it is not mass produced and there is no clearinghouse from which to preview and order it. However, teacher-developed software is more likely to be appropriate for the user (Hummel & Farr, 1985). The teacher is able to develop software focusing on specific skills needed by students while considering their unique learning styles and characteristics. From a learning theory approach, teacher-made software should be developed in a hierarchical format proceeding from knowns and unknowns. Teacher-developed software can supplement commercial software by meeting students' special needs.

PERSONAL COMPUTER APPLICATIONS

A mathematics curriculum typically includes the areas of operations and applications. Proficiency in these areas implies that ability to apply computational and operational concepts to the solution of real life problems. Excellence in computation is achieved through the drill and practice of correctly learned mathematical concepts and principles. According to Ashlock (1976), erroneous computational skills result from faulty skill development or lack of mastery of mathematical concepts. A careful analysis of errors helps to formulate a pattern of mistakes, and many programs keep both a log of errors and a description of errors. With this information, teachers know which concepts need to be acquired and, thus, can plan instruction accordingly. There are numerous programs that aid the student in the acquisition of mathematical concepts leading to good computational skills. Many of these programs are self-paced and utilize appropriate multisensory techniques commonly associated with the LD student.

A language arts curriculum develops skills in reading and related areas (Thompson, 1980). Many types of programs have been developed that emphasize reading skills such as word analogies, sentence completion, vocabulary building, identifying main ideas, identifying supporting details, and phonics development (Rosegrant, 1985). For many LD students, the language experience approach appears to be an effective instructional approach. The language experience approach uses the student's own dictated stories as part of the reading material, thus stimulating interest, building expressive language skills, and providing the security of a familiar vocabulary and structure. Speaking, listening, reading, writing, and spelling skills are employed. In using this approach on a personal computer, the teacher and student may sit at the computer together with the teacher keying in words as the student dictates them. An alternative strategy using a word processing program, would be for the teacher to copy the dictated story on paper for the student to key into the computer. These stories can be saved so that the student can read and edit what he or she has written.

Another diagnostic technique often used with LD students is the "cloze" procedure. Using this approach, the student is asked to fill in a missing word from a sentence or brief passage. This aids the student in learning to use contextual clues when faced with unfamiliar words. Many personal computers employ a cloze procedure. Some are programmed to accept a variety of answers that are spelled incorrectly as well as correct answers.

SOFTWARE EVALUATION

The first step in purchasing software is for the teacher to develop a list of instructional needs (Stearns, 1986). After doing so, Hannaford and Sloane (1981) suggested that teachers "identify and use systematic criteria that will allow (them) to wisely select software that meets learner/teacher

needs, has instructional integrity, and is technically adequate and usable"
(p. 54). Thus, schools should develop their own criteria for evaluating software, based on their specific instructional needs and the population they
serve. Evaluation of software should continue after purchase, to guide in
future software acquisition (Berkell, 1984; Smith & Tomkins, 1984).

Tables 5-1 through 5-5 were developed specifically to determine
whether particular software was appropriate for use with LD students. The
tables evaluate content areas: language arts, mathematics, social studies,
science, and miscellaneous areas. Additional information is provided in
narrative form. It should be emphasized that addresses may have changed.

Definition of terms used in the tables follow.

Appropriate length. (15 to 25 minutes) The software is divided into
small segments appropriate for the attention span of most LD students.
The 15- to 25-minute segment serves as a guideline; the actual length may
vary based on the needs of the population and the specific task.

Required reading level. It is important to determine the reading level of
a screen presentation so that it can be matched with the reading level
of students.

Purpose clearly stated. A clearly stated purpose will allow the teacher to
determine whether or not a program is appropriate to the curriculum and
the abilities of students.

Appropriate objectives. The objectives clearly state what the program will
accomplish and what can be achieved with successful completion of the program.

Logical progression. The program employs a task-analysis approach,
progressing from easier (known) to harder (unknown) concepts.

Peripherals required. The program requires the use of additional software (e.g., a graphics tablet, tape recorder, and light pen).

Interest level. The interest level is high enough to motivate the student
to attend to the task until its completion. The teacher should compare the
interest level to the required reading level. For LD students, it is advisable
to have interest level exceed reading level.

Adaptable to special needs. Some aspects of the program can be
changed to meet students' needs. These aspects may include reading level,
speed of presentation, mode of response, and screen presentation.

Diagnostic-prescriptive format. The overall format of the program is
based on the diagnostic-prescriptive process. In a broad sense, this implies
that the program will either progress through a hierarchy or branch to a
tutorial section to offer additional training and reinforcement.

Varied response mode. The program allows the user to interact with the program through switching devices or more than one keystroke on the keyboard.

Prerequisites defined. The program clearly states what skills or other requirements the student needs to bring to the learning situation. These prerequisites may be defined in an accompanying manual or an introductory section
of the program.

Appropriate response intervals. This is an important user-friendly characteristic. The program offers feedback to the user at a rate that will encourage continued participation and maintain motivation.

Log of errors. The program tracks how many errors the student had made and displays them at the conclusion of the program.

Description of errors. At the conclusion of the program, a summary delineates the types of errors the student made.

Color and graphics cues. To enhance motivation and maintain a high level of student interest, the program design incorporates the use of color and graphics. These factors are used throughout the program to help students focus on important and/or difficult concepts.

Auditory cues. To offer added stimulation during the program and to help emphasize feedback, auditory cues have been included.

Appropriate screen presentation. The screen has been designed so that the student can easily interact with the computer. Factors that should be considered include the amount of printed matter on the screen at any given time, the size of the print, spacing between lines and words, and the use of color.

Validity. The content is appropriately matched to the stated objectives.

Usefulness. Completion of this program indicates that the student has achieved certain prescribed academic goals.

Content-objective match. The content corresponds to the stated objectives.

Multi-user capabilities. The program is designed to accept input from more than one student through cooperative or competitive interactions.

Accommodates cooperative peer interaction. The program allows more than one student to interact with it. Students can discuss possible answers before responding.

Accommodates competitive peer interaction. The program offers the option of competitive peer interaction and can maintain records of each student's responses.

Accommodates individual response. The program allows for single student responses. The design of the program is such that only one student's responses can be tracked at a time since it is measuring a specific skill.

Language Arts Programs

Information about the programs listed in Table 7–1 follows. Addresses and phone numbers for manufacturers can be found in Appendix 7–2.

Vowels. The objective is to acquire skills in identifying and discriminating vowel presentations in the area of long and short vowels, double vowels, diphthongs, r-controlled vowels, schwa sound, and other related skills. The intended users are kindergarten through tenth-grade students. A major benefit is that the teacher can adjust the stimulus words to accommodate students' curricular needs. It can be ordered from Hartley Courseware, Inc.

TABLE 7-1

Language Arts Programs

Characteristics	Vowels	Compu-Read	Four Basic Reading Skills, Unit 1	Magic Spells
General				
Appropriate length	Yes	Yes	Yes	Yes
Reading level (grade)	K-10	1-4	5-6	2-7
Purpose clearly stated	Yes	Yes	Yes	Yes
Appropriate objectives	Yes	Yes	Yes	Yes
Logical progression	Yes	No	Yes	Yes
Peripherals required	No	No	No	No
Interest level (grade)	2-10	-5	3-4	2-8
Adaptable to special needs	Yes	Yes	No	Yes
Methodology				
Diagnostic-prescriptive format	No	No	Yes	No
Varied response mode	No	No	No	No
Prerequisites defined	Yes	Yes	Yes	Yes
Appropriate response intervals	Yes	Yes	Yes	Yes
Log of errors	Yes	Yes	Yes	Yes
Description of errors	Yes	Yes	Yes	No
Curricular				
Color & graphics cues	No	No	Yes	Yes
Auditory cues	Yes	No	Yes	Yes
Appropriate screen presentation	Yes	Yes	No	Yes
Validity	Yes	Yes	Yes	Yes
Usefulness	Yes	Yes	Yes	Yes
Content-objective match	Yes	Yes	Yes	Yes
Multi-user capabilities	Yes	Yes	No	Yes
Student-Computer Interaction				
Accommodates cooperative peer interaction	Yes	Yes	Yes	Yes
Accommodates competitive peer interaction	No	No	No	No
Accommodates individual response	Yes	Yes	Yes	Yes

Compu-Read. The objective is to enhance reading ability and build skills in speed and comprehension. Compu-Read consists of a series of four programs of increasing difficulty from simple letter recognition, identification of rapidly presented words, and vocabulary practice to high-speed sentence presentations. The intended users are first through fourth graders. The teacher can adjust the speed of the presentation and the number of problems presented and can create lists of words and vocabulary. It can be ordered from Edu-Ware Services, Inc.

Four Basic Reading Skills, Unit One. The objective is to gain proficiency in the following skill areas: (a) how to recall details; (b) how to identify main ideas; (c) how to draw conclusions; and (d) how to put things in order.

Within each area, there are 10 reading passages followed by a series of questions. The student receives visual reinforcement for correct answers. The student has unlimited opportunities to respond until questions are answered correctly. However, since there are only two response choices, the student can correct responses without learning the concept involved. Pressing a response key other than the two requested responses is interpreted as an incorrect response, thus penalizing accidental responses. After the student completes all four reading areas, a quiz requires the student to identify the skill needed to answer the question, and then to give factual information. A teacher's guide is included which encourages the teacher to plan lessons corresponding to the program. It is available from Brain Box: The Computer Tutor.

Magic Spells. The objective is to develop spelling skills and visual and mental agility in unscrambling words. The teacher's guide gives explicit instructions on how to play the game, create word lists, and use existing activities already on the disk. The program not only has ready-made word lists for use with elementary age students, but also allows the teacher to create word lists. Letter presentations are in both upper-case and lower-case letters. If the student answers incorrectly, he or she is given clues as to where the errors are. The student has unlimited opportunities to correct responses. Incorrect responses are reinforced more than correct responses, as a demon appears with lively music. This game incorporates both color and graphics and has an on-off music option. It is available from Advanced Learning Technology, Inc.

Mathematics Programs

Information about the programs listed in Table 7–2 follows.

Alligator Mix. The objective is to reinforce, through drill, basic addition and subtraction operations with sums and remainders of less than 20. The intended users are elementary-age students. It generates a random series of

TABLE 7-2
Mathematics Programs

Characteristics	Alligator Mix	Soccer Math	Math Ideas With Base Ten Blocks	Q.E.D. Arith-Magic
General				
Appropriate Length	Yes	Yes	Yes	Yes
Reading level (grade)	N.A.	2	2-3	4-5
Purpose clearly stated	Yes	Yes	Yes	Yes
Appropriate objectives	Yes	Yes	Yes	Yes
Logical progression	Yes	Yes	Yes	Yes
Peripherals required	Optional	No	No	No
Interest level (grade)	1-4	1-5	1-8	7-10
Adaptable to special needs	Yes	Yes	No	No
Methodology				
Diagnostic-prescriptive format	No	No	No	No
Varied response mode	Yes	No	No	No
Prerequisites defined	No	No	Yes	Yes
Appropriate response intervals	Yes	Yes	Yes	Yes
Log of errors	Yes	Yes	Yes	No
Description of errors	No	No	No	No
Curricular				
Color & graphics cues	Yes	Yes	Yes	Yes
Auditory cues	Yes	Yes	No	No
Appropriate screen presentation	Yes	Yes	Yes	Yes
Validity	Yes	Yes	Yes	Yes
Usefulness	Yes	Yes	Yes	Yes
Content-objective match	Yes	Yes	Yes	Yes
Multi-user capabilities	Yes	Yes	Yes	Yes
Student-Computer Interaction				
Accommodates cooperative peer interaction	Yes	No	Yes	Yes
Accommodates competitive peer interaction	No	Yes	No	No
Accommodates individual response	Yes	Yes	Yes	Yes

addition and subtraction problems. A major benefit is that it can be used with nonreaders. The teacher can adjust the level of difficulty, speed of presentation, duration of activity, and response mode (e.g., responses can be made through keyboard or paddles). The graphics enhance student concentration and attention to task. It is available from Developmental Learning Materials, Academic Skill Builders in Math.

Soccer Math. The objective is to reinforce addition, subtraction, and multiplication facts through drill. Soccer Math offers a competitive math teaching program, in which students score a soccer goal for each correct response. It can be played at 10 different skill levels, with computations involving numbers 1 through 99. The intended users are first through fifth graders. The teacher can adjust the level of difficulty, and students can compete at different skill levels. The teacher may also adjust the number of problems needed to complete the program. It has an on-off music option. The computer is able to record the skill levels of 35 students, so that a student begins at the correct level each time. This program uses graphics that enhance student concentration and attention to task. It is available from Compu-Tation.

Q.E.D. Arith-Magic. The objective is to strengthen skills in addition, subtraction, and multiplication. Reinforcement of these objectives helps the student see relationships and patterns in math puzzles. To be successful in these activities, the student needs to use logic and deductive reasoning skills. A major benefit of Q.E.D. Arith-Magic is its high interest level. It emphasizes logical and deductive reasoning, but requires relatively low reading skills. The program enhances cooperative peer interaction and problem-solving skills. It is available from Cuisinaire Company of America.

Math Ideas With Base Ten Blocks. The objective is to reinforce skills in counting and comparing as well as in addition, subtraction, multiplication, and division. The intended users are first through eighth graders. The program generates a random series of problems. The teacher can adjust the number of problems presented and the level of difficulty. Math Ideas includes record-keeping sheets to monitor student progress. The program promotes concentration and attention to task. It is available from Cuisinaire Company of America.

Social Studies Programs

Information about the programs listed in Table 7–3 follows.

States and Capitals. The objective is to drill states and their capitals. The program generates a random series of states, and the student is expected to type the corresponding capitals. It also lists capitals, and the student is required to type the names of the corresponding states. Students must be able to read and spell the names of all states and capitals to be successful.

TABLE 7-3

Social Studies Programs

Characteristics	States and Capitals	Elementary Social Studies, Vol. 1
General		
Appropriate Length	Yes	Yes
Reading level (grade)	4+	6+
Purpose clearly stated	Yes	Yes
Appropriate objectives	Yes	Yes
Logical progression	No	Yes
Peripherals required	No	No
Interest level (grade)	2–3	6–12
Adaptable to special needs	No	No
Methodology		
Diagnostic-prescriptive format	No	Yes
Varied response mode	No	Yes
Prerequisites defined	Yes	Yes
Appropriate response intervals	Yes	Yes
Log of errors	Yes	No
Description of errors	No	No
Curricular		
Color & graphics cues	Yes	No
Auditory cues	Yes	No
Appropriate screen presentation	Yes	Yes
Validity	Yes	Yes
Usefulness	Yes	Yes
Content-objective match	Yes	Yes
Multi-user capabilities	Yes	Yes
Student-Computer Interaction		
Accommodates cooperative peer interaction	Yes	Yes
Accommodates competitive peer interaction	Yes	Yes
Accommodates individual response	Yes	Yes

Each incorrect answer prompts a one-letter cue. States and Capitals can be ordered from Micro Learningware.

Elementary Social Studies, Volume I (M.E.C.C.). The objective of this volume is to use drill and practice, as well as other methods, to recognize states by their shapes on a map and to develop skill in recalling corresponding states and their capitals. The Civil War section of the program offers randomly produced simulations of 14 battles. The other four sections of this program deal with simulations that teach economic concepts. The student must learn to make decisions using mathematics, money management, and business skills. These programs appear to be too difficult for most elementary-level students. Elementary Social Studies is available from Sunburst Communications.

Science Programs

Information about the programs listed in Table 7–4 follows.

Rocky's Boots. The objective is to acquire the ability to use logic in creating unique electronic "machines." Players build animated logic machines to score points. The intended users are aged 7 and older. However, since third- to fourth-grade reading levels are required to operate the program independently, students reading below those levels will need assistance. The program serves to enhance student concentration and attention to task with color graphics, music and sound effects. The auditory components have an on-off option. It can be ordered from The Learning Company.

The Human Body. This is a two-disk program. The objective is for students to identify the six major systems of the body, the major function of each system, and some of the major body parts. The manual provides activities for the teacher to use in the classroom and offers discussion questions. A review test is provided at the end of each lesson. The program can be ordered from Brain Box: The Computer Tutor.

Science, Volume 3 (M.E.C.C.) The program has two primary objectives. The first objective is for the student to acquire scientific knowledge, which the program provides, about types of fish, minerals, lakes, and earthquakes. The second objective is for the student to simulate this newly-acquired knowledge and make decisions. To make appropriate decisions, the student needs to rely on past knowledge in mathematics, science, and other related areas. This program provides the opportunity to learn by using logic and simulated events. The program includes a manual of lesson plans that the teacher may use to augment the computer instruction. It is available from Sunburst Communications.

Miscellaneous Programs

Information about the programs listed in Table 7–5 follows.

TABLE 7–4

Science Programs

Characteristics	Rocky's Boots	The Human Body	Science, Vol. 3
General			
Appropriate Length	Yes	Yes	Yes
Reading level (grade)	3–4	5+	5–7
Purpose clearly stated	Yes	Yes	Yes
Appropriate objectives	Yes	Yes	Yes
Logical progression	Yes	Yes	Yes
Peripherals required	No	No	No
Interest level (grade)	7+	6+	6–8
Adaptable to special needs	No	No	No
Methodology			
Diagnostic-prescriptive format	No	Yes	No
Varied response mode	Yes	Yes	Yes
Prerequisites defined	Yes	Yes	Yes
Appropriate response intervals	Yes	Yes	Yes
Log of errors	No	Yes	No
Description of errors	No	Yes	Yes
Curricular			
Color & graphics cues	Yes	Yes	Yes
Auditory cues	Yes	Yes	No
Appropriate screen presentation	Yes	Yes	Yes
Validity	Yes	Yes	Yes
Usefulness	Yes	Yes	Yes
Content-objective match	Yes	Yes	Yes
Multi-user capabilities	Yes	Yes	Yes
Student-Computer Interaction			
Accommodates cooperative peer interaction	Yes	Yes	Yes
Accommodates competitive peer interaction	No	No	No
Accommodates individual response	Yes	Yes	Yes

TABLE 7-5

Miscellaneous Programs

Characteristics	Apple Logo	Apple Pilot*	Shell Games: Educational Series*	Gertrude's Puzzles
General				
Appropriate Length	Yes	Yes	Yes	Yes
Reading level (grade)	3–5	1–12	1–12	2–3
Purpose clearly stated	Yes	Yes	Yes	Yes
Appropriate objectives	Yes	Yes	Yes	Yes
Logical progression	Yes	Yes	Yes	Yes
Peripherals required	No	No	No	No
Interest level (grade)	7–10	1–12	1–12	5–7
Adaptable to special needs	No	Yes	Yes	Yes
Methodology				
Diagnostic-prescriptive format	No	Yes	No	No
Varied response mode	Yes	Yes	Yes	Yes
Prerequisites defined	Yes	Yes	Yes	No
Appropriate response intervals	Yes	Yes	Yes	Yes
Log of errors	No	No	Yes	No
Description of errors	No	No	No	No
Curricular				
Color & graphics cues	Yes	Yes	No	Yes
Auditory cues	No	Yes	No	Yes
Appropriate screen presentation	Yes	Yes	Yes	Yes
Validity	Yes	Yes	Yes	Yes
Usefulness	Yes	Yes	Yes	Yes
Content-objective match	Yes	Yes	Yes	Yes
Multi-user capabilities	Yes	Yes	No	Yes
Student-Computer Interaction				
Accommodates cooperative peer interaction	Yes	Yes	Yes	Yes
Accommodates competitive peer interaction	No	Yes	No	No
Accommodates individual response	Yes	Yes	Yes	Yes

Apple Logo. This is a self-contained language system that aids the student in acquiring and refining skills in deductive reasoning, mathematics, reading, spelling, and logical progression. Logo allows students to quickly become familiar with programming. It is best known for its graphics environment, called "turtle geometry." A white triangle, the turtle, appears in the center of the computer screen. The student controls the movement of the turtle by using commands. The progression goes from simple lines and shapes to intricate designs, incorporating color cues and newly defined commands. Logo can be used with students of all ages and abilities. The program uses concrete experiences to foster abstract thinking. It is available from Apple.

Apple Pilot. This is an authoring system that allows the teacher to develop unique lessons by incorporating color and graphics presentations, auditory presentations, and screen presentations. The teacher is not restricted to any content area or special formatting guidelines. The teacher can adjust required reading level, acceptable responses, and appropriate reinforcements. The two manuals provide explicit instructions on the authoring language and procedures. Apple Pilot is available from Apple.

The Shell Games: Educational Series. The objective is to provide the framework for developing three types of activities: matching, multiple choice, and true/false. Included in the framework are explanations about how each progrm is used, how the test is formatted, how reinforcement is given, and how responses are recorded. The teacher needs to consider the following factors when developing activities: (a) content area, (b) reading level, (c) screen presentation, and (d) stimuli and required responses. A manual clearly describes how to design lessons within the program's format. Shell Games is available from Apple Computer Company.

Gertrude's Puzzles. The objective is to use deductive reasoning and problem-solving skills to solve any of three types of puzzles that are included in the activity. For example, to solve one puzzle, the student must determine how to place objects of varying shapes and colors into a series of boxes in a 3 × 3 matrix in such a way that there is no duplication of color and shape in any row or column. The program can be used with students who have limited reading skills. The teacher can make shapes more similar, thus increasing the level of difficulty, or less similar, thus decreasing the level of difficulty. Each of the three puzzles has two levels of difficulty. Gertrude's puzzles is available from The Learning Company.

SOURCE LISTS

Appendices 7-1 and 7-2 list professional publications about personal computers and addresses of software publishers. These lists are not inclusive and represent only a small sample of what is available. Address, publicaton cycle, cost, and a brief description are included for each publication. Please note that all information is subject to change.

APPENDIX 7-1

Source List

AEDS Journal, 1201 16th Street, NW, Washington, DC 20036. This publication focuses on original research, projects, and theoretical or conceptual positions related to the field of educational computers. It is published quarterly, and a subscription costs $25.00.

BYTE, Byte Publications, Inc., 70 Main Street, Peterborough, NY 03458. This journal is published by McGraw–Hill, Inc., and contains many technical articles, software reviews, and a "catalog" of hardware, software, peripherals and reviews of computer publications. It is published monthly and a subscription costs $19.00.

Classroom Computer News, 341 Mt. Auburn Street, Watertown, MA 02172. This magazine is designed for the classroom teacher and focuses on computer-assisted instruction. It is published bi-monthly, and a subscription costs $12.00.

The Computing Teacher. Dept. of Computer & Information Science, University of Oregon, Eugene, OR 97403. This journal is published by the International Council for Computers in Education (ICCE) and is written specifically for educators. It is published nine times a year, and a subscription costs $14.50.

CourseWare Magazine, 4949 North Millbrook, Suite 222, Fresno, CA 93726. This is a computer magazine with a program cassette or diskette and supporting material, including a teacher's guide and pupil worksheets for the Apple II (16K), Pet (8K), and TRS-80 (16K). Programs concentrate on curriculum areas: business, consumer economics, English, fine arts, foreign languages, industrial arts, mathematics, physical education, science, and social studies. It is published monthly, and a subscription costs $449.00.

Educational Technology, 140 Sylvan Avenue, Englewood Cliffs, NJ 07632. This is a professional journal for educators. It covers all types of educational technology and includes product and book reviews. It is published monthly, and a subscription costs $17.00.

Interface Age, 16704 Marquardt Avenue, Cerritos, CA 90701. This journal provides hardware and software comparison tables, new product information, book reviews, tutorials, and applications for personal computers. It includes a monthly column on education, and at least one issue each year focuses on education. It is published monthly, and a subscription costs $18.00.

Journal of Educational Technology Systems, Baywood Publishing Co., Inc., 120 Marine Street, Farmingdale, NY 11735. This journal is published by the Society for Applied Learning Technology (SALT). It focuses on techniques and approaches for using technology in all types of educational systems. It is published quarterly, and a subscription costs $51.00.

Personal Computing, PO Box 13916, Philadelphia, PA 19101. This publication is nontechnical and concerns computer applications and hardware for business, school, and home use. It is published monthly, and a subscription costs $18.00.

School MicroWare Directory, Dresden Associates, P.O. Box 246, Dresden, ME 04342. This publication includes information on instructional software available for major personal computers and a catalog that lists more than 1,200 products from over 100 suppliers. Each entry includes title, topic, grade level, system and computer language requirements, cost, source, and the instructional technique used in the program. It is published twice yearly, and a subscription costs $25.00.

APPENDIX 7–2

Software Publishers

American Guidance Service, Publishers' Building, Circle Pines, MN 56223; (612) 786-4343, (800) 328-2560.

Apple Computer, Inc., 20525 Mariani Avenue, Cupertino, CA 95094; (408) 554-5152.

Atari, Inc., Home Computer Division, 1196 Borreagas Avenue, Sunnyvale, CA 94086; (408) 554-5152.

Compu-Tations, Inc., P.O. Box 502, Troy, MI 48099; (313) 689-5059

Control Data Corporation, 8100 34th Avenue, South, P.O. Box 0, Minneapolis, MN 55440; (612) 853-8100

Creative Computing Software, 390 East Hanover Avenue, Morris Plains, NJ 07950; (800) 631-8112

Cuisenaire Company of America, 12 Church Street, Box D, New Rochelle, NY 10805; (914) 235-0900

Cybernetic Information Systems, Box 9032, Upper Union Street, Schenectady, NY 12309

Developmental Learning Materials, One DLM Park, Allen, TX 75002; (214) 248-6300

Educational Courseware, 3 Nappa Lane, Westport, CT 06880; (203) 227-1438

Educational Software & Marketing Company, 1035 Outer Park Drive, Suite 309, Springfield, IL 62704; (217) 787-4594

Edu-Ware Service, Inc., 28035 Dorothy Drive, Agoura Hills, CA 91301; (213) 706-0661

Encyclopedia Britannica Education Corp., 425 N. Michigan Avenue, Chicago, IL 60611; (311) 321-7330

Ex-Ed Computer Systems, Inc. 71-11 112th Street, Forrest Hills, NY 11375; (212) 268-0020

Gamco Industries, Inc., P.O. Box 1911, Big Springs, TX 79720; (915) 267-6327

Hartley Courseware, Inc., Box 431, Dimondale, MI 48821; (616) 942-8987

Insight Unlimited, Inc., 3600 East Memorial Drive, Suite 3, Muncie, IN 47302; (317) 747-1015

Instant Software, Route 101 and Elm Street, Peterborough, NH 03458; (800) 258-5473, (603) 924-9471

K-12 Micromedia, Inc., 172 Broadway, Woodcliff Lake, NJ 07675; (201) 391-7555

Krell Software Corporation, 1320 Stony Brook Road, Suite 219, Stony Brook, NY 11790; (516) 752-5139

Laureate Learning Systems, Inc., 1 Mill Street, Burlington, VT 05401; (802) 862-7355

The Learning Company, 4370 Alpine Road, Portola Valley, CA 94025; (415) 851-3160

Learning Tools, 686 Massachusetts Avenue, Cambridge, MA 02139; (617) 864-8086

MCE Inc., 157 South Kalamazoo Mall, Suite 250, Kalamazoo, MI 49007; (617) 345-8681

Media Materials, Inc., 2936 Remington Avenue, Baltimore, MD 21211; (301) 235-1700, (800) 638-1010

Micro-Ed, P.O. Box 24156, Minneapolis, MN 55424; (612) 926-2292, (800) 642-7633

Micro Learningware, P.O. Box 2134, North Mankato, MN 56001; (507) 625-2205

Microcomputer Education Applications Network (MEAN), 256 North Washington Street, Falls Church, VA 22046; (703) 536-2310

Microcomputer Software Systems, Inc., 4716 Lakewood Drive, Metairie, LA 70002; (504) 887-8527

Microcomputers Corporation, 34 Maple Avenue, Box 8, Armonk, NY 10504; (914) 273-6480

Milton Bradley Company, 443 Shaker Road, East Longmeadow, Massachusetts, MA 01028; (413) 525-6411

Minnesota Educational Computing Consortium (MECC), 2520 Broadway Drive, St. Paul, MN 55113; (612) 638-0612

MUSE Company, 347 North Charles Street, Baltimore, MD 21201; (301) 659-7212

Quality Educational Designs, 2924 NE Stanton Street, Portland, OR 97212; (503) 287-8137

The Reading Laboratory, Inc., P.O. Box 28, Georgetown, CT 06829; (203) 544-9233

Scholastic Inc., 50 West 44th Street, New York, NY 10036; (212) 944-7700

Spinnaker Software Corporation, 215 First Street, Cambridge, MA 02142; (617) 868-4700

Sunburst Communications, 39 Washington Avenue, Pleasantville, NY 10570; (914) 769-5030, (800) 431-1934

Tamarack Software, Water Street, Darby, MT 59829; (406) 821-4596

The Teaching Assistant, 22 Seward Drive, Huntington Station, NY 11746; (516) 499-8397

Teaching Pathways, Inc., P.O. Box 31582, 121 East 2nd Avenue, Amarillo, TX 79120; (806) 373-1847

Terrapin, Inc., 380 Green Street, Cambridge, MA 02139; (617) 492-8816

Texas Instruments, Inc., Personal Computer Division, P.O. Box 10508, Lubbock, TX 79408; (800) 858-4565

TSC/Houghton Mifflin Company, P.O. Box 683, Hanover, NH 03755; (603) 448-3838

Vocational Bibliographies, Inc., P.O. Box 31, Sauk Centre, Minneapolis, MN 56378; (612) 352-6516

Teaching Tools: Microcomputer Services, P.O. Box 50065, Palo Alto, CA 94303; (415) 493-3477

CHAPTER 8

Computer Applications

Gregory Church

I t has now been several years since the personal computer entered the school and home market, and there appears to be consensus that computer literacy is and will continue to be important to everyone (Taber, 1983). The mass-media approach of many computer companies appears to have achieved the short-term goal of computer awareness and is now moving toward promoting the concept of computer necessity. With this approach, advertising is directed, in part, to showing how much we need a specific computer, peripheral, or software package. The concept of novelty and computer games is rapidly fading. It now appears to be time to move toward evaluating and/or developing educational software and systems that act as tools in teaching and solving learning problems. It is somewhat ironic that a great amount of the initial resistance to incorporating computer technology into school programs has not come from students but from the very professionals who are charged with teaching them. This fact has often been justified with excuses that include (1) lack of hardware, (2) poor software, (3) lack of training, and (4) lack of time.

Without question, hardware development is significantly ahead of software development, and the gap appears to be widening. Each day, new

This chapter originally appeared as an article by **Michael Bender** and **Gregory Church** in *Learning Disabilities: An Interdisciplinary Journal* (Vol. III (8), 91–102, 1984) and was adapted by permission of Grune & Stratton for inclusion in this *Handbook*.

equipment is advertised, often with a more competitive price than in the months before. In-service training, with the exception of basic computer-literacy courses, has almost stagnated. Teaching of BASIC (a computer language) continues to be stressed in many school training programs, despite the fact that BASIC is often inappropriate for classroom use. Drill and practice are still the preferred computer activities in the elementary schools whereas computer programming is emphasized in the secondary schools (Becker, 1983). Software programs for LD students are often the same ones used in regular classes, despite the fact that the content and vocabulary level may be too high, too low, or age inappropriate (Flynn, 1985).

If, a Harvey (1983) said, teaching *just* computer literacy is the wrong idea, what is the right idea, or are there many right ideas? Maybe one of these right ideas is to demonstrate to students that computers can be used to enhance their lives (Hummel & Balcon, 1984). Computers can represent a major breakthrough for LD students. A child may suddenly find success in using a word processor or computerized dictionary, or a student who has difficulty writing may be helped by using a graphics tablet or touch-sensitive screen. The increasing quality of voice synthesizers has also opened up new avenues to those disabled adults and children who have been educationally restricted due to communication problems. For many LD students who have difficulty with positive self-concept, the computer can provide nonjudgmental interactions when appropriate, while at the same time providing needed instruction.

It is now certain that computers will be integrated into almost every conceivable facet of education by the next decade. Concepts involving artificial intelligence (Halpern, 1984), which once seemed foreign and remote, are already being assimilated into programs for the disabled at all levels.

Negative aspects have become associated with this new technological era. The inclusion of computers in some school districts has become merely a public relations vehicle to demonstrate that a specific school or region has kept pace with other systems. Too often, there are few objectives and little substance behind the actual computer programs, especially when the same inappropriate software is used daily. It is these types of unidimensional programs that eventually fall prey to critics who are quick to point out that the novelty of computers is already waning. Feeding into this atmosphere are poorly trained software salespeople who continue to push any product as part of a quota or planned-obsolescence strategy.

A pilot study of microcomputer use given to teachers of the learning disabled (Church & Bender, 1984) produced some interesting facts regarding training needs: (1) teachers continue to think they need to be programmers to use computers with their students; (2) school-based computer-training programs are minimal; and (3) software companies are targeting schools and teachers as part of their marketing plans. Often, product validity is only superficially addressed.

It is now clear that a systematized computer-training program is needed rather than the cafeteria-type workshops now being offered to many school programs. This chapter, therefore, will address (1) the development of a computer-training program (COMP-TREX), and (2) some suggested classroom applications that have proven successful with LD students.

USE OF A COMPUTER TRAINING PROGRAM

The training needs of professionals in special education are vast and often overwhelming. With the advent of microcomputers, exigency and resources have come to a crossroad — a dynamic period with the potential of revolutionizing the course of education and the roles of educators as active participants in this new technological era. Microcomputers have the ability to become powerful instructional resources. However, there are the bewildering problems of training, program implementation, and classroom applications. Teachers need to know what computers are, how they can be implemented in a variety of educational settings, and what technical and material support is required for developing a computer-based instructional program. The self-imposed mandate of teacher literacy through computer programming has done much to stagnate the use of computer technology in the classroom. With many teacher-training programs focusing their energies on technical computer-programming activities, the results have been regurgitory programming classes in secondary school settings and developmentally poor computer learning experiences such as drill and practice at the elementary level. Training emphasis needs to shift toward integrating practical computer applications into the classroom through the exploration of word processing, videodisc/microcomputer technology, computerized student-information networks, authoring utilities, computer-facilitated social-interpersonal skills development, innovative career and vocational programming, and effective life skills development.

Consequently, the major challenge facing the LD field today is the development of an interactive training system that capitalizes on the latest advances in microcomputer technology and utilizes these developments in a responsive and nonthreatening instructional manner.

THE COMP-TREX MODEL

The Computer Training Experience (COMP-TREX) model (Figure 8–1) is a systemized approach for implementing a computer-based educational training program, with a primary focus on teacher training through practical hands-on systems development. The training process becomes a series of applications training modules that are teacher specific and allow highly

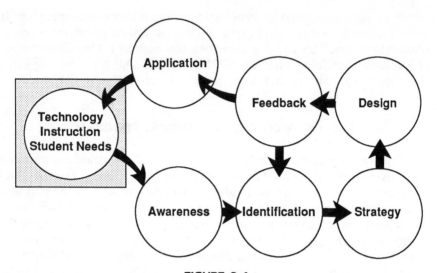

FIGURE 8–1
COMP-TREX: six-phase sequence of activities
for developing staff competencies.

specialized staff experiences. The development of computer applications as a method of teacher training becomes a continuous process — an exercise in contriving new instructional initiatives and, at the same time, extending the applicability of computer technology to teachers. COMP-TREX is designed as a dynamic and interactive process; that is, information and program(s) evolve through interacting with the environment, with the training program's structure contingent on the configuration of the environment. As a result, the model's subsystems, which provide training content, are continuous, occurring in both the predevelopmental and postdevelopmental phases, although each may vary in scope and function at various points of the process.

The environment comprises factors that directly or indirectly affect the structure and processes of the COMP-TREX model but are beyond the direct control of its associated participants. At the heart of this environment are three external influences: technology, instruction, and student needs. Together, these causative agents play important roles as delineators in developing timely and accurate information on emerging computer technologies, changing instructional designs, and individualized needs of children. These critical influences must be realized and anticipated, especially when developing a computer training program for teachers that pursues technological familiarity and responsive approaches to computer instruction.

The emphasis of the COMP-TREX system is on assembling and maintaining subsystems as a means of planning for short- and long-term computer goals. These subsystems divide the process into steps, stages or phases of work or categories of information development. The model becomes a guide in an attempt to describe the step-by-step process through which teacher training and developmental projects can be carried out.

Subsystems

The awareness subsystem is an integral part of the organizing component. This phase becomes the receptor of all incoming external influences in terms of identifying participant problems and issues, organizing participant roles and communication processes, outlining program goals, and reviewing similar projects.

As a preliminary step in this information-processing system, it necessary to appraise the attitudes and concerns of all staff members involved in the program. A need-analysis survey for gathering this information is used to help administrators make better decisions regarding the computer-training programs they wish to implement. The survey considers problems, needs, and goals and includes questions that address basic computer issues. Answers to these questions can provide unique insights into how a staff feels about technology. Frequently, the success or failure of a program hinges on the ability of administrators to recognize any confounding issues or specific needs that may become impediments as a program develops.

The organization of participant roles and communication processes will vary depending on the complexity and resource needs of the program. Getting specific people involved during the planning stage and assigning them specific tasks is crucial. Not only should assignments be clearly stated, but administrators must be sure each task responds to the overall program plan.

A major emphasis in staff involvement is determining who should be part of the training and how to structure that involvement in various stages of the process. Every effort should be made to include as many staff subgroups as possible, because people with different views are valuable resources in conceptualizing participant roles. Figure 8-2 provides an example of this type of involvement.

Creating a communications network among those involved in individual training projects and between the program and the rest of the school or district is essential. Information should be directed toward all those who are in any way involved in the training process. They must be kept informed of how their individual efforts fit into the overall training plan.

One of the simplest means of communication is a periodic memorandum or newsletter reporting progress, reminding people of upcoming meetings, and indicating the next steps. Equally important are communication links with other information sources: electronic networks (Table 8-1).

Whether just a few participants get together to carry out a training project or a large number work together through task groups, the need to

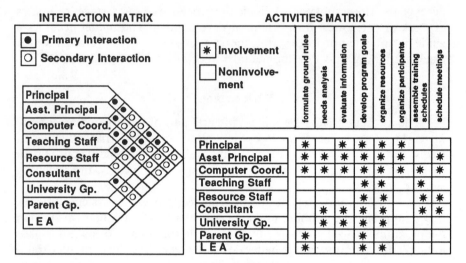

FIGURE 8–2
COMP-TREX participant involvement matrix.

	formulate ground rules	needs analysis	evaluate information	develop program goals	organize resources	organize participants	assemble training schedules	schedule meetings
Principal	*		*	*	*	*		
Asst. Principal	*	*	*	*	*	*		*
Computer Coord.	*	*	*	*	*	*	*	*
Teaching Staff				*	*		*	
Resource Staff				*	*		*	*
Consultant		*	*	*	*		*	*
University Gp.		*	*	*	*			
Parent Gp.	*			*				
L E A	*		*	*				

establish some type of organizational structure is necessary. Essentially, the organization is the structure that develops and holds the various committees and working groups together and keeps the entire program and associated projects coordinated and on track. The organization and committee structure should be kept simple, and task groups, subcommittees, and other administrative units should be developed as the need arises. Too often, large organizational structures require time and organizational maintenance at the expense of implementation of training and applications projects.

Most training and application projects continue over a period of time from a few weeks to a few months. Each objective reached not only gives teachers a feeling of progress toward program goals, but provides an opportunity to assess whether a project is on the right path to a program's eventual goals. Nothing is more important for achieving objectives than developing a logical step-by-step plan. Establishing goals and subgoals and setting target dates are a good start in this direction. Figure 8–3 provides an example of a goal formulation model.

The goal formation model consists of the external environment and the COMP-TREX system. Existing within the COMP-TREX system are a series of program goals that are conceptualized and developed during the initial awareness subsystem phase. Program goals are divided into long-term objectives that are systemized jointly with long-range training goals. These long-term objectives are then arranged into a subsystem of short-term objectives. Existing within this subsystem of objectives are specific training modules that address specific instructional and training needs.

TABLE 8-1
Communication Links

Item	Description
Electronic Networks	
SpecialNET	Electronic mail/bulletin board on computer applications in education
Bibliographic Retrieval Services (BRS)	Online database search service, including education (SPIF and SPIN)
Source	Information and communication database
Handicapped Educational Exchange (HEX)	Bulletin board and database of information resources for the handicapped
DIALOG	Information retrieval service (behavioral and educational psychology, special education)
DATA SPAN	Primarily a resource for science, math, and computer applications
Human Services Networks	
Computer Use in Social Services Network (CUSS)	Quarterly newsletter providing information on computer usage in the social services
Technology And Media (TAM)	National professional organization promoting computer usage in all areas of education
The International Council for Computers in Education (ICCE)	International professional organization promoting educational computing
Microcomputer Education Applications Network (MEAN)	General computer users information newsletter
Association for Special Education Technology (ASET)	Promotes educational computing for the learning disabled
Educational Resources Information Center (ERIC)	Provides access to education research through nationwide network
Periodical References	
AEDs Bulletin/JRNL/Newsletter	Professional/academic quarterly publishing computer research
Educational Technology	Offers a collection of articles examining classroom technologies
Closing The Gap	Explores computer usage with the handicapped
Classroom Computer News	Computer-based learning and applications for teachers
The Computing Teacher	General and technical articles on instructional uses of computers
T.H.E. Journal	Reviews publications and projects dealing with educational technology
The Catalyst	Bimonthly newsletter for computers in Special Education

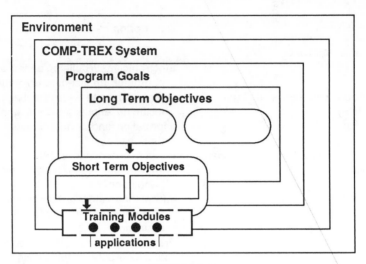

FIGURE 8–3
Goal formation model.

Another important resource tool in developing an awareness of training needs is the review of similar projects. By evaluating similar projects, developers can assess the relative effectiveness and efficiency of different program strategies, policies, or interventions within programs. Similarly, program review can provide information regarding the amount of program resources, staff time, and computer equipment involved in similar programs. Finally, by reviewing these programs, the staff can evaluate interventions and develop meaningful comparisons as to what objectives are successful and integrate them into their own programs.

As part of the organizing mechanism, the identification subsystem involves organizing materials and identifying training needs. The procedures include (1) analyzing development areas, (2) organizing directives, and (3) identifying sources of help. In determining what teachers and support staff want to know, hope to gain, or are willing to do, a useful approach is an informal, continuing planning process. This develops the training focus and suggested strategies. This process is largely a series of discussions among key staff members and administrators producing a reasonable consensus on the type of objectives to pursue. However, the planning process must adapt to the constraints of the environment, with its structure contingent on current student needs, available hardware and software, and specific instructional objectives.

Once training activities have been identified, it is necessary to outline various courses of action. This is accomplished by generating as many alternatives as possible, and by looking at each of the alternatives in terms of cost, time, feasibility, and training objectives. It is also important to review existing resources and the availability of outside resources to determine if they are adequate to successfully carry out the training program.

An essential part of any computer-development activity is the identification, evaluation, and recruitment of the resources needed to attain the desired training objectives. In developing resources, it is necessary to consider three levels of support: (1) human resources, such as professional associations, universities, local user groups, or private consulting firms (sources of technical information support); (2) equipment resources, including computer hardware, software, peripherals, communications, and various support materials and tools for actual training and applications development; and (3) funding resources such as grants, fundraising activities, and associated flexible funds. It is important to assess carefully the kinds and amounts of resources that are likely to be needed and to develop a timetable for their use.

As part of the transitional phase, the strategy and design subsystems create a developmental framework for applying needs and resources to relevant training experiences. These experiences take the form of hands-on skills acquisition through practical classroom applications projects. These projects, conceptualized jointly with program objectives, provide participants with the opportunity to explore computer usage and instructional methods for specialized student-needs development. Techniques and tools necessary for this effort include (1) defining project objectives, (2) organizing specific needs modules, (3) allocating resource support, and (4) scheduling activity times.

It is important to reiterate program goals when defining project objectives. This may seem elemental, but it is necessary to have a clear and agreed-upon agenda of what is to be accomplished. A priority list based on specific training needs should be developed, both for equipment familiarization and software support. Along similar lines, training should address the particular instructional needs and interests of teachers, because the results will be translated into a greater understanding of technical equipment usage and applied instructional presentation in the classroom.

Organizing specific-needs modules provides an appropriate sequencing of activities based on those that can be performed independently and those that are dependent on the results of others. This functional-training sequence should consider overlaps in responsibility, simultaneous performance, and sequential interdependence. These modules provide an outline for coordinating tasks and accomplishing objectives in a timely, efficient manner. Figure 8–4 provides an example of one type of implementation model. All training modules should be provided with current computer and instructional information and properly organized resources, and should be presented in an orderly and meaningful manner. Similarly, each module should be specific in terms of training and applications development, avoiding resource and equipment overlaps.

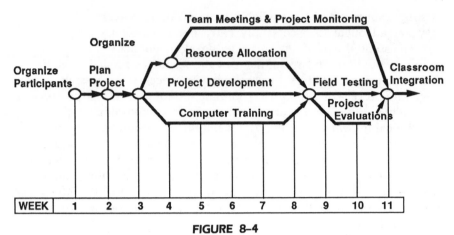

FIGURE 8-4
Sample implementation schedule for a training module.

In allocating resource support for each training module, it is important to determine the types of resources needed for performance and appropriate quantities of professional and technical support personnel, computer time usage, support materials, and actual equipment cost estimates. It is also important to develop a resource-use schedule, which includes a short- and long-term projection of potential alternative uses due to functional changes in planned growth, anticipated developments, and predicted training needs.

Because scheduling is a means of determining the appropriate use of staff time and resources to accomplish various project activities, a schedule should include a listing of tasks, time estimates, and a sequence of interdependencies. Scheduling also provides a formula for determining the duration of activities, important events or dates, and functional sequences. A schedule can correlate other considerations such as potential delays, unforseen circumstances, and project changes.

The design subsystem integrates program objectives into a structure for training and classroom-applications development. The design phase and its system structure will vary in scheme depending on the complexity of the objectives. The design process is primarily intuitive and interpretive. The application can be as simple as developing a supplemental class lesson for LD students on an authoring system or as complex as developing a multimedia student-access network. The following model (Figure 8-5) presents a basic design cycle and delineates the major linkages across the system.

As a preliminary step in the design process, it is necessary to define specific student learning objectives for the applications project and to

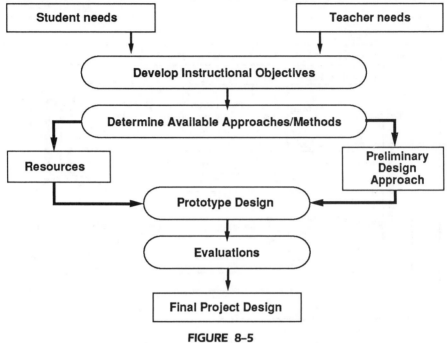

FIGURE 8-5
Design model for applications development.

integrate the associated teaching skills needed to apply the application in a classroom setting. For example, teachers of the learning disabled may want to develop student skills in the style and form of writing business letters while exploring the uses of word processors.

In determining the available approaches for designing a project, it is necessary to evaluate required resources (support software, training, and computer time) and the instructional approach. As a preliminary design approach, teachers should become familiar with writing and editing modes, text manipulations, and specific file-handling sequences. Then, an instructional approach that is user specific for the student population should be developed. Finally, the prototype design should be evaluated in light of the specific software and the associated effectiveness of the instructional approach in terms of student objectives.

Thus far, continuous planning sessions have been used to develop, analyze, and organize information and to produce training and program decisions. The feedback phase provides the opportunity to evaluate the training process and review the appropriateness of applications developed during each of the training modules. Evaluating a training program is

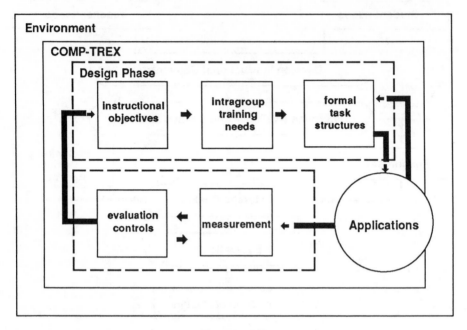

FIGURE 8–6
Feedback evaluation model.

basically an attempt to determine to what extent the project and training methods accomplished what they were developed to do. These evaluations seek to provide answers that will guide future decisions and actions (see Figure 8–6).

The feedback and evaluation model provides a setting for monitoring and assessment. In evaluating any training module, the external environment acts as an indicator for ascertaining the adequacy of the process. The design and feedback systems act on the applications project (developed during each training module), forming an iterative development cycle. Assessments are made on instructional objectives, training tasks, and the continuity in curriculum content of the applications.

The first part of the program review is referred to as a formative evaluation. Its purpose is to help formulate and examine the adequacy of the training process used to plan and carry out the project. The evaluation process should involve as many of the program's participants as possible. Regularly scheduled staff meetings provide an excellent monitoring system for making decisions or corrections.

Also included in the review process is the summative evaluation. This focuses primarily on summing up the project's outcomes or results. Evaluations should should reflect both short- and long-term consequences. Again, the project evaluation should be carried out by those people involved in the planning process and those people who actually conducted the project. When possible, the LD student should be included in this evaluation process.

The feedback phase is an integral part of each training module. This process should be systematic and iterative, addressing such issues as the justification of the present use of resources to accomplish objectives, the need for additional or continuing resources, and the effectiveness of current policies and program process methods.

During the applications phase, computer projects developed during the training module are integrated into the classroom, completing the COMP-TREX cycle. However, maintenance and requirements reviews are necessary to stay current with microcomputer technology and instructional needs. By monitoring instructional procedures, both administrators and teachers can provide consistency and continuity in curriculum content, an awareness of special-needs development, and a greater understanding of the problems involved with the conceptualization of computer projects.

Applications are developmental in nature because external influences (technology, instruction, needs, etc.) are constantly placing new pressures on the developmental cycle. As a result, all applications are cycled back into the COMP-TREX system — beginning the training and development cycle again.

INTEGRATED CLASSROOM APPLICATIONS

The microcomputer is becoming a familiar sight in many classrooms across the United States. By January 1983, nearly 70% of all middle and junior high schools had one or more microcomputers, and elementary usage had increased over 40% (Becker, 1983). The influx of computers into the classroom is likely to continue in the coming years. The need for support courseware and practical computer applications has surfaced as a dominant issue in the wake of the microcomputer profusion. For special educators, the need has become a real dilemma in terms of planning computer instruction.

In reflecting on the use of computer applications in the area of teaching the learning disabled, it is necessary to outline some of the important student needs that should be considered when developing or purchasing software systems. Some critical considerations should include (1) providing a failure-free system, (2) developing social-interpersonal skills, (3) providing immediate positive reinforcement, (4) developing practical survival skills, (5) increasing the child's sense of competence, and (6) providing a multisensory instructional format.

As a general rule, computer literacy among schools has meant computer programming — BASIC language instruction — in most middle school settings. By January 1983, nearly 98% of all schools that offered students more than 30 hours of programming instruction used BASIC. The trend is similar for those schools (1 to 3 years of using microcomputers) in elementary and secondary settings (Becker, 1983).

The BASIC language programming approach for elementary and middle school special education students is inappropriate as a preferred computer-programming method. The fundamental and higher-order skills necessary to use the language in an efficient manner are often self-defeating in terms of the needs of LD students. In providing flexibility, creativity, pattern development, and outlining information, BASIC fails many criticial considerations of LD children. That is not to say that the BASIC language is poor in design or effectiveness in regular school settings; BASIC has proven its worth in many application areas. However, the language structure of BASIC provides little success for LD children exploring the world of programming.

The argument against the use of BASIC lies in many of the assumptions we have about special education students. At the elementary and middle-school levels, LD children have had prolonged histories of failure in exploring their learning environments. As a result, many of these children have little self-confidence. The BASIC language is void of the many intrinsic properties vital to the success of first-time special-needs users.

The BASIC environment was designed as a system for doing scientific computational work and data processing. As a result, complex subroutines and file structures are needed to develop programs. Similarly, BASIC has no modular structure built into the language — a confusing factor for children often needing task analysis and sequential teaching. As an early developmental computer awareness tool, BASIC is everything but a failure-free system in terms of learning and exploration for LD students. Handling textual informatioin can become a complex process for students using BASIC and the results are often hours of tedious debugging and personal frustrations.

The BASIC language provides little or no immediate positive reinforcement for a child's programming efforts. Children naturally like to explore the many facets of computer programming — text manipulations, graphics, and sound generation. However, the concepts of PEEKS, POKES, and binary files do much to mystify and frustrate the LD student's creative programming desires. Beyond simple program applications like printing one's name on the screen or even rudimentary smiling faces in low-resolution graphics, many computer applications using BASIC are unattainable for special-needs children. This is primarily due to the student's need for advanced programming instruction, and the obdurate nature of the concepts involved in the language's structure.

Typically, in elementary and secondary schools, students get between 15 and 45 minutes of computer time per week. Furthermore, because most elementary schools with microcomputers currently have only one or two units, many schools try to give access to as many students as possible (Becker, 1983). These schools typically use their equipment during only one-half of the school day; hence, a student user is not likely to receive much time on the computer, much less any advanced computer programming.

Similarly, LD students need a formula for concept development that is straightforward, especially when dealing with complex programming structures. Consequently, students tend to lose many of the reinforcing qualities programming has to offer when their creative desires cannot be realized due to the extensive training needed to accomplish advanced programming applications. BASIC, with its complex tasks of manipulating strings, branch statements, and other format conventions, has done much to stifle the success-oriented learning environments of LD children. Learning-disabled students should concentrate on the creative process, developing logical thinking and systematic approaches to problem solving rather than worrying about complex language patterns and sophisticated data-processing mechanisms.

What programming language is appropriate for children? The answer depends largely on the tasks and user needs of the learning environment.

LANGUAGE PROCESSING FOR LEARNING-DISABLED USERS

In developing an approach for utilizing language-processing applications for LD users, it is necesary to provide students with (1) a flexible text-search system, (2) an interactive input/output device, (3) a modular system for developing specific tasks, and (4) a conceptually specific and efficient programming process.

The Super Pilot software system has been used as an introductory approach to computer programming for LD students. This software system is classified as an authoring language designed as a simple programming language for creating computerized lessons or programs. The system is flexible, allowing individuals to structure their own interpretive framework for program development. The modular format of Super Pilot provides students with individual editors for developing specific text files and special effects files. The author mode combines these files with a minimal amount of student effort (one or two letter instructions), keeping the program process success oriented and focusing student efforts on creative endeavors rather than on technical processing mechanisms. The processing concept for Super Pilot is well suited for the LD student because it is accurate yet user friendly. Students can design and implement the programming process easily using Super Pilot's command instructions and modularity. Typically, such applications can be conceived and realized in 2 to 3 hours of programming lab time and are exceptional as approaches for developing a sense of technical competence in LD children.

Developing social interpersonal skills in LD children has been a perpetual need among special education teachers. The process has been hampered by such factors as students' poor self-concepts and poor written communication skills. Recently, Super Pilot was used as a student programming exercise in developing varied social and written skills. As part of a computer-literacy class during special holidays, it was decided that students would develop programs that generated greeting cards for relatives and friends. The Super Pilot language provided a systematic process for developing this applications project. The programming tasks were separated into distinctive activities by the students and developed by the students based on their understanding of the Super Pilot programming structure. See Figure 8–7 for an example of the Super Pilot programming process.

The Super Pilot programming environment provided an efficient means of developing the student's conceptualized process. As a group, the students defined a specific routine of activities for accomplishing the exercise. The Super Pilot systems provided a flexible setting with specific modules that facilitated a success-oriented learning environment. The developmental cycle included the following activities: (1) developing specific

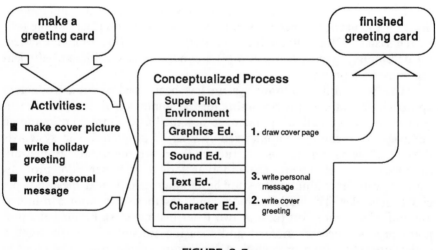

FIGURE 8–7
Student programming model.

graphic pictorials, (2) organizing written text materials, and (3) integrating each of the various programming tasks.

The introductory programming phase utilized the graphic editor, one of four main modules within the Super Pilot language system, in designing the graphic pictorials. The computer's keyboard, joystick, and paddles were integrated into the graphics process by the teacher. Consequently, the activity became a highly motivating environment for the children using the multiple-input modes. As a result, even children with severe attention deficits showed increases in activity awareness and attending during the programming sequence. By using these various modes, students developed an awareness of the different capabilities of the computer/software system. The students were operating in a success-oriented environment during this lab phase. Graphics, both simple and complex, were developed with amazing ease. Positive reinforcement was immediate — one input command resulted in direct color-graphic responses to the screen. The failure-free learning approach was fostered by the simple yet efficient manipulation of graphic designs; students had the ablity to save, edit, and manage the process in quick, easy steps. This was especially true for students desiring to improve and develop their original pictorial concepts after sharing design ideas with other students.

The second phase of the programming process involved the creation of a character set for writing the holiday greeting on the cover page. Again, a user environment was created for students to think and act in an independent creative manner. The character set editor's programming structure is similar to the graphics editor. As a result, students were famliar with the design process and assimilated the previous success orientations and motivational behaviors into their new programming phase.

Briefly, the character set module allows students to create their own set of characters corresponding to the keys on the keyboard. In developing the actual greeting phrase, students had the choice of using standard phrase banks or developing their own greeting phrases (birthday and special-events wishes, etc.). Students clearly preferred developing independent greeting banks. The character set module has the flexibility of designing up to 96 characters/set. Again, teachers can use the multiple input modes as students develop new symbols. Joysticks in combination with the scratch pad offer students greater flexibility in designing characters. This mode appears to have a profound impact on children with motor problems, especially in the area of writing ability. Many students often go to extravagant lengths to develop new letter characters. The process also seems to eliminate the frustration and embarrassment that LD students often convey when organizing written work, notably in the areas of orientation and spatial relationships.

The final programming stage involved writing personal messages for the greeting card and the actual programming process. This activity is handled directly through the text editor of Super Pilot. In the text editor, students can insert, delete, change, or replace phrases and duplicate or move portions of programming instructions.

Super Pilot's programming structure is straightforward and very easy to write. Most of the commands used in the programming structure are one or two letters in length. Subsequently, students can read each other's programs and logic structures with little difficulty, vastly increasing the child's sense of technical competence. Also, the instruction format is effective for many children who are severely limited by visual perception problems, such as transposals or sequencing processes. The user environment is success oriented and does not facilitate uncomfortable or initimidating feelings when dealing with intricate language-processing instructions.

Apart from general computer literacy or drill-and-practice activities, computer instruction can become a rewarding experience for first-time LD elementary and middle school students. However, the student's needs must be matched closely with the abilities of individual software programs. With proper teacher planning and careful implementation, the needs of both the student and the special-education teacher can be realized.

SUMMARY

A word of caution is in order for those proponents who have become convinced of the benefits of computer technology as a tool for helping the disabled learner. Computers are not a panacea for those teachers searching for instant help in changing the complex behaviors of their students (Salend & Salend, 1985). Too often in education, we rush toward new ideas without careful analyses (Hofmesiter & Thorkildsen, 1982). Initial positive results are often tempered by long-term realities. Because of this, computer-training programs must be well thought out and carefully planned. Efficacy studies comparing computer utility with existing approaches (Trifiletti, Frith, & Armstrong, 1984), must be addressed. We cannot afford to move so quickly that we overlook sound educational methodology when integrating technology into existing programs. We must be cautious of software that is unproven, and of those technological entrepreneurs who place monetary success over educational values. The plethora of new software companies promoting poor, untested, and incompatible products is a vivid example of the latter.

In essence, developing any educational computer program takes thought and planning. There are few shortcuts, although staff can visit successful programs and learn a great amount. Overriding any and all technical prerequisites is the commitment that must be made by the administration of a school or program, the teacher and the student. Without this collaborative commitment, it will be difficult for a computer program to be successful and fulfill its great promise.

PART IV

Adult Consequences of
Learning Disabilities

T his section looks at what happens when the LD child grows up. If LD is a pervasive problem, then what does it mean for the LD child? There is a growing awareness that LD is not a short-term problem, and efforts have been directed at studying LD over the long-term. The two chapters in Part IV provide insight into the status of the child as an adult.

What about postsecondary education for an LD student? This intriguing question is addressed in Chapter 9 which surveys the nature and emergence of programs for LD students at 4-year institutions of higher learning. Information regarding the characteristics of LD students in higher education, admission policies, program services, and suggestions for preparing high school LD students is summarized to provide a comprehensive overview of this new phenomenon.

The final chapter reviews the longitudinal research in LD to provide an answer to the question: What are the long-term consequences of LD? Follow-up studies are summarized so professionals may be in a better position to answer the question frequently asked by parents, "What will happen to my child?"

CHAPTER 9

College Opportunities

Charles T. Mangrum
Stephen S. Strichart

$\mathbf{T}$his chapter discusses the emergence and nature of programs for LD students at 4-year colleges and universities. Topics discussed include the reasons why college programs for the learning disabled emerged, the characteristics of students who attend them, the steps by which the programs were developed, admission policies, program services, and recommendations to high schools for preparing LD students for college.

EMERGENCE OF COLLEGE PROGRAMS

Special programs and services to meet the needs of LD students in colleges and universities are a relatively new phenomenon. Efforts of this nature extend back no further than the early 1970s, when a few colleges set out to develop and implement the necessary conditions for LD students to succeed in college (Mangrum & Strichart, 1984). Today, nearly 300 colleges and universities provide programs for LD students with college potential (Mangrum & Strichart, 1985). However, many more colleges and universities are giving serious thought to developing such programs. The authors identified

This chapter originally appeared as an article by **Charles T. Mangrum** and **Stephen S. Strichart** in *Learning Disabilities: An Interdisciplinary Journal* (Vol. II (5 & 6), 57–81, 1983) and was adapted by permission of Grune & Stratton for inclusion in this *Handbook*.

five factors that have been instrumental in the emergence of existing programs and that have heightened interest in developing new ones: extension of high school programs, LD students' desire to attend college, pressure from advocates, college financial crises, and federal legislation. Enumeration of these factors follows.

Initially, the field of learning disability focused on the needs of young children. Although there was initial optimism that early and intensive intervention would cure learning disabilities, it soon became obvious that learning disabilities persist into adulthood. As these young children moved beyond elementary school, LD programs were extended to the junior and then the senior high school levels. The increased emergence of college programs for LD students was the next logical step in this sequence.

Many LD students are interested in attending college. A recent survey reported that 67% of young adults who were diagnosed as learning disabled by their schools, at some point during their elementary or secondary school programming had plans for future education (White, Alley, Deshler, Schumaker, Warner, & Clark, 1982). If all these students actually entered college, it would mean approximately 35,000 LD students would enter each year. Although not all of these students actually pursue college, an increasing number have, and this has brought pressure on colleges to develop programs for them.

Increasing pressure from parents, adult groups, and concerned professionals is another factor that brought about the emergence of college programs for LD students. Breakthroughs in educational services for disabled students have historically been stimulated by the unyielding activities of nonprofessional and professional advocates organizing their efforts through various associations. History has repeated itself on behalf of the young LD adult. This is evident by the formation of a number of adult-oriented groups consisting of LD individuals and their advocates. Many of the activities of these groups have focused on inspiring and convincing more colleges and universities to offer appropriate opportunities for LD students.

A fourth, and practical factor, is economic reality. Most colleges throughout the nation are facing financial crises due to declining student enrollment. Private and public institutions are searching for ways to increase student enrollment to generate needed revenue for maintaining programs and faculty. Learning-disabled high school students with potential for college success represent a significant source of new enrollments for these colleges. More and more colleges are providing programs to attract these students.

Possibly the most important factor affecting college programs for LD students is federal legislation. The Education of All Handicapped Children Act of 1975, Public Law 94-142, requires that all handicapped children between the age of 3 and 21 be given the opportunity to receive an appropriate education through the secondary school level. As a result of being educated with nonhandicapped students, many LD students developed the same academic aspirations for postsecondary study as their peers.

Although Public Law 94-142 does not apply to the college level, Section 504 of the Rehabilitation Act of 1973 does apply, based on the implementing regulation appearing in the *Federal Register* of May 4, 1977. The regulation states:

> No qualified handicapped person shall, on the basis of handicap, be excluded from participation in, be denied the benefits of, or otherwise be subjected to discrimination under any program or activity which requires or benefits from Federal financial assistance. (p. 22678)

Providers of services are required to make programs accessible to handicapped persons and to operate their programs in a nondiscriminatory manner. By the definition of Section 504, handicapped persons include those with a physical or mental impairment substantially limiting one or more life activities. "Specific learning disabilities" is one of the disorders constituting physical or mental impairment. Miller, McKinley, and Ryan (1979) noted that although a learning disability is not as obvious as other handicaps encompassed by Section 504 (e.g., sight or mobility handicaps), assurances for equal opportunities for LD individuals are uncompromised.

Subpart E of Section 504 specifically refers to postsecondary education. Subpart E prohibits discrimination against qualified handicapped persons in admissions, recruitment, and treatment after admission.

Admissions

Qualified disabled persons may not be denied admission or be subjected to discrimination in admission policies on the basis of their disability and the regulations specifically prohibit any quotas for the number of disabled individuals admitted to a program. The regulations also prohibit the use of tests or other criteria for admission that have a disproportionate, adverse effect on disabled persons. Further, they require assurance that admission tests be accurately selected to reflect an applicant's aptitude or achievement level, rather than reflect the disability. Only when an institution is taking mandated or voluntary remedial action to correct the effects of past discrimination against the disabled may the institution make preadmission inquiry as to whether an applicant has a disability. Even in this case, such information is restricted to use to matters directly concerned with the remedial action, and disclosure is voluntary on the part of the applicant.

Vogel (1982) described the inherent dilemma for college officials since, although it must be known which students are disabled to be in compliance with Section 504, the officials are dependent on voluntary disclosure by disabled applicants. Many of the applicants withhold such information in fear it may be used against them. To avoid this problem, many professionals advise LD students to provide information about their disability to ensure their access to needed services.

Recruitment

Recruitment is defined as those activities intended to influence students to attend a given institution (Redden, Levering, & DiQuinzio, 1978). Given that disabled students must have the same opportunity to learn about an institution as nondisabled students, Redden and colleagues suggested that colleges and universities expand their recruitment activities to include schools and special classes attended by disabled students. They also suggested that training be provided to make recruitment personnel more aware of services required by these students. Such training would assist recruitment personnel to identify qualified disabled students.

Treatment

Part E of Section 504 requires institutions to modify academic requirements so that qualified disabled students are not discriminated against on the basis of their disabilities. Suggested modifications include changes in the length of time permitted to complete degree requirements, substitutions of specific required courses, and adapations of the manner in which specific courses are conducted. Academic requirements that a college or university demonstrates are essential to a specific program, or to any directly related licensing requirement, are not regarded as discriminatory. As observed by Ross and O'Brien (1981), Section 504 does not require that essential program requirements be modified or waived.

Part E of Section 504 also prohibits imposing any rules on disabled students that limit their participation in a program or activity. Course examinations must measure a student's achievement rather than reflect a disability. Also, disabled students must be provided with appropriate auxiliary learning aids. These stipulations paved the way for special provisions and support services, such as the use of tape recorders to record class lectures, untimed and/or oral examinations, and taped texts.

The significant and enhancing effect of Section 504 on college opportunities for the learning disabled is easily perceived. Given a fairer opportunity to be admitted to programs, being made more aware of these opportunities, and receiving appropriate assistance within the programs, increasing numbers of LD individuals have seriously considered and pursued a college education. A guarantee of nondiscriminatory consideration for financial assistance, another element of Part E, has added to the effect of these provisions. Section 504 requirements are being taken seriously by colleges and universities. As Chesler (1980) surmised, the teeth of the law consist of stipulations that will inevitably lead to curtailment of federal funding for any institution found to be discriminating against disabled individuals.

Over the past 10 years, there has been a modest increase in the number of programs for the learning disabled available for qualified college students. There is still a need for additional comprehensive college programs to assist young LD adults to realize their dreams of a college education. The number of such students with the desire to go to college currently far exceeds the capacity of appropriate college programs to serve them. The factors that have inhibited the growth of college programs for the learning disabled, although significant, are not insurmountable for the college or university that is committed to meeting the needs of all qualified students. The five factors we identified as bringing about the emergence of college learning-disability programs will, we believe, result in more and more colleges taking on this commitment.

CHARACTERISTICS OF STUDENTS

With the recentness of college programs for the learning disabled and the historical emphasis of the LD field on the needs and characteristics of school-age children, little is known about the specific characteristics of LD students at the college level. Information concerning characteristics of these students is just now beginning to accrue. The characteristics presented below were derived from an analysis of various written accounts and from discussions with directors of college programs for LD students. Before presenting the characteristics, several points should be noted. First, the authors focused specifically on characteristics descriptive of students attending learning-disabilities college programs. Characteristics reported for LD adults in general, or for those in adult basic education programs, were not included. Second, most reports of characteristics were based on observation and clinical work with these college students and not on empirical research. Third, as expected in a field that focuses on disabilities, most reports were of deficits rather than of strengths. Therefore, although the characteristics presented are, unfortunately, negatively toned, it should be kept in mind that LD college students have many positive attributes. Finally, all the characteristics do not apply to any one student. Each student has a different pattern of these characteristics.

Although there is some unavoidable overlap, the characteristics have been organized into seven categories: cognitive, language, perceptual-motor, academic, work and study habits, social, and personality. Specific characteristics were primarily derived from the following sources: Barbaro, 1982; Brown, 1982; Chesler, 1980; Cordoni, 1979, 1980, 1982a, 1982b; Vogel,

1982; Vogel and Adleman, 1981; Vogel and Moran, 1982; Vogel and Sattler, 1981; Webb, 1974; Worcester, 1981; and R. W. Barsch, personal communication, July 21, 1982; I. Götz, personal communication, September, 1982; J. McGuire, personal communication, October, 1982; R. Nash, personal communication, June 17, 1982; P. Quinlan, personal communication, July 16, 1982; and D. Saddler, personal communication, July 14, 1982.

Cognitive

It is difficult to generalize about the overall cognitive ability of the LD college students. IQ levels varied as a function of each program's view of the IQ level needed for success. Where it was felt that these students needed above average intelligence to be successful in college, reported IQs were in the high-average range. Where IQ was not deemed to be as important for success in college, reported mean IQs were lower. The only possible generalization is that where IQ scores were reported for students in learning-disabilities college programs, they were no lower than 85.

Some specific accounts of LD students' functioning on the Wechsler Adult Intelligence (WAIS) were available (Cordoni, 1979; Cordoni, O'Donnell, Ramaniah, Kurtz, & Rosenshein, 1981; D. Saddler, personal communication, July 14, 1982). These accounts indicated that verbal IQ was higher than performance IQ, with higher scores on Bannatyne's (1974) spatial factor (comprising the picture completion, block design, and object assembly subtests) and verbal conceptualization factor (comprehension, similarities, and vocabulary subtests) factors. Performances on the digit span subtest and coding subtests) and acquired knowledge (information, arithmetic, and vocabularly subtests) factors. Performance on the digit span subtest was particularly low.

Other reported cognitive characteristics included (a) poor abstraction; (b) inflexible thought patterns; (c) poor ability to spontaneously employ cognitive strategies; (d) poor deductive reasoning; (e) little awareness of cause-and-effect relationships; and (f) deficits in long- and short-term auditory and visual memory.

Language

Language difficulties are the core of learning disabilities. Consequently, it was no surprise to find that deficits in both spoken and written language were characteristic of college LD students. Spoken language was characterized by poor receptive language, resulting in a failure to understand assignments or to grasp important points, immature syntax, limited vocabulary, difficulties with word retrieval, and inappropriate use of words. Written language was characterized by imprecise and unclear expression, immature syntax, poor style reflected in a relatively unvaried sentence structure and word selection, lack of organization, incorrect use of punctuation, use of a limited number of words, compositions limited in length and sentence structure, infrequent use of long words (i.e., more than three syllables), and underutilization of verbs, adjectives, and adverbs.

Perceptual-Motor

Perceptual-motor problems were still found among some LD college students. Specific characteristics included reversals, rotations, and inversions of letters and numerals, unestablished laterality and/or directionality, poor spatial awareness, poor visual discrimination, difficulty forming a visual gestalt, inaccurate visual sequencing, and imprecise fine motor coordination, manifested by awkward writing.

Academic

Reported achievement levels for basic skills ranged from third grade to college level. Reading, spelling, handwriting, and mathematics were variously cited as the primary area of deficit.

Reading deficits included gaps in phonics and other word attack skills, poor comprehension, poor ability to determine main ideas, slow reading rate, and failure to adapt reading rate to reading purpose.

Spelling deficits included transposition of letters, omission or substitution of sounds, attempts to phonetically spell irregular words, and avoidance of writing words that are difficult to spell.

Handwriting was characterized by awkward writing, slow rate of writing, tendency to use manuscript rather than cursive, poorly formed or illegible letters, overly large writing, writing that varied in size throughout the same paper, sloppy appearing papers, difficulty keeping writing within the margins, paper and/or pencil held improperly, overuse of uppercase letters, and deterioration of writing quality when time limits were imposed (e.g., timed tests or notetaking).

Mathematics deficits included underdeveloped computational skills, incomplete mastery of multiplication tables, inadequate mathematical reasoning, poor problem-solving ability, difficulty recalling the sequence of an operational process, and failure to understand and retain terms representing quantitative concepts.

Work and Study Habits

As LD students progress through school, efficient and effective work and study habits become increasingly important. At the college level, these work and study habits are of crucial significance. Learning-disabled college students were described as lacking good work and study habits. Specific characteristics included poor organization and budgeting of time, difficulty meeting schedules, problems in initiating and sustaining effort, difficulty establishing short- and long-term goals and objectives, inability to identify essential task requirements, difficulty integrating information from various sources, unfamiliarity with the use of library resources, difficulty using dictionary and other reference tools, poor notetaking and outlining skills (notes were typically sparse, incomplete, and inaccurate), and excessive test anxiety.

Social

Cordoni (1982b) identified social functioning as the major problem area for LD college students. Increasing emphasis was given to social aspects in descriptions of this population. Specific characteristics included difficulty establishing good relationships and making friends, difficulty working with others, poor family relationships, difficulty reading body language and facial expressions, inappropriate social behaviors, problems expressing thoughts or feelings, regretting what was said or done, uncertainty about what to say in a situation, misunderstanding humor and sarcasm, difficulty engaging in "small talk," few hobbies and interests, insufficient attention to personal appearance, and difficulty relating to authority figures (e.g., professors, counselors).

Personality

A range of personality characteristics were reported in descriptions of LD college students. Specific characteristics included low self-esteem, insecurity, inferiority feelings, lack of self-confidence, overdependence, vulnerability, hypersensitivity, frustration, pessimism, suspicion, impulsiveness, self-centeredness, and defensiveness.

An examination of the above characteristics of LD college students enhances an understanding of their nature and needs. Although this information is just beginning to accrue, it is obvious that many of these students have the cognitive ability to do college level work. They have, however, many deficits that, if not attended to, will make it difficult for them to realize their potential. College programs need to assist such students in developing more effective spoken and written language skills, compensating for residual perceptual-motor difficulties, increasing achievement in basic skills, improving work and study habits, and fostering social and personality development.

The characteristics reported for LD college students suggest that to meet their needs, programs must be flexible, comprehensive, and interdisciplinary. Flexible programs provide LD students with alternative ways to meet course and degree requirements without lowering standards. A comprehensive program provides differentiated testing for admission, remediation of basic skills, assistance in learning course content, and counseling. An interdisciplinary approach involves learning-disability specialists, reading specialists, psychologists, counselors and subject area professors, all working cooperatively to help LD students succeed in college.

DEVELOPING A PROGRAM

College programs for LD students have almost invariably come about through the inspired efforts of single individuals commited to the goal of providing higher education for students with learning disabilities. These individuals served as the necessary catalysts for initiating the steps to bring these programs to fruition at their institutions.

Convincing the Administration

Individuals who served as catalysts for successful programs typically started by convincing their administrators of the need to provide higher education for qualified LD students. Usually, they began by citing Section 504 of the Rehabilitation Act of 1973 and arguing for compliance. Next, they tied the program to the mission of their college or university. This was easiest to do in small colleges where the primary mission was teaching and serving the community. Another argument, to which many administrators were receptive, proposed the learning disabilities college program as another way of recruiting students.

Typically, administrators had to be convinced that the program would not alter the image of their colleges. Administrators were fearful that their institutions would become known as colleges for LD students and, thereby, reduce the primary population. This was a greater concern for small colleges than for large universities. Some institutions, such as Southern Illinois University, already had an established reputation for helping disabled students. The consensus of the program directors we interviewed was that there was no change in a college's image as long as the population of LD students did not exceed 10% of the base population.

Administrators were also concerned about the cost effectiveness of the programs. Advocates of programs for LD college students must help administrators understand that their colleges cannot immediately expect to earn additional dollars for the general fund through such programs. Learning-disabilities college programs are expensive to operate due to the high cost of providing special services. However, where necessary, parents of LD students were willing to pay an additional fee for the special services. These fees ranged from a few hundred to several thousand dollars per year. Parents did not object to paying for quality services that helped their children succeed in college.

Identifying the Director

Once the administration was commited to starting a program for the learning-disabled, the first task was to identify a program director. Frequently, the administration selected the individual who had been the initial catalyst for the program to serve as the director. The director became the driving force behind all aspects of program development. In addition to being knowledgeable about learning disabilities, the director had to be able to help faculty members and administrators understand the nature of learning disabilities and the types of services LD students needed to succeed in college. It was important for the director to possess the necessary experience and skills to promote and achieve a comprehensive program.

Convincing the Faculty

It was more difficult for program directors to convince faculty members than it was to convince administrators of the need for these college programs. Program directors documented spending hundreds of hours winning the support of faculty members. This was an activity that often began a year or more before the first LD student arrived on campus and continued throughout the program's existence. It appeared to be one of the most challenging and frustrating jobs the program director had. L. Martin (personal communication, June 29, 1982) reported that she started her program before she had solid faculty support and, as a result, had to spend considerable time backpedaling to develop the support needed to make the program a success.

Every program director reported that the learning-disabilities college program must have the support of the faculty or it will fail. J. D. Barsch (personal communication, July 21, 1982) stated, and others agreed, that the key to winning over faculty was personal contact. Barsch started with department-level meetings to explain the program and its services. He followed these meetings with individual faculty conferences, usually over coffee. It was the unanimous recommednation of program directors that faculty-awareness programs should have the director's personal touch rather than rely on typical modes of communication such as memos, forms, and large group meetings. S. A. Vogel (personal commuication, June 16, 1982) recommended providing orientations for new faculty members and renewal workshops at the beginning of each semester to keep the faculty educated and involved.

Although many program directors spend considerable time explaining their programs to faculty members, only half to three-quarters of the faculty were receptive. The remainder had beliefs that ranged from perceiving LD students as "just lazy" to total rejection of college for LD young adults.

Cordoni (1982b) created a slide/tape presentation and showed it at faculty meetings when developing and promoting her program. She designed the presentation for "consciousness raising" and used special education majors to play the roles of LD college students. Her presentation answered three basic questions: What are learning disabilities? What can be done about learning disabilities? How do LD students fit into a university setting? Other program directors have used Cordoni's slide/tape presentation to promote such college programs on their own campuses.

Cordoni (1982b) reported that she distributed to interested faculty members articles that explained what LD students were like and what they needed to succeed in college. She found that these articles sometimes broke through a professor's preconceptions in a more convincing manner than she could.

Many program directors reported that it was important to explain to faculty members that having LD students in their classes would not lower class standards. They reassured their faculties that these students would be required to meet the same standards as all other students and the degrees they earned would be equivalent to the degrees earned by other students studying the same curriculum. The directors further assured faculty members that they would not be required to spend additional time working with LD students, realizing that faculty were protective of the time they needed for class preparation, research, and community and college service. Program directors recognized that if faculty members were to perceive working with LD students as a burden, they would not support the program.

Among every faculty there are key members who influence the actions of other faculty members. It is very important to single out these influential individuals for special, intensive contact. Winning over an influential faculty member may provide access to an entire area, department, or even a college. Most directors were acutely aware of the influential faculty members at their colleges and made every effort to keep them apprised of the services and accomplishments of the college program for LD students.

Faculty members who know nothing about learning disabilities are probably easier to enlist than those who have some familiarity with learning disabilities. Faculty with limited perceptions usually know only the common myths, and erasing these from their minds is a difficult task. Erroneous views in which learning disabilities are seen as another name for retardation, or are believed to be caused by emotional factors, impede acceptance of the need to provide a college opportunity for LD students.

Learning-disabled students are a valuable resource in the effort to convince faculty of the need for a learning disabilities college program. Successful LD students, through their performance in courses, will help convince the faculty of the worthiness of the program. To facilitate this,

S. A. Vogel (personal communication, June 16, 1982) recommended beginning the program with a small, carefully selected group of students with a high probability for success.

Planning Team

During the process of developing a college program for the learning disabled, some program directors formed a planning team. Under the director's leadership, the team worked to realize the program. The planning team's major objectives were (a) to learn about the nature of LD college students; (b) to acquire an understanding of the services needed by these students to succeed in college; and (c) to formulate the generalizations upon which a learning disabilities college program could be developed at their institution.

When a special education teacher-training program already existed, directors began looking for planning-team members among the teaching faculty. S. A. Vogel (personal communication, June 16, 1982) suggested that the search for team members be extended to the office of the dean of students, English department, office of handicapped student services, guidance and counseling department, evaluation center, health services, library, and media center.

Once the planning team members were identified, the program director circulated materials to assist them in understanding the characteristics of LD students, as well as the characteristics of successful programs at other colleges. Some planning team members were sent to professional conferences and others visited ongoing learning-disabilities college programs. Planning-team members were also given opportunities to meet LD college students. When the team members had acquired sufficient knowledge, the program director met with them to formulate the specific program. Once the learning disabilities college program was implemented, some planning teams continued to work with the program as advisory boards.

Staffing the Program

The critical variable in all of the programs we examined was the director. As noted above, the director was the driving force behind all aspects of the learning disabilities college program and its development. As G. M. Webb (personal communication, July 15, 1982) pointed out, "You need a good leader — a leader who has fun with it, works well with her staff, and supervises them heavily." K. Chandler (personal communication, June 9, 1982) perhaps best exemplified the intensity of the work of the director when she said that she and her assistant "viewed themselves as mothers to the students." She reported that one day she went to a baseball game and took the pitcher off the mound because he had not attended tutoring sessions. The point is clear. To directors, what they do is more than a job — it is their lives.

Most programs had an assistant director to work along with the program director. The assistant director's primary responsibility was qualifying new students for the program. This responsibility included answering telephone and letter inquiries, which in some cases were as many as 30 per day. In addition, the assistant director also had to assemble records, schedule prospective students for campus visits, arrange for or complete individual testing needed for incoming students, prepare reports, and participate in admission conferences. As secondary responsibilities, the assistant director scheduled students for classes or tutoring, regularly met with staff members to discuss the progress of individual students, dealt with special problems the students had, gathered books and made arrangements to have them recorded, and spoke to groups of high school students and teachers regarding the learning-disabilities program. Assistant directors strongly supported the philosophical position of the director and were equally strong advocates for the program, sharing the same degree of commitment to the program's success.

Any additional personnel needed to operate these college programs were a function of the services that constituted the program. Most programs provided diagnostic testing to identify specific educational needs. For this function, training psychoeducational diagnosticians were employed. The students were usually provided with remediation of basic skills by trained learning disabilities specialists. For subject tutoring, non-LD college students, outside professionals, or college faculty members were hired. Other adjuncts were hired to provide assistance in test proctoring, notetaking, taping of study materials, and to serve as taped-text librarians. Advising and counseling were usually done by the program director or assistant director.

Staff members from other college agencies were utilized when appropriate. They included staff working in basic skills centers, diagnostic centers, guidance and counseling centers, and media centers. Because these non-program staff members were trained to work with the regular population and not specifically with LD students, they were not systematically employed by the programs. Most services required by LD students were provided directly by the program staff.

It is important to note that people were the major resource of these programs. Although some equipment and materials were necessary, the success of the programs largely rested on securing a well-trained and enthusiastic staff.

Housing the Program

These programs were typically housed in one of three areas within a college. Where a program was housed seemed to depend on which area in the college demonstrated the initial enthusiasm for the program, and location of the program appeared to be unrelated to program effectiveness.

In most cases, programs were started by professionals involved in learning disabilities teacher-training programs. As a result, the programs they developed were housed within special education departments. This was advantageous to these programs because undergraduate and graduate students provided tutoring, counseling, and supervision as part of their coursework and practica. This is an example of how such a program can benefit LD students and students in teacher-training programs.

Some programs were housed in the offices of handicapped student services, particularly at larger colleges or universities, or those with a history of services to disabled students. Often, the office of handicapped services had professionals who were attuned to developments in the learning disabilities field. Because of their acute sensitivity to trends and their commitment to meeting the needs of all disabled students, these professionals often provided a supportive atmosphere for the development of the programs. They fostered the development of the program and in some cases the program remained housed within their office.

Occasionally, the impetus for program development came from a staff member in the office of the dean of students who recognized the need for providing services to LD students already on campus. Usually, the staff member in conjunction with a colleague knowledgeable about learning disabilities initiated a program that remained housed in the office of the dean of students.

Funding the Program

Program directors reported varied sources of funding. Some programs were fully supported by their sponsoring institutions and no fee was charged to students beyond the usual tuition and fees. Other programs were supported by additional fees ranging from several hundred to several thousand dollars a year. A few programs received some federal funding.

Of those programs with an additional fee, some charged a flat fee for each semester the student was in the program. In other cases, the fee was graduated with a high fee charged for the first year, and reduced fees for subsequent years. The theory behind this policy was that as services to students were reduced year by year, the fee should be correspondingly reduced.

College learning disabilities programs came to fruition through the efforts of determined professionals who had the ability to focus on a problem and inspire other professionals to participate in its solution. Behind every successful program was a director who had rallied the administration and faculty to the support of LD college students. In all programs, the staff was the major resource for meeting the needs of these students. Directors hired staff members who shared their enthusiasm and point of view. It is clear that the growth and success of these college programs has been due to the efforts of such dedicated professionals.

ADMISSION POLICIES

The 1977 regulations implementing part E of Section 504 of the Rehabilitation Act of 1973 forbade discrimination in admissions policies in institutions of higher learning. As fully described earlier, nondiscrimination in admission policies means that colleges may not require different standards for LD applicants than they do for other applicants. Further, they may not use for admission decisions test results that reflect the disabilities of applicants rather than their potential for doing college work.

Learning disabled applicants are likely to encounter three types of admission policies: open admission, regular admission, and special admission. Open admission requires an applicant to have only a high school diploma or its equivalent to be granted admission to a college. For regular admission, an applicant must have a high school diploma or its equivalent and provide grade point average (GPA), rank in graduating class, and scores on standardized tests such as the SAT or ACT. Special admission is a case-by-case approach using flexible entrance criteria and varied sources and types of information.

Section 504 has had an impact on all three admission policies. It is clear that where open admission policies are in effect, LD applicants with high school diplomas or the equivalent must be admitted with the same ease as other applicants. For regular admission, the implications are not as clear. Standard requirements such as GPA, rank in graduating class, and SAT or ACT test results may not be indicators of ability and knowledge to do college work. Rather, they may be reflections of learning disabilities and, therefore, discriminative against LD applicants. To circumvent the problems of regular admission, many colleges admitted LD applicants by special admission. In the learning, disabilities college programs the authors visited, special admission was clearly the predominant procedure used to admit students.

Cooperative Admission

Applicants to learning disabilities college programs were considered for admission by both the college and the program. In the case of the college, the admission decision was made by the director of admission or the college admission committee. For the learning disabilities program, the admission decision was made by the program director or the program admission committee.

In the typical chronology, the learning disabilities college program staff made decisions about applicants and forwarded the recommendations to the college director of admissions. The recommendations of the learning disabilities college program staff were supported by the college directors of admission or college admission committee. The authors were not told of any instances where a student recommended for admission to a college by the learning disabilities program staff was not subsequently admitted by the college. Because both looked for intelligent, knowledgeable, and emotionally and socially mature students who could succeed in college, the recommendations of applicants from the learning disabilities programs were highly regarded by college admission personnel.

Because of the possible discriminatory nature of the regular admission procedure, a special admission procedure was frequently used to identify applicants who qualified for admission to the college and learning disabilities program. The responsibility for developing and implementing the special admission procedure rested with the directors of the programs.

Special Admission

The special admission procedure can be viewed as a series of key questions in the minds of learning disabilities college program staff as they considered the applicants. Each key question helped the program staff to gather the information they needed to make admission decisions. The key questions considered by the staff and the ways in which they sought answers follow.

Does the Student Have the Ability To Do College Work?

Colleges must be able to obtain information on the academic aptitude of their applicants. They must be able to differentiate between those applicants with the ability to do college work and those applicants whose parents hope college will transform them into scholars (Webb, 1974; G. M. Webb, personal communication, July 15, 1982). To make judgments regarding the ability of non-LD applicants, college admission officials used GPA, high school rank, and SAT or ACT results. Since these indexes were believed to reflect learning disabilities, program staffs used the results of individually administered intelligence tests such as the Wechsler Adult Intelligence Scale (WAIS), Wechsler Adult Intelligence Scale-Revised (WAIS-R), Peabody Picture Vocabulary Test, Slosson Intelligence Test, and the Ravens Standard Progressive Matrices to obtain information from which they made judgments regarding applicants' abilities.

Most program directors preferred the WAIS or WAIS-R to other intelligence tests. Vernoy (personal communication, 1982) looked for a full scale IQ of 115 or a verbal or performance IQ of 120. Götz (personal communication, September, 1982) reported that students in the learning disabilities program at Hofstra University had WAIS/WAIS-R IQs between 115 and 120. G. M. Webb (personal communication, July 15, 1982) looked for college-level thinking ability as evidenced by scaled scores of 13 or higher on the comprehension, similarities, and block design subtests of the WAIS/WAIS-R. Cordoni, O'Donnell, Ramaniah, Kurtz, and Rosenshein (1981) suggested that the ACID cluster (arithmetic, comprehension, information, digit span subtests) on the WAIS/WAIS-R could be very useful for making decisions about college potential. Some of the program directors believed that LD students with IQ scores as low as 90 could succeed in college if they had sufficient motivation.

While it is clear that LD students with a wide range of abilities are being admitted to college, it is also clear that learning disabilities programs are designed for students with at least average intellectual ability. Variations in IQ levels accepted for admission appeared to be related to the intellectual ability of the student body at a specific college.

What Knowledge Has the Student Acquired?

Grade point averages (GPA), rank in graduating class, and SAT or ACT scores were used to answer this question for non-LD applicants. Since the GPA of LD applicants was largely a function of the quality of special-education services provided by high schools, D. Saddler (personal communication, July 14, 1982) regarded GPA as meaningless for making admission decisions about these applicants. By the very same logic, we assume that class rank may have very little relevance.

College-program directors for LD students obtained information about their applicants' background knowledge in three ways, singularly or in various combinations. The first was to require applicants to take the SAT or ACT without a time limit. The applicants were encouraged to use readers or audio casettes to reduce the reading requirements on these standardized tests. The second was to request letters from English, math, science, and other high school teachers describing the applicants' knowledge in these subject areas (Vernoy, 1982). The third was to assess knowledge during an interview with the LD applicant.

Does the Student Have a Learning Disability?

Applicants to learning disabilities programs were required to provide evidence of a learning disability. Usually an applicant's former learning disabilities teacher wrote a letter or completed a form to substantiate the learning disability. At Adelphi University, an applicant also had to submit a copy of an IEP that had been used to provide services in high school (Barbaro, 1982). Letters or reports from psychologists, medical doctors, and school counselors were also used to verify a learning disability.

Can the Student Succeed in College?

To answer this question, staff of virtually all learning disabilities programs conducted personal interviews with applicants. The interviews were sometimes conducted by the director or assistant director (G. M. Webb, personal communication, July 15, 1982). At other times, the interviews were conducted by the program staff (Bireley & Manley, 1980), or by a team comprised of such specialists as the program director, admission counselor, and a psychologist (I. Götz, personal communication, September, 1982).

There was considerable agreement on what the program staff sought to learn from the interviews (Vogel & Adelman, 1981; K. Chandler, personal communication, June 9, 1982; I. Götz, personal communication, September, 1982; J. McGuire, personal communication, October, 1982; P. Quinlan, personal communication, July 16, 1982; D. Saddler, personal communication, July 14, 1982; G. M. Webb, personal communication, July 15, 1982). Basically, interviewers were looking for indications of (a) college level thinking ability; (b) accumulated information about the world; (c) high motivation to succeed in college; (d) productive use of high school years; (e) insight into one's learning disability; (f) awareness of academic strengths and weaknesses; (g) emotional stability; and (h) assertiveness. Parents or guardians were often interviewed by the program staff to verify facts and to obtain additional information. Staff members also sought assurances that parents or guardians would fully support the goals of the program.

At Adelphi University, all applicants to the learning disabilities program were required to attend a 5-week summer session before they were officially admitted to the university (Barbaro, 1982). The summer session was used to assess applicants' motivation, maturity, and ability to handle college classes. Students who succeeded were then recommended for admission to Adelphi University.

When the key questions had been answered, the program staff reviewed the information and formed a recommendation that was forwarded to the college director of admission for action. Admission is a long procedure and program directors recommended that interested LD applicants begin looking for a college with a learning disabilities program in their junior year of high school. Significantly, as Cordoni (1980) pointed out, there is not a well-designed program for college LD students that does not have a waiting list.

Our examination showed that although there were three college admission policies that applicants encountered, they were typically considered for entrance using a special admission policy. Through special admission procedures, colleges could, in a nondiscriminatory way, obtain information they needed to determine the probability of the applicants' success in college. Responsibility for implementing special admission procedures rested with the programs. The staff of these programs sought answers to key questions by obtaining information from professionals, parents, and applicants. Admission decisions reached by the program staff were consistently supported by the college admission officials. The flexibility shown by colleges in admission procedures and the good working relationship between learning disabilities staff and admission officials has allowed many students the opportunity to realize their potential.

PROGRAM SERVICES

At colleges with learning disabilities programs, grading standards and graduation requirements were the same for LD students as they were for other students. Cordoni (1980) identified two important reasons for supporting these requirements in her program: (1) the university at which her program resides, Southern Illinois University, would not support the program if course and degree requirements were modified substantially; and (2) the LD student would not accept a different set of standards that would make them feel less competent than their peers.

In the learning disabilities college programs we examined, the curricular for the LD students were not substantially different from that for their peers. For the most part, program modifications permitted for LD students were the same as those normally permitted for other students. Special modifications were occasionally necessary. At the College of the Ozarks, when it became apparent that a student's learning disability precluded satisfactory performance in a required course, the course was waived by the academic dean (Ben D. Caudle, 1981). Webb (1974) reported that at Curry College, LD students with severe language problems were often exempted for foreign language requirements.

Learning-disabled students were generally neither encouraged nor discouraged from pursuing specific majors (P. Quinlan, personal communication, July 16, 1982). Cordoni (1982a) reported that students in her program were in every major from anthropology to zoology. This latitude stemmed from the belief that given the necessary support, there was no limit to what LD students could be. Cordoni reported that three of her program graduates were in medical school and another was in law school.

Most formal services provided by learning disabilities college programs were delivered during the freshman year. Students participated in the programs on an as-needed basis beyond the sophomore year. The overall desire of the program staff was for students to achieve independence from the program as quickly as possible. In no programs were students terminated from services before they were ready to proceed independently. The procedure described by R. Nash (personal communication, June 17, 1982) at the University of Wisconsin–Oshkosh, was representative. Once students were accepted into the program, they could participate as long as they felt necessary. In some programs, students progressed through program phases in which the amount of services they received was gradually reduced.

College learning disabilities programs offered an array of services to students. In this chapter, program services are grouped into five categories: (a) diagnostic testing and prescriptive planning; (b) program advisement; (c) instructional assistance; (d) instructonal aids; and (e) counseling.

Diagnostic Testing and Prescriptive Planning

In many learning disabilities college programs, students were diagnostically tested during their first semester on campus. The test results were used to plan basic skills remediation, course tutoring, and counseling.

Test batteries varied from program to program. However, certain areas of functioning were routinely examined, including intelligence, academic skills, oral and written language, auditory and visual-perceptual processes, study habits and skills, persnality, and self-concept. Because of the lack of standardized tests normed on adult populations, tests normally used with younger LD students were frequently used with LD college students (Cordoni, 1980). Standardized tests typically used in diagnostic batteries included the Wechsler Adult Intelligence Scale and its revised form (WAIS-R); the Peabody Picture Vocabulary Test; the Slosson Intelligence test; the Ravens Standard Progressive Matrices; the Peabody Individual Achievement Test; the Wide Range Achievement Test; the Key Math Diagnostic Arithmetic Test; the Woodcock-Johnson Psycho-Educational Battery; the Detroit Tests of Learning Aptitude; the Test of Written Language; the Specific Language Disability Test; the Wepman Test of Auditory Discrimination; the Bender-Gestalt Test; the Developmental Test of Visual-Motor Integration; and the Tennessee Self-Concept Scale. Each program also used informal tests and devices to gather data not provided by standardized tests.

The data from the diagnostic testing were used to formulate individualized educational programs (IEPs) for the students. The IEPs identified the goals and objectives for remediation in reading, spelling, writing, mathematics, and related language and perceptual areas. The IEPs also included tutoring strategies and specified areas in which students needed counseling.

Advisement

Careful academic advising was important for LD college students. Swann (1982) found that students frequently enrolled in courses that were too difficult for them. He also discovered that when students felt an instructor was understanding, they enrolled in as many courses as possible with that instructor, even when the courses were out of sequence or not part of their degree programs. Similar experiences on the part of program directors led to the following set of guidelines for advising LD college students.

Consider strengths, weaknesses, and specific disabilities when planning students' programs (Bireley & Manley, 1980; Vogel, 1982). Learning-disabled students were advised not to take courses that required higher-level basic skills than the student possessed. Similarly, they were advised not to take courses where their learning disabilities would make it difficult for them to master the content and/or profit from the method of instruction. Therefore, Vogel recommended that before placing students in courses, the courses should be analyzed for difficulty level, prerequisite knowledge, and method of instruction.

Advise students to take fewer than the usual number of credits per semester (Bireley & Manley, 1980; Vogel, 1982; Vogel & Sattler, 1981; F. Leonard, personal communication, June 23, 1982; J. McGuire, personal communication, October, 1982; P. Quinlan, personal communication, July 16, 1982). Students in learning disabilities programs were advised to take reduced course loads so they would have extra time to prepare for courses and to participate in tutoring, remediation, counseling, and other program services. G. M. Webb (personal communication, July 15, 1982) advocated encouraging students to move through their degree programs at a pace appropriate for them. K. Chandler (personal communication, June 9, 1982) suggested that GPA be used as a criterion for increasing the students' course loads. She routinely told new students in her program that they would find it difficult to complete their degrees in a conventional 4-year period.

Work out a balanced course load with respect to difficulty (Bireley & Manley, 1980; Cordoni, 1980; Vogel & Sattler, 1981; F. Leonard, personal communication, June 23, 1982). Vogel and Sattler recommended examining reading, writing, and other course requirements to determine course difficulty. Once the difficulty of the courses had been determined, they recommended planning students' programs so that the difficulty factor was taken into account. For example, Bireley and Manley recommended that in a four-course load students take one difficult course, two courses of moderate difficulty, and one course of minimal difficulty.

Consider the frequency and length of class meetings (Vogel, 1982; Vogel & Sattler, 1981). Vogel observed that students with long-term memory deficits did better in courses that met several times a week than in those that met once a week. We believe that length of class meetings is also important. Students with attention deficits will find it difficult to sustain attention in classes that exceed 1 hour in length. These logistical factors should be considered when planning students' programs.

Know who is teaching the course. Program directors reported that not all faculty members had the desire and/or skills to meet the needs of LD students. It is important to consider who is teaching a course before advising students to take it.

Arrange for cooperative academic advisement. At Barat College, LD students were advised by the program director or one of the program specialists in consultation with faculty members from academic departments (S. A. Vogel, personal communication, June 16, 1982). In contrast, at the College of the Ozarks, advisement was done by academic department faculty in consultation with the program director (Ben D. Caudle, 1981). Who has primary responsibility for academic advisement of the students is not as important as ensuring that the program and academic departments work together in a facilitative manner. The program staff knows more about the student, whereas the academic faculty knows more about courses and programs of study. Both are critical for effective advisement of LD college students.

Instructional Assistance

Most learning disabilities college programs provided basic skills remediation and course tutoring for program participants. In some cases, the programs offered special courses designed to help the students adjust to and succeed in college. When appropriate, program staff members conferred with course instructors to advocate on behalf of the students.

Remediation

The focus of basic skills remediation was on reading, mathematics, and written language. Attention was also given to developing study skills and compensatory learning strategies. Sessions were often one-to-one and were usually conducted two to three times a week by trained learning disabilities specialists. In some programs, other specialists were used to provide specific assistance in reading and study skills. Economic considerations sometimes required remediation to be provided in small groups rather than with individual students. G. M. Webb (personal communication, July 16, 1982) saw this circumstance as desirable because she believed that the students benefited from group interaction. She observed that because LD students had so much individual remediation in the past, this was no longer a stimulating approach for them.

The goal of basic skills remediation was to assist the students in meeting the reading, mathematics, and written language requirements of courses they took as part of their degree program. The focus was on improving basic skills and was not on tutoring in course content. Intensive instruction was provided to fill gaps in the students' basic skills' profiles and to raise their overall achievement levels.

The students were helped to develop effective study skills and strategies that could be applied across all courses. Students were taught how to prepare study schedules, organize notes, meet course requirements, select appropriate themes for term papers, and use library resources.

Because of their disabilities in cognitive, language, and perceptual-motor areas, LD students were taught the use of compensatory learning strategies. These strategies enabled them to use their learning strengths to meet the demands of their college courses.

Tutoring

The primary goal of tutoring was to help the students get through their courses. Tutors helped students understand and master the content of subject-area courses. In most programs, the amount of tutoring LD students received varied with their ability to handle course content and requirements. R. Nash (personal communication, June 17, 1982) saw the role of tutors as reviewing course content and keeping students responsive to course requirements. K. Chandler (personal communication, June 9, 1982) viewed tutoring as the most important component of the learning disabilities college program. Her tutors attempted to "stuff" their students with the information they needed to succeed in courses. Swan (1982) noted that as the content of courses became more difficult, students became increasingly manipulative and tried to get their tutuors to do their work for them. Although some students were reluctant to engage in reme-diation activities, Vogel (1982) found students responded favorably to tutor-ing directly related to their course work.

Vogel (1982) stated that subject-area tutors must know their content area and be aware of their tutee's learning styles. She added that tutors must be accepting, supportive, and mature individuals who conduct them-selves in a professional manner. R. Nash (personal communication, June 17, 1982) observed that the relationship between tutors and tutees often became intense and required a careful matching of personalities. As he noted, the tutors often became friends and counselors to the students. Cor-doni (1980) found that having tutors attend group counseling sessions with the students improved interpersonal relationships between tutors and tutees. Cordoni (1980) included a formal tutor-training component in her program. She required tutors to meet with learning disabilities program staff on a weekly basis. Initial sessions addressed logistics and later sessions dealt with specific problems and tutuoring techniques.

Most programs used non-LD students as peer tutors. Tutoring was most effective when peer tutors had completed or were enrolled in the courses for which they served as tutors (Vogel, 1982). Because this gave the tutors first-hand experience with the courses, they were readily able to review lecture material, clarify important points, ensure that notes were complete, review study-guide questions, help students prepare for exams, and regularly review course material. However, Vogel recognized the need for the program staff to supervise peer tutors very carefully.

There were two basic sources of peer tutors. One source was students enrolled in learning disabilities teacher-training programs, and the other was students from subject-area majors. An ideal peer tutor was a student in a learning disabilities student-training program with expertise in a subject area. As S. A. Vogel (personal communication, June 16, 1982) observed, these tutors brought a double set of skills to the tutoring effort — knowledge of learning disabilities and subject matter. Tutors with these double skills did not abound.

To ensure adequate knowledge of subject matter among his tutors, Vernoy (1982) required a minimum GPA of 2.5 and at least a *B* in the courses they tutored. When peer tutors were not learning disabilities or special education majors, Cordoni (1980) suggested that they needed to be sensitized to the nature and needs of the students. R. Nash (personal communication, June 17, 1982) used juniors and seniors as tutors because he believed they were more knowledgeable, mature, and responsible than freshmen and sophomores. Most programs did not have problems obtaining peer tutors. Vernoy obtained all the tutors he needed by writing invitational letters to work-study students.

Some programs preferred to use learning-disabilities and/or subject-area teachers to tutor the students in subject-area courses. Although this tended to be a more expensive arrangement than peer tutors, it provided for more program continuity and brought a higher level of training to bear upon the problems of the students. When assisting the students, these trained professionals did not have competing responsibilities to meet their own course requirements, as did the peer tutors. For example, peer tutors frequently found it difficult to give LD students the time and assistance they required at exam time since the peer tutors also had to spend time preparing for their own exams.

Special Courses

Some learning disabilities college programs offered special courses. In some cases, these courses were offered for credit. Some colleges averaged the grades for these courses into students GPAs. The program at the College of the Ozarks offered *Fundamentals of Communication,* which taught entry-level skills for the college's freshmen composition course (D. Saddler, personal communication, July 14, 1982). All students in the program at the University of Wisconsin–Oshkosh were required to take Language Remediation (R. Nash, personal communication, June 17, 1982).

Here they learned to use the Orton-Gillingham Trimodal Simultaneous Multisensory Instructional Procedure to meet the reading and writing requirements of regular courses. At Metropolitan State College, M. Bookman and E. Dyer (personal communication, October 25, 1982) developed a series of courses in basic skills and language development. Vogel and Adelman (1981) noted that most learning disabilities programs offered an orientation/study skills course to help students adjust to the academic demands of college. These courses typically emphasized time- and stress-management and organizational skills.

Some programs offered special sections of regular courses for LD students. At Southern Illinois University the English department offered a special section of English Composition 101 for the students (Cordoni, 1980). The special section contained the standard course content, but the text and teaching style were adjusted for the learning disabilities of the students. The section was team-taught by the program staff and the English department faculty.

Advocacy

Another service provided to LD students was advocacy. Program staff members helped college instructors understand the needs of the LD students in their courses. This was difficult when instructors believed that students sometimes tried to get out of assignments and responsibilities on the basis of faked handicaps (I. Götz, personal communication, September, 1982). Once he confirmed the validity of his students' learning disabilities. Götz found that instructors were very cooperative.

Program staff members requested lists of required texts for taping, permission for LD students to tape record lectures, and opportunities for students to take tests in alternative ways. When students needed more time to complete a course, arrangements were made for an incomplete grade. When extra time was not the answer, consideration was given for allowing the students to withdraw without a grade penalty (Vogel & Adelman, 1981). Vogel (1982) found that college instructors were particularly flexible when the program advocate was also a member of the teaching faculty.

In most programs, LD students were encouraged to act as their own advocates. In these programs, staff members intervened only when students had unusual difficulties with their instructors (S. A. Vogel, personal communication, June 16, 1982; G. M. Webb, personal communication, July 15, 1982). Cordoni (1980) provided a range of options to her students. Students could (a) go to instructors on their own; (b) take a staff member along; or (c) request a staff member to go instead of them. R. Nash (personal communication, June 17, 1982) used a modeling technique in which the students observed staff members interact with instructors until the students were ready to assume the advocacy role.

When the students did not want instructors to know of their learning disabilities, the advocacy function was suppressed. F. Leonard (personal communication, June 23, 1982) found that students with mild learning disabilities preferred to remain anonymous, whereas those with more severe learning disabilities wanted instructors to be aware of their difficulties.

Instructional Aids

The reading and written-language deficits of LD college students made it difficult for them to take lecture notes, read text materials, and take tests. Frequently, the students' potential for achievement in courses was inhibited by these difficulties. Learning disabilities programs responded by providing tape recorders, notetakers, taped texts, and alternative testing procedures.

Tape Recorders

Learning-disabled students who had difficulty taking written notes during lectures were encouraged to use tape recorders. Before they used a tape recorder in their classes, the students were advised to obtain permission from their instructors. Few instructors objected to having their lectures taped. When instructors objected to the use of tape recorders, Brown (1982) recommended having students sign a form indicating that the taped lectures were only for use by the student.

P. Quinlan (personal communication, July 16, 1982) portrayed the use of tape recorders as the professor's "defense" against LD students. The use of tape recorders allowed the students to participate normally in classes and have a second chance to listen to the lectures. Vogel (1982) noted that the use of this technique provided the students with opportunities for unhurried listening, integration, organization, and coherent writing of complex ideas. I. Götz (personal communication, September, 1982) voiced concern with the time required to listen a second time to an entire lecture. Vernoy (1982) described how a steno-mask could be used to reduce this time. The steno-mask is essentially a microphone within a mask that enables one to talk into a tape recorder without being heard. This allowed the students to selectively dictate the important points as they listened to a lecture. The process is analogous to taking written notes.

Notetakers

Many programs provided notetakers for students. Most often these were non-LD students who were taking the same classes as the LD students and who were identified as good notetakers. Occasionally individuals were hired to sit in classes and take notes for students. K. Chandler (personal communication, June 9, 1982) paid non-LD students a nominal fee to take duplicate notes using carbon paper. She then had the notetakers leave the duplicate pads with her to distribute to the LD students. In this way, the LD students were able to remain anonymous. Chandler found that paying the notetakers a nominal fee encouraged them to be more active and careful notetakers. Cordoni (1980) had LD students rewrite the furnished notes in their own words to ensure that they understood the content.

Where programs did not provide notetakers, the LD students were encouraged to ask fellow students for copies of their notes. The National Technical Institute for the Deaf[1] produces a special notetaking pad that facilitates making duplicate copies. Vernoy (1982) recommended that LD students offer to pay for all paper used by fellow students who agreed to share notes.

Taped Textbooks

To facilitate textbook reading, LD students were provided with audio-taped textbooks. Learning disabilities programs had textbooks used by their students taped by Recordings for the Blind.[2] Because the taping process took several months, programs had to obtain textbooks to be taped far in advance of the beginning of a semester. G. M. Webb (personal communication, July 15, 1982) automatically had all textbooks used in freshman and sophomore classes at Curry College taped. Programs established audio libraries from which students checked out books or specific chapters of books. When students required books that had not been previously taped, programs taped them using their own equipment and personnel.

Not all LD students used taped testbooks (I. Götz, personal communication, September, 1982). Some students did not need them and others did not like to use them. Others found taped textbooks difficult to use because of the requirements made on auditory memory and listening comprehension skills. For these students, it was helpful to have a program staff member summarize on tape the important information from textbooks. Vogel (1982) suggested that students be taught ways to enhance their comprehension and retention of taped materials.

Alternative Test Procedures

All learning disabilities college programs the authors examined made arrangements for their students to take tests in alternative ways when necessary.

---

[1] Available from the Bookstore, Rochester Institute of Technology, 1 Lomb Memorial Drive, Rochester, NY 14623.
[2] Recordings for the Blind, Inc., 215 E. 58th Street, New York, NY 10002.

These alternatives included untimed tests, oral tests, take-home tests, objective tests instead of essays or vice versa, and special projects. Students were also allowed to type or tape their answers to test questions. Proctors sometimes read tests to the students, clarified or rephrased questions, defined words, and/or wrote the students' dictated responses. Typically, instructors sent their tests to the learning disabilities program and the tests were administered there. To ease the concern of leery instructors, some program directors even agreed to supervise the testing personally at whatever site the instructors preferred.

Counseling

Learning disabilities programs provided a variety of counseling services. The most common were individual counseling, group counseling, and informal rap sessions. The major counseling goal was to reduce the students' anxiety associated with the demands of college life. Swan (1982) identified three additional goals: building self-confidence, promoting socialization, and teaching life skills such as goal-setting and time- and stress-management. Barbaro (1982) suggested the counseling goals of helping students to become assertive, to clarify their values and attitudes, and to develop trust in others.

Counseling sessions were usually held once a week. This allowed program personnel to assess students' needs on an ongoing basis and use the counseling sessions to provide timely corrective actions.

Group sessions were particularly effective because of the mutual support they fostered. Swan (1982) observed that group counseling encouraged students to share successful adaptive techniques. Cordoni (1982b) reported that rap sessions were often the first opportunity LD students ever had to talk to other LD individuals about their problems and feelings. Students talked about problems they had in common, such as dealing with the effects of medication and the pressure of having no free time. The sessions were useful for helping the students better understand their own problems.

Few specific guidelines exist for providing counseling services to LD college students. Miller, McKinley, and Ryan (1979) proposed a four-step communication-interaction model. The four steps are (a) interact with students to assess their perceptions of immediate problems; (b) focus on problems students encounter in their courses; (c) help students understand their disabilities; and (d) develop plans for solving the problems. Miller et al. believed that as anxiety and tensions were reduced, academic performance would improve, and this would lead to a more positive self-concept. Brown (1982) provided additional strategies for counseling LD college students.

Learning-disabled college students require a wide range of program services to succeed in college. The services begin with careful diagnostic testing and prescriptive planning. Based on IEPs, LD college students are given program advisement, instructional assistance, and counseling. They are also taught how to use a variety of instructional aids. These services represent the core of learning disabilities college programs. It is essential that these program services be provided by dedicated and competent personnel who follow the strategies and techniques to be successful with LD college students.

RECOMMENDATIONS FOR HIGH SCHOOLS

Directors of learning disabilities college programs told us that students entering their programs were poorly prepared to meet the demands of college. Learning-disabled students graduated from high school with an insufficient background for college in English, math, science, and social studies. They lacked study skills, and deficits remained in reading, writing, spelling, and spoken language. All this was compounded by their lack of understanding of their learning disabilities.

In this section, we offer recommendations to help high schools prepare LD students for the college experience. These recommendations, if implemented, will help LD high school students profit from a learning disabilities college program and function in college without any special assistance at an earlier date.

Recommendations for Counseling

High schools must provide counseling as a normal part of their services to all LD students. Learning-disabled students with college aspirations should be counseled regarding their potential for college. Those with college potential should be given information on college programs and assisted in selecting and gaining admission to specific colleges.

High school counseling can help LD students to realistically assess their potential for college. It is important to determine if an LD student has the ability for college studies. Sometimes as a result of success experienced in high school learning disabilities programs, students develop inflated perceptions of their cognitive ability. As a result, they may erroneously believe they can succeed in college. High school counselors must help the students to compare their abilities to the abilities of non-LD college-bound high school students. As a result of this comparison, LD students will be able to make realistic decisions as to whether or not they should pursue a college education.

Counselors should provide information on learning disabilities college programs. Information on learning disabilities college programs is not readily available. Most high school counselors are unaware of the few directories that identify colleges with such programs. These high school counselors need to obtain copies of these directories and become familiar with the nature and location of the college programs. They should contact program directors to learn what the programs can offer the high school LD students with whom they work. Finally, they must share the information with the students and their parents/guardians.

High school counselors should help students and their parents or guardians select learning disabilities college programs. K. Chandler (personal communication, June 9, 1982) noted that parents must be very careful when selecting programs for their college-bound children. She cautioned that although some colleges provide programs designed to help LD students, others suggested they did, but actually provided very little more than the services available to all college students. It is important that LD students and their parents verify that programs claiming to meet the needs of these students actually do so. Our examination of the services offered by comprehensive learning disabilities college programs leads us to believe that the following questions should be used for this verification: (a) Is diagnostic testing used to generate an individualized educational program for providing services?; (b) Is the program staff trained to work with LD students?; (c) Do college faculty members support the efforts of the program? How?; (d) Does the program provide for remediation of deficits in reading, writing, spelling, and mathematics?; (e) Does the program provide tutuors to assist students in mastering the content of their college courses?; (f) Does the program provide taped textbooks?; (g) Are provisions made for notetakers or for taking class notes using tape recorders?; (h) Can arrangements be made to take course examinations in alternative ways?; and (i) Is individual or group counseling available?

Students should be encouraged to apply to college early. Learning-disabled students need to begin thinking about college in their sophomore year of high school. Most learning disabilities college programs admit qualified students on a first come, first served basis. The admission process takes considerable time; consequently, if students wait too long, they are apt to find themselves at the end of a very long waiting list. Program directors suggested that students make formal application to these college programs during their junior year. High school counselors must encourage students to apply early, help them gather information, and complete application forms.

High school counselors should prepare students for the college admissions interview. An important part of the admission procedure for learning disabilities college programs is a personal interview. Learning-disabled students have very little experience participating in interviews. As a result, there is a danger that they will not present themselves in a representative manner. To assist these students in accurately portraying themselves, high school personnel can conduct mock interviews with the students, asking the types of questions they are likely to experience during an admission interview. From the authors' discussions with learning disabilities college program directors (K. Chandler, personal communication, June 9, 1982; R. Nash, personal communication, June 17, 1982; P. Quinlan, personal communication, July 16, 1982; D. Saddler, personal communication, July 14, 1982; S. A. Vogel, personal communication, June 16, 1982; G. M. Webb, personal communication, July 15, 1982), and an analysis of application forms (Application for Admission, undated; Barat College, undated; Project Achieve, undated), the authors have identified questions that might be asked during an interview: Why do you want to attend college? What do your parents think about your going to college? What would you like to major in? What are your plans after college? What kind of a person are you? What kind of learning disability do you have? How does your learning disability affect you? What are your academic strengths and weaknesses? What kinds of things are easy for you to learn? Which are difficult? What things have helped you to learn in the past? What help do you need from our program to make it in college? Are you prepared to spend extra time and effort to make it in college?

Recommendations for Instruction

Most non-LD students entering college have the basic content-area information, study skills, and learning strategies to be successful. Program directors told the authors this is not true for LD students entering their programs. The following suggestions should help high school personnel deliver more effective instruction to LD college-bound students.

Provide content-area instruction by specialists. In some cases, LD high school students receive content-area instruction from learning disabilities teachers who are not certified or trained in specific content areas. This staffing pattern reduces both in quantity and quality the information to which LD high school students are exposed in important areas such as social studies, science, English, and mathematics. It is important that college-bound LD students receive their content-area instruction from teachers who are trained specialists and interested in meeting their special needs.

Provide college-type assignments. College-bound LD high school students need experience with assignments similar to those they will encounter in college. It is important that they be required to do such things as write research or term papers, present oral reports, read novels, prepare book reviews, and complete other independent assignments. It is unrealistic to expect that these students will be able to do such things in college without extensive instruction and practice while in high school.

Prepare LD students to function independently. As college-bound LD students progress through high school, they must be given increasing responsibility for meeting requirements and resolving problems on their own. Many learning disabilities college program directors reported that their students were overly dependent on program staff as a result of a history of excessive assistance from teachers, parents, and/or siblings. This was often exacerbated by overly structured and supportive high school learning disabilities programs. S. A. Vogel (personal communication, June 16, 1982) stated that the most impressive learning disabilities college program applicants were those who demonstrated that they had taken responsibility for their own lives by requesting application forms, writing letters, and making phone calls.

Many LD college-bound students have a difficult time reading textbooks. They can be helped to develop this crucial college skill by learning to use textbook reading strategies. Robinson (1974) suggested the use of the SQ3R study strategy for reading social science text material, and Spache (1963) recommended the PQRST study strategy for reading physical science text materials. These and similar strategies will help LD students achieve higher levels of comprehension and retention.

Teach graphics skills. College texts contain many graphs, tables, charts, diagrams, flow charts, and maps. These graphic aids are used by textbook authors to explain facts and trends more simply than can be done with text discourse. High school teachers need to ensure that LD college-bound students possess the necessary skills to use and understand the graphic material in their textbooks.

Teach study skills. Success in college requires that students have highly developed study skills. College-bound LD students must be taught how to take notes efficiently and accurately from lectures and textbooks. They must also be taught how to prepare outlines, write reports, proofread, and memorize facts.

Teach how to organize for learning. Directors of learning disabilities college programs frequently indicated that students did not know how to handle their unscheduled time. High school teachers must show college-bound LD students how to prepare schedules that allow time for both studying and fun. These students also need to be shown how to arrange their home and school study areas for maximum on-task behavior. They should be shown the value of working with study partners as a strategy for monitoring and completing assignments.

Teach the use of instructional aids. Learning disabilities college programs typically provide a variety of instructional aids to help students compensate for their learning difficulties. Students can make better use of these instructional aids in college if they are exposed to them in high school. Therefore, college-bound LD students should be taught to use tape recorders to record lecture notes, taped textbooks to assist them with reading assignments, and typewriters to facilitate their performance with written assignments.

Teach how to prepare for and take tests. Most college courses include quizzes and examinations in a variety of forms. College-bound LD students need to be taught how to organize and study for quizzes, midterms, and final examinations. They must also be taught how to take multiple choice, essay, and cloze-type tests, since these are the most common forms of tests used by college instructors. (In cloze-type tests, every fifth, seventh, or ninth word is deleted in the printed discourse; the student must fill in the blanks.)

SUMMARY

College learning disabilities programs assist students to earn degrees in their chosen fields of study. Learning-disabled students arrive on college campuses with many skill and knowledge deficiencies. To the extent that high school programs can reduce these deficiencies and build awareness of what college is like, learning disabilities college programs will achieve their goal with more students. Recommendations were provided for counseling and instructing LD college-bound students in the high school setting. Efforts of this nature will contribute heavily to the continued growth, development, and success of college learning disabilities programs.

CHAPTER 10

Adult Outcomes

W hen faced with a diagnosis of learning disability for their child, parents frequently ask about the child's future. Although information can be provided about the short-term consequences of learning disabilities (placement options, remedial methods, auxillary services, and the like), it is difficult to answer questions about long-term consequences. The situation reflects the lack of knowledge about the outcome of the condition and about the factors affecting the prognosis for individual children. These concerns about the natural history of learning disabilities are of more than theoretical interest since they reflect directly on the validity and effectiveness of treatment programs. Furthermore, examination of the natural history of LD provides insight into whether or not observed changes are due to treatment effects or maturation. Long-term assessments, in addition to providing information about treatment efficacy, also provide insights into the extent to which the consequences of LD may be attenuated or accentuated by associated factors.

It is surprising that the natural history of learning disabilities has been so poorly described. Learning disabilities as a diagnostic entity emerged not much over two decades ago, but has become the category containing by far the most children receiving special education. More than two in five disabled children are considered LD (USDE, 1987), which is more than 4% of all school-age children. The number of children identified as learning disabled has increased more than 100% since federal legislation (PL 94-142) mandating special education first took effect. This rapid growth has been a source of consternation since LD is the category most open to vague diagnostic interpretation and most likely to contain children who do not require special services. The problems are, at least, partially attributable to inconsistencies surrounding definition, etiology, and treatment (see Kavale & Forness, 1985) and to the lack of information about LD's natural history. The need for follow-up research has long been acknowledged (Bateman, 1966). Recently, there has been increased emphasis on LD at the secondary level (Deshler, 1978), but a significant gap in understanding the long term consequences of learning disabilities remains (Cronin & Gerber, 1982).

LONGITUDINAL RESEARCH

Long-term follow-up studies of LD do exist, but they come from diverse sources that differ markedly in their purposes, methodologies, and populations. For example, Robins (1977, 1979) discussed the common methodological problems found in follow-up studies. Conflicting findings appear to be the result of (1) failure to define precisely the sample included in the study; (2) failure to provide a control group for legitimate comparisons; (3) failure to control for attrition; (4) failure to provide sufficient data in the original assessment, which prevents systematic comparison; (5) failure to provide consistent data across subjects by relying on whatever data is available; (6) failure to provide equivalent data at different assessment points; and (7) failure to predict adult outcomes for individual children rather than for a group of children. The diversity and methodological difficulties make it difficult to arrive at an integrated picture of outcomes. This leads to widely variant claims about the ultimate fate of the LD child, including the possibility of (1) having persistent academic problems, (2) dropping out of school, (3) developing emotional problems, (4) becoming delinquent, and (5) being in lower socioeconomic occupations. However, these findings have all been challenged; no consensus exists regarding the long-term consequences of learning disabilities. Many findings are marked by enough equivocation to render them tentative, at best.

The many and varied findings appear to be related to the nature of longitudinal research. The diversity seems to be related to methodological variables and the difficult pragmatic demands in conducting long-term studies. Because of the relative recency of the identification of learning disabilities, its course is still being chronicled. This is generally accomplished first by case histories. Although interesting, case studies usually lack the rigor necessary to generalize findings. Individual case studies are typically followed by more systematic research designs found in either retrospective studies or, less common, prospective studies. The latter two designs can be differentiated by the time at which the child becomes a subject. Retrospective studies diagnose children as LD after the fact, and then assess these children and (usually) a control group to determine how the LD group differs. Prospective designs identify LD subjects in early childhood and study subsequent behaviors as they occur. Again, a control group is generally used and may be either a comparison group of non-LD children or the LD sample as its own control, comparing subsequent status with baseline data. Prospective studies are difficult to design and to implement, so their numbers are small. Retrospective studies are more numerous but, when compared to prospective designs, possess a variety of problems that limit interpretation.

Early Studies

Learning disabilities was established as a major category of special education during the 1960s. The 1970s saw the first appearance of follow-up literature with LD children as subjects. Hinton and Knights (1971), in a 3-year follow-up of 67 LD children, found a consistent pattern; early failure was highly related to later academic difficulties. In fact, Wide Range Achievement Test (WRAT) scores for reading, spelling, and arithmetic were correlated about .60 between diagnosis and outcome assessment. This finding was later verified by Ackerman, Dykman, and Peters (1977a) who followed 93 LD boys classified in grade school to age 14. The LD group remained seriously deficient in reading, spelling, and arithmetic when compared to non-LD achievers. The LD students who had the poorest outcomes at follow-up were those who had the most severe early reading problems and who scored poorly in the information, arithmetic, digit span, and coding subtests of the Wechsler Intelligence Scale for Children (WISC). The later achievement levels of the LD group were independent of both earlier classification by activity level and neurological maturity.

Koppitz (1971) conducted a 5-year follow-up study of 177 LD children aged 6 to 12 years. Most subjects had been experiencing school difficulty since kindergarten. Information was attained about school district, sex, age, IQ, visual-motor perception, academic levels, behavior, developmental and medical history, and social background. For the sample studied (1) the ratio of boys to girls was 6:1, (2) subjects had a mean IQ of 92, (3) 77% had visual-motor perceptual difficulties, (4) a majority showed behavior problems (which had been the major reason for referral to special class), (5) 84% were from unstable home environments, (6) 45% had mild behavioral disorders, and (7) 97% were hyperactive. At the end of 5 years, 40% remained in special classes, 15% had been referred for hospital or residential programs because of autism or psychosis, 24% had returned to regular classes, and 3% transferred to other special classes for the deaf or educable mentally retarded. The remaining 18% had either been withdrawn by their parents or moved.

It was found that among those returned to regular classes, success was more contingent upon behavior than achievement (although their reading levels were better from the beginning and their mean IQ was 98 versus 87 for those remaining in LD classes). Age appeared significant: the younger the LD subject, the more impaired and the longer special services were required. It was also noted that better progress was made if the LD child's deficit was restricted to a single area. For example, a child with only impaired visual-motor difficulties was able to better compensate for the problem and show better progress. An LD child, however, with both visual-motor and auditory-perceptual deficits (or any other combination of deficits) usually exhibited a more severe learning disability and exhibited little gain, if any. In fact, the LD sample as a whole displayed little improvement in academic achievement; the average gain was only 3–5 months for each year spent in the special class. Koppitz (1971) suggested that many reported gains were spurious and that academic progress typically levels off. Therefore, LD pupils require not just 1 or 2 years of remediation, but rather long-term remedial efforts. Additionally, it was suggested that the value of intervention programs may be in improving self-concept and instilling more positive attitudes.

The Koppitz (1971) study, although widely cited, possessed difficulties, especially in sampling, that limit conclusions. The lack of a control group, of course, is a problem since no comparisons can be made. The criteria used for sample selection, however, do not seem to discriminate LD children from other conditions, as evidenced by the inclusion of subjects who later became psychotic, mentally retarded, deaf, or required other special placement. Furthermore, the initial population may have included many subjects with behavioral disorders since a large majority were referred for behavior difficulties, came from unstable home environments, and were placed outside their school districts. Consequently, it is questionable whether this study included a "typical" LD population (even given the difficulties in defining what that might be). The characteristics and findings attributed to this sample may be unique and not applicable to the LD population at large.

Gottesman (1978, 1979) followed 43 LD children, who were referred initially between ages 7 and 14 years, for a period of 5 to 7 years. Over half the sample received special help after evaluation, or were referred to special classes or to special schools for LD children. When their reading achievement was assessed at follow-up, the LD sample, as a group, showed very small gains; they progressed, on average, at the rate of 4 months per year. The students in special education placements were more likely to have lower IQ levels and to score lower on the achievement outcome assessment. Again, these findings must be approached with caution because of possible sampling difficulties. As a group, the selected sample revealed a higher incidence of neurological, psychiatric, and language disabilities. Additionally, their mean IQ level (88) fell within the low-average range.

Although reading achievement appears to be a major disability area for the LD child, several follow-up studies reported generally favorable outcomes. Abbott and Frank (1975) studied the outcome for 139 LD students who had formerly attended a private school but who had since returned to regular class placement. Of the 139 LD students, about 75% were rated as making satisfactory progress, with about the same percentage showing improved social and emotional status. It should be noted, however, that 50% required psychological counseling after leaving the special school.

In a 10-year follow-up, Edgington (1975) found that, of 25 LD children, 22 were still enrolled in school or had since graduated and 3 had dropped out (2 were working full time and 1 was planning to re-enroll). Five students had not repeated a grade during their school history whereas 19 had repeated a grade prior to or concurrent with enrollment in a special program. Only one student had repeated a grade after enrollment in the special program. It was concluded that high-school-age LD children are "rather indistinguishable from regular students in so far as successful completion of secondary school is concerned" (Edgington, 1975, p. 60). Although these findings are positive, they must be approached with caution because of the large attrition rate. The original group consisted of 47 LD subjects, but follow-up data were gathered on only 25, which represents a self-selected group. Conceivably, the other 22 subjects might present a different outcome picture.

A positive tone was also found in a follow-up study reported by Lehtinen-Rogan and Hartman (1976), who assessed the adult attainments of 91 LD individuals who had received special education for an average of 3 years between the ages of 6 and 13. They found that 69% graduated from high school, 36% completed college, and 8% either completed or were pursuing graduate study. About 70% were employed, with the following breakdown: professional (13%), clerical (33%), unskilled (23%), and the remainder (31%) in other employment categories. Approximately 55% were independent of parental supervision. Only 6% showed evidence of delinquency. All IQs were in the average range, but achievement levels were still depressed, with mean grade scores of 10.4 in reading, 8.4 in spelling, and 6.7 in arithmetic. Although these are positive outcomes, almost 75% of the group reported some therapeutic or counseling experience. Personality testing showed them to be particularly vulnerable to stress, to possess low self-esteem, to be highly sensitive, and to be unable to form close interpersonal relationships. These were seen as the hidden handicaps of LD, but were partially off-set by a strong motivation toward academic achievement and productive work. Although positive, the findings should be approached with some caution given the possible sampling bias caused by the selection of a private school population where families were supportive and sought remedial services.

In summary, a review of early longitudinal studies produced the following conclusions. Learning disability is a persistent problem that adversely affects both academic and behavioral functioning and is highly related to early school failure. Studies appeared to show a relationship with age; the younger the LD child, the more severe the disability and the more likely remediation will be required over a longer period. Better progress is made by an LD child with a deficit in only one area (as opposed to multiple deficits), and better outcomes are associated with greater gains in behavioral functioning, although academic remediation is also important. A child with a learning disability is likely to need long-term services, even after specific remedial efforts cease, but generalizations are difficult given the heterogeneous nature of the LD samples used.

Later Studies

Generally favorable outcomes have been reported in later investigations. For example, White, Schumaker, Warner, Alley, and Deshler (1980), in a retrospective study comparing young adults diagnosed as LD during their elementary school years with a group not labeled LD, found a relatively small number of differences. Members of both groups were holding approximately the same number of full-time jobs and were earning about the same amount of money. Members of both groups had a number of friends and had frequent contact with parents and relatives. Generally, the LD group appeared to be adjusting as well as the non-LD group. There were, however, several differences. In the area of vocational adjustment, the LD young adults were holding jobs with less social status and were less satisfied with their employment situation. Socially, the groups differed primarily with respect to degree of involvement in recreational and social activities.

Similarly, Fafard and Haubrich (1981) found that unemployment was not a problem at follow-up for 21 young adults who had received LD services. Most had graduated from high school and were involved in a variety of social relationships. However, most still had residual reading disabilities and the vocational area was marked by concern and frustration. Fafard and Haubrich concluded that an important component of LD programming is vocational education. Motivation was not the problem, but assistance was needed in determining how to get a job, identifying the types of available jobs, and understanding what constitutes economic independence. These findings suggest a cautious optimism, but also a cause for concern, as suggested by White et al. (1980):

Although LD young adults are "making it" in a number of important areas, they seem to be much less satisfied with at least some areas of their lives. Personally, this can be related, in part, to the way in which past experiences have shaped their present attitudes and values, the difference between their expectations for adult life and what they have encountered, or a combination of these. In any case, the schools have neither adequately prepared the LD young adults for the social/affective facets of adult life nor taught them what to expect when they leave school. (p. 17-18)

In a 10-year retrospective study, Major-Kingsley (1982) attempted to analyze the achievement, adjustment, and aspirations of 40 LD boys as young adults. By the age of 12, most LD subjects recognized that they had learning problems, evidenced by academic difficulties, especially in reading. In many cases, they reported feeling frustrated, depressed, hostile, inferior, alienated, and discouraged by their school difficulties. The LD group, when compared to a non-LD comparison group, was far more likely to have received special education services. However, nearly 80% felt that they continued to have a learning problem. These problems were described as primarily in reading, math, and writing. Most felt uneasy about their current reading ability (average reading score at ninth grade level) and tended to avoid situations that required reading. About 25% continued to experience feelings of low self-esteem, inadequacy, or frustration. Despite the persistence of some academic difficulties, very few LD boys dropped out of school prior to high school graduation and more than half planned to complete college. (Similar positive achievement findings were reported by Leone, Lovitt, and Hansen, 1981, in a follow-up of 10 LD boys 5-6 years after enrollment in an LD program.) It was found that initial reading deficits (average 2 years below grade level in fourth and fifth grades) did not prevent the LD group from being successful in high school. When compared to a control group, few differences were noted on general measures of high school performance (grade point average, attendance, class rank). The free-time activities and occupational interests of both groups were also similar. As found in previous follow-up reports (e.g., Fafard & Haubrich, 1981; White et al., 1980), Major-Kingsley (1982) concluded that, "The overwhelming impression from this study is that individuals with learning disabilities in childhood function in young adulthood in much the same way as do individuals who achieve adequately in school during childhood" (p. 116). Few differences between groups were found in either vocational or personal-social outcomes. Although generally setting lower educational and vocational goals than the non-LD group, the LD group, when considering the severity of their learning problems in childhood, was judged to have done remarkably well.

Positive conclusions were also drawn by Cobb and Crump (1984) in a retrospective follow-up of 100 young adults born before 1964 who were classified as LD. That total sample included 25 identified as LD but not placed in an LD program and 75 identified and placed in an LD program. Although the placed and nonplaced groups differed relatively little on outcome measures, the placed group had poorer grades and seemed to evidence poorer coping skills. However, as a group, the total sample appeared to be functioning reasonably well as adults. About 85% were employed and a majority graduated from high school, with many obtaining postsecondary training and education. A wide variety of jobs were represented, but a majority were in the skilled and semi-skilled areas. Reported incomes were generally low (averaging $10,000 per year), but interviews revealed the sample was generally satisfied with their vocational choices. A majority reported that they no longer experienced reading problems, although about 5% revealed that reading continued to be a source of difficulty. Although the LD students rated their regular class placement as beneficial, they were much more positive about LD classes and, especially, vocational education. In summary, Cobb and Crump concluded that, "The overall impression presented by the data is that these persons are fulfilling their adult roles quite well; they are, by and large, decent, productive citizens" (p. 143–144).

Levin, Zigmond, and Birch (1985) reported results of a 4-year follow-up of 52 LD adolescents who entered a special education program in the ninth grade. At follow-up, the group should have been in the 12th grade; but 16 were still enrolled in a special education program, 7 were in a regular class, and 24 had stopped attending high school (5 could not be located). Academic skills were assessed in 34 students (all those in school, plus 11 dropouts). Although school status was below expectation, academic gains over the 4-year period were impressive. Reading gains averaged about 2 years and math gains averaged about 1 year. Further analyses, however, showed that about half of the achievement growth had taken place during the ninth grade, with the remaining half spread over the following 3 years. Thus, after an initial spurt of academic growth, achievement tended to level off. Interviews with the 11 dropouts found that only 4 felt the decision to leave school had been their own. The remainder reported that they had been encouraged to leave school because of persistent academic and behavior problems.

In summary, a review of later longitudinal studies produced the following conclusions:

1. There tended to be an initial spurt of academic gain after remediation, which leveled off over time.
2. Most LD subjects possessed residual academic difficulties as young adults but appeared to be well-adjusted.
3. The LD group did not have a higher drop-out rate, and most members expressed a desire to attend college.

4. In terms of vocational adjustment, LD individuals possessed jobs with less social status and appeared less satisfied with their employment than non-LD individuals.
5. Considering the severity of their initial disabilities, most LD subjects appeared to be doing well, although most felt uneasy about their reading ability and avoided situations that required reading.
6. Most LD subjects, although finding the regular class beneficial, reported that LD classes and vocational education were especially beneficial.

Efficacy Studies

The LD follow-up literature has focused on treatment approaches and assessed treatment efficacy. A large proportion of LD remedial services were delivered in a mainstream situation with resource room programming. For example, the positive findings reported by Edgington (1975) were based on a resource room model where daily attendance ranged from 25 to 90 minutes and small group instruction was scheduled throughout the school day. Weiner (1969) evaluated the effectiveness of a resource room for 72 LD children. Results indicated significant growth in reading, spelling, and arithmetic over a 10-month period. Similarly, Sabatino (1971) investigated the use of a resource room as an alternative to the special class for 114 LD children. Resource room programming, especially for students who attended daily, was found superior to either biweekly resource programming, the regular class, or the special class. Other efficacy studies (Pepe, 1974; Sindelar & Deno, 1978) have also shown the effectiveness of the resource room in increasing academic achievement and appropriate behaviors. These studies suffer from a short follow-up period, which suggests caution in interpretation because of the possibility that the results may be due more to novelty effects than to any program variables (see Silberberg & Silberberg, 1969).

Bloomer (1978) reported the results of a 6-year follow-up of 163 LD children in grades 4 through 10 who were enrolled in a resource room. Bloomer concluded that the resource room was an effective alternative special education service. The mean rate of gain in both reading and arithmetic was significantly greater than the rate of gain in the regular classroom after treatment. There was also a relationship with length of treatment: the greater the gain, the shorter the period of resource programming. Additionally, benefits from the resource room were associated with less severe learning disabilities, higher IQ level, and more perceptual integrity. It was found that the first year in the resource room was most important in terms of later status. Students who did best later, achieved at a rate of 1-month of gain for every month of treatment during the initial year. Nevertheless, the average reading gain during the first year back in the regular classroom revealed a regression in reading achievement.

This result was supported by Ito (1980, 1981), who found that, although resource room programming was effective for increasing reading rates of LD children, the increased rates were not maintained in the regular classroom. Herr (1976) studied the effects of mainstreaming on the academic achievement of seven LD children and concluded that, "mainstreaming had a serious detrimental effect on the academic achievement of six of the seven subjects. Although these subjects made significant gains during their enrollment at the Easter Seal Learning Center, they made no significant academic gains in the three years in public school and in some instances the data show that individual subjects lost ground on one or two of the WRAT subtests" (p. 27). Similarly, Ritter (1978) found, that although gains in reading and arithmetic made by 20 LD subjects in a learning disabilities program were maintained during the mainstreamed year, there was a significant decrease in gains for spelling. Ritter concluded that regular classroom instruction alone may not be sufficient for LD children, and supplemental programming seems necessary if prior learning rates are to be maintained. Ito (1980, 1981) suggested the following possibilities for supplemental programming: systematic fading of resource room services; follow-up services by the resource room teacher during the year following resource room placement; training regular classroom teachers to work more effectively with the returning LD child; and continued support of former resource room children through the itinerant/consultant teacher model.

Besides evaluating the resource room, the LD follow-up literature has also evaluated other intervention programs. One option was the special class and program. Foster (1972), for example,followed 33 LD students between 5 and 10 years after enrollment in a perceptual development program. About 67% had attained a level of functional literacy and 30% were reading at or above their expectancy level. About 33% continued to experience reading problems. On the social side, the results were positive and most subjects showed significant school involvement. Generally, the students held realistic perceptions of their abilities and possessed appropriate levels of aspiration.

Gershman (1976) followed 295 LD students originally enrolled in a perceptual development program in 1971. By 1975, about 50% were in regular classes. Most appeared to be coping adequately in the regular class but generally remained in the bottom third of the class. They were rated, however, as similar to students of the same age and sex by teachers.

A self-contained special class for LD was evaluated by Winter and Wright (1983) in a 5-year follow-up of the progress of 255 LD students. Significant gains were noted in reading, spelling, and arithmetic. Teachers noted that individualization was an integral part of their programs. Positive changes in reading were related to teaching methods that emphasized motor development and perceptual activities.

Precision teaching (Beck, 1977), structured phonetic and multisensory interventions (Mitchell, 1981), and team teaching (Schwartz, 1977) have also been effective in producing remedial gains. With the exception of precision teaching, however, the remedial gains tended to "wash out" over time, and LD students generally continued to experience some academic difficulties. To prevent this regression in achievement, Silver, Hagin, and Beecher (1981) described an interdisciplinary school-based preventive program for LD students (TEACH). Results from both 2- and 5-year follow-up studies suggested that academic and behavioral gains can be sustained over the long-term with a program for secondary prevention, so that former LD students become indistinguishable from their "normal" peers.

In a comprehensive longitudinal analyses, McKinney and colleagues (McKinney & Feagans, 1984; McKinney & Kreuger, 1974; McKinney & Speece, 1983) attempted to follow identified LD children over the early elementary school years. In Project MELD (Models for Educating the Learning Disabled), McKinney and Kreuger (1974) reported follow-up data on 97 LD children and found that Project MELD had a significant impact on both academic and social competence. The models offered two alternatives: a deficit model that emphasized remediation of specific weaknesses through one-to-one instruction by a resource teacher and an eclectic model that emphasized teacher consultation and attempted to build on strengths as well as remediate weaknesses. Follow-up data, however, indicated that during the second year the LD group failed to progress academically at the same rate. Thus, again there is an indication of a slowing of achievement gain and the necessity of continued support if the LD child is to maintain the same rate of gain.

McKinney and Speece (1983) followed 43 LD students who were identified in grades 1-3 during their second year of special education service. Teachers completed a behavior inventory on the 43 LD students, who were found to exhibit the same pattern of classroom behavior reported previously (Feagans & McKinney, 1981). Generally, teachers rated LD students as deficient in behaviors that reflected academic competence (i.e., task-orientation, independence, verbal expression) as opposed to those reflecting social adjustment, which also showed a consistency across time (McKinney, McClure, & Feagans, 1982). Findings from the Schedule of Classroom Activity Norms (SCAN) showed some consistency over time, as evidenced by results showing that LD children interacted with teachers more often than classmates. LD students were shown to exhibit a relatively stable pattern of classroom behavior that distinguishes them from average students. It appears that task-oriented behavior, independent functioning, and socially appropriate behavior are important elements in understanding the achievement difficulties of the LD child.

In a 3-year follow-up, McKinney and Feagans (1984), using teacher rating scales, a classroom observational system (SCAN), and achievement tests, found that LD children fall progressively further behind their normal peers in reading comprehension. In math, the LD group remained about the same distance behind their peers. The LD group exhibited more off-task and less on-task behavior, which suggests their classroom patterns were less efficient than normal peers in optimizing the learning situation (McKinney, Mason, Perkerson & Clifford, 1975). Thus, LD children do fall progressively further behind their peers, despite intervention aimed at making them approximate the academic status of their normally achieving peers. Although the behavior of the LD group improved over time, this improvement was matched by the normal comparison group. The LD students continued to exhibit the same maladaptive behaviors, particularly distractible, impulsive, and dependent/aggressive behaviors, in year 3 as they did in year 1.

These findings suggest caution in interpreting the earlier, more optimistic findings. In fact, it appears that LD symptoms, particularly in academic and behavioral areas, are longstanding and possibly not as amenable to treatment as previously believed. The differences may be related to sampling differences. The McKinney group carefully selected their LD sample by specifying identification criteria in advance and assessing the extent to which the sample met those criteria. Consequently, this LD group probably does include a large portion of children who do manifest primary symptoms of reading disorders and hyperactivity among the constellation of factors contributing to their learning disabilities.

Prospective Studies

Prospective reports provide support for a more tempered view of the long-term outcomes of learning disabilities. The Kauai Longitudinal Study (Werner, Blerman & French, 1971; Werner & Smith, 1977, 1979, 1982) suggested that the long-term detrimental consequences of learning disabilities may be more debilitating in adulthood than other forms of exceptionality. The study followed a large cohort of births which were scored on a 4-point scale for severity of perinatal complications. By age 10, 3% of the sample had been diagnosed as LD because of severe reading and language problems (despite average or above-average WISC IQs), visual-motor impairment, hyperactivity, and difficulty in attention and concentration (Werner, Simonian, & Smith, 1967). Members of the LD group, at age 1, were rated by their mothers as "not cuddly," "not affectionate," "not good-natured," and "fretful." At 2 years, psychologists rated the LD group as "awkward," "distractible," "fearful," "insecure," "restless," and "withdrawn." Additionally, IQ differences were found and developmental ratings placed them "below normal." When evaluated at age 18, the LD group was still underachieving in reading, writing, and language. The persistent academic difficulties were accompainied by behavioral difficulties (e.g., school misbehavior, frequent absences, delinquent behavior). A majority of the LD group members exhibited an external locus of control (i.e., lack of faith in the effectiveness of one's own actions) that prevented them from using their intellectual resources in scholastic achievement and influencing positive change in coping behavior. The LD group revealed persistent and chronic deficits across two decades that did not seem to be affected significantly by either short- or long-term service, especially when based on strong biological and temperamental underpinnings.

In another prospective study based on a total cohort of 30,000, Nichols and Chen (1981) followed a subgroup of 2,476 children classified as LD based on behavioral, cognitive, perceptual-motor, academic, and neurological identification variables during 7-year follow-up examinations. A factor, analytic study identified learning disabilities as a factor and sample selection was based on variable scores falling in the extreme 8% of the distribution. These factor scores were then associated with more than 300 antecedent variables including socioeconomic studies and maternal, pregnancy, delivery, neonatal, infancy, preschool, and medical histories. These were all determined prospectively, whereas some measures of physical and neurological status were determined concomitantly.

Analysis revealed that learning disabilities were stongly related to socioeconomic status, and demographic variables, particularly large family size, low socioeconomic status, and frequent residence changes. Most of the 62 variables related to pregnancy, labor, and delivery periods were not significant except for hospitalizations and low blood pressure during pregnancy. Two infancy discriminators of the LD group were small size at 1 year and an "unkempt" appearance at 8 months (independent of socioeconomic status). Additionally, 1-minute Apgar score, Bayley Score, and intensity of social response were other neonatal variables related to LD, but which were no longer significant when later performance measures were included. Finally, the LD children in this sample of first and second graders had started school at a younger age than the non-LD comparison group.

The 4-year examination revealed variables with strong associations to the LD. The LD group had more failures on the Porteus Mazes, shorter attention spans, and greater activity levels than the comparison group. At age 7, LD discriminators included difficulty with right-left discrimination, refractive error, anemia, and a history of measles. Given the importance socioeconomic status and demographic characteristics, LD was found to run in families, with the best predictor being the average LD factor score of siblings. Because risks of LD siblings of affected children were nearly identical, and since risks to other relatives did not vary systematically by degree of relationship, the strong familial association appeared to be environmentally rather than genetically determined.

A subgroup of the LD group with hyperactivity were found, at age 4, associated with ratings of hyperactivity, impulsivity, and short attention span, which were also related to hyperactivity at age 7. The hyperactivity subgroup, like the LD sample, also tended to fail the Porteus Maze test and had difficulty with right-left discrimination. There were also a variety of demographic, perinatal, and early developmental antecedents associated with later hyperactivity. Thus, these findings support the suggestion of Alberman (1973) that LD was more strongly related to socioeconomic status than with perinatal complications.

Identification Studies

The early identification of learning disabilities has been investigated in several other follow-up studies. For example, Gottesman (1979) found that the best predicator of final achievement level was initial achievement level. Excluding initial and subsequent scores, WRAT outcomes were best predicted by initial age at testing, educational placement, and neurological history. Thus, the older child with a negative neurological history in a regular class was most likely to show the best reading performance. For the other outcome assessment (Adult Basic Learning Examination), final status was most related to initial age at testing, educational placement, and IQ. Thus, an older child with a relatively high IQ in a regular class would most likely show the best outcome. Initial status as predictive of later status was confirmed by Francis-Williams (1976) in a 5-year follow-up of 42 LD children who had been identified during the preschool period. When compared to a control group, the LD group scored more poorly on reading and arithmetic outcome assessment in which they had scored poorly in the preschool period. In fact, 11 of the 42 subjects were unable to read and 13 were retarded in reading by, at least, 12 months. Only 9 LD subjects were reading at or above expected age levels, compared to 22 of the controls. During the preschool assessment, the LD group was poorer than, the control group in language, copying ability, and concept formation, and follow-up assessments revealed a high correlation with initial scores in these areas.

Behavioral status has also been found predictive of later learning disabilities Forness and Esveldt (1975), using direct observation of kindergarten classes, were able to predict educationally high-risk children. At the end of first grade, Forness, Guthrie, and Hall (1976), through teaching ratings and achievement scores, found that the high-risk children were doing poorly. Later on, Forness, Hall, and Guthrie (1977) found that, in second grade, the high risk group continued to experience academic difficulties and had more special education assistance. The high-risk group had been rated as more inattentive, more disruptive, more hyperactive, and more impulsive in kindergarten. These same off-task behaviors were predictive of later underachievement by McKinney and Speece (1983). A multiple regression analysis indicated that behavioral ratings were predictive of academic progress over time. These findings suggest that LD has antecedents in early behavioral functioning and that off-task behaviors are predictive of later academic difficulties.

SUMMARY

The deficits associated with learning disabilities (both academic and behavioral) were generally persistent. However, the outcome picture was guardedly optimistic. This was partially due to sampling bias caused by the difficulties in defining learning disabilities and specifying identification criteria. Nevertheless, although a positive bias may have been inherent because of overrepresentation of mild learning disabilities, those studies using LD subjects selected early tended to include more severely disabled subjects. In these studies, the age factor tended to influence outcomes: the youngest children at diagnosis generally showed the poorest outcomes, whereas older children at diagnosis revealed better outcomes. There also appeared to be a relationship with age at follow-up. Those studies that followed LD children into adulthood (i.e., beyond 25 years of age) generally had more positive outcomes. Unfortunately, a majority of the LD follow-up studies had subjects that were still in elementary school, high school, or only a year or so out of school. Thus, these outcomes are restricted in scope and may not reflect accurately the outcome picture for LD students beyond the school years.

Besides age, outcomes appeared to be related to follow-up assessments. General measures of educational and vocational status based on level of schooling completed or occupational status, for example, revealed positive outcomes for LD students. These global assessments yielded a majority of findings suggesting average or better attainment levels for LD subjects at follow-up. The positive picture did not emerge, however, when more specific academic assessments (e.g., achievement tests, reading tests) were the outcome measures. When the WRAT, MAT, or SAT were the measures used, for example, the LD samples showed continued deficits in reading, spelling, handwriting, and arithmetic. Some studies not only found significant deficits, but also found that deficits increased with age relative to age and grade placement. Basic skills deficits appear to be persistent and enduring for the LD child, with no indication that they "catch-up" with normal peers. In the area of social and behavioral functioning, the follow-up literature presented a mixed picture: the studies were about evenly split between positive and negative outcomes. This finding appeared relatively independent of either educational, vocational, or basic skills outcomes. Thus, outcome measure is an important variable in LD follow-up studies since findings seem to be partially related to the type of outcome assessment used.

With respect to treatment, no one remedial practice appeared to be superior. All treatment practices appeared to result in some gain, particularly in the short term. Regardless of the intervention, those initial gains tended to wash out over time and, if they were to be sustained, required support service over the long-term. The actual effectiveness of LD treatment was difficult to ascertain, however, because of the extensive variability encountered in LD samples. Additionally, samples were not usually randomly separated into treatment and nontreatment conditions, which limits any conclusions about positive or negative effects of intervention. Studies generally reported group statistics for either treatment effects or predictive antecedents, which tended to mask individual outcomes that usually fell along a wide continuum. Although some LD subjects did well, others did not. If global educational or vocational outcomes were positive and basic skills deficits persisted, then some LD subjects had to develop strategies to compensate for the range of individual differenes found. The nature of these strategies was not evident in the group statistics provided.

The LD follow-up literature needs to be approached with caution because of several methodological problems. Attrition appeared to be a problem; several studies approached a 50% attrition rate. These high rates always raise the question of whether the follow-up sample was similar to the sample selected at diagnosis. If the sample composition is altered significantly by attrition, then the outcome findings are not generalizable to the LD population as a whole but only to the specific sample assessed. Few LD follow-up studies, however, addressed the issue of attrition. It is necessary for future research efforts to analyze follow-up to determine whether attrition has introduced a systematic bias.

A majority of the LD follow-up literature did not include a control group, which limited interpretation since it is never certain if the outcome is related to the LD condition alone or to other factors. For example, Hinton and Knights (1971) required a control group in which almost half of the subjects had significant behavior problems so the effects behavioral disorders could be controlled. A common method of control in LD follow-up studies is to compare LD subjects' progress to estimated growth based on expected normal gain or test norms. Such a procedure is not recommended because these expectations are hypothetical and do not take into account variables that may influence outcomes such as IQ or socioeconomic status. Additionally, the use of estimated growth is likely to ensure that regression effects will influence outcome findings. Because LD subjects are diagnosed on the basis of discrepancy scores (expected versus actual achievement), any improvement in achievement levels at follow-up is likely to reflect, at least partially, regression toward the mean. When actual rates of achievement gain are compared to expected rates, regression effects are likely to confound outcomes, since expected achievement gains are based on the assumption that LD subjects will maintain the level of discrepancy seen at diagnosis. If the same level is not maintained, especially for LD subjects with the largest initial discrepancies, regression effects would probably overestimate improvement.

In some studies (e.g., Ackerman et al., 1977), even though a control group was included, it is likely that a bias in the control group confounds comparison. When classroom teachers are asked to recommend non-LD children from the same classroom from which the LD sample was selected, it is possible that teachers may nominate children who differ from the LD group not only in terms of the learning disability but also along other dimensions (e.g., behavior, IQ) that confound the effects of the learning disability. This problem can be overcome by random selection of the non-LD group, which eliminates any potential bias introduced by the nominating process. Biasing factors may also be eliminated through the epidemiological approach (e.g., Nichols & Chen, 1981; Werner & Smith, 1977) wherein entire populations are studied rather than samples. The population is divided at diagnosis into LD and non-LD groups. Through this procedure, biasing factors are minimized and any resulting group differences can be considered to have been based on valid comparisons.

The long-term consequences of learning disabilities defy a unilateral interpretation. Although many findings were similar to those found for reading disorders and hyperactivity, many were not similar. Consequently, answers to questions about LD outcomes remain tentative. The many and varied findings suggest that more longitudinal research is called for if the natural history of LD is to be fully understood. The present conflicting results makes it difficult to resolve basis policy issues for LD.

Robins (1979) identified questions that follow-up studies can address. Most prominent are questions about the natural history of a disorder like learning disabilities: What are the symptoms? How early do they occur? How long do they last? Are there age-related exacerbations and remissions? Do symptoms change with age? Does childhood LD presage academic and behavioral difficulties later on? Another group of questions involves treatment: Does treatment alter the course of LD? Which treatments are most effective? What can parents do to ameliorate a learning disability? What can teachers do? A related set of questions involves etiology: Is childhood LD in part a genetic disorder? What is the role of sociocultural factors? What part do educational circumstances play in the development of learning disablilties? Finally, questions about epidemiology can be addressed: What are the incidence and prevalence rates? What individuals or groups are at risk?

Despite the variability and imperfections of method, the LD follow-up literature provided answers to some of the above questions. There is some consensus, for example, that children diagnosed as LD continue to show impairment in those functions initially assessed as deficient. On the average, reading progress shown by LD children is below normal expectation. For those LD children with hyperactivity, it appears that they continue to be somewhat more active than the average child. Even for bright and successful subjects residual difficulties in reading and spelling were reported. When neuropsychological functions were assessed at follow-up, LD subjects often showed reduced but still significant deficits in some areas (e.g., figure-ground discrimination, visual-motor skills). Although the evidence is scanty, the LD child probably continues to have more difficulties coping with ordinary life stresses. There is likely to be lowered self-esteem accompained by the development of self-critical reactions.

There appears to be some consensus that children diagnosed as LD have a great deal of difficulty keeping up with their peers. Several studies found only a minority of the diagnosed LD children in the appropriate grade for age at follow-up. These findings appeared to be independent of treatment effects, since no appreciable differences emerged among intervention approaches. Although all treatments appeared effective in the short-term, their efficacy tended to wane over time. Social and vocational adjustment after school years appeared highly variable from study to study. It does seem safe to conclude, however, that LD children have an elevated risk of later emotional and behavioral difficulties, but the ultimate impact of these problems on other aspects of the LD child's life (e.g., work, marriage) is unclear.

Prediction of later adjustment and status for a child diagnosed as LD is highly uncertain at present. Findings suggest, however, that an LD child with a high IQ, high socioeconomic status, and intensive systematic educational efforts has a relatively good prognosis for both academic achievement and vocational success. Conversely, LD children with more modest IQ and socioeconomic status do not necessarily have a poor prognosis, but are likely to attain lower levels of achievement and occupational status. Prediction for LD children is probably more difficult than for children in general, because of the range restriction of scores for many predictors implicit in LD diagnosis and the generally more diffuse structure of abilities in LD children (see Wallbrown, Wherry, Blaha & Counts, 1974). Individual LD children may be idiosyncratic, so attempts to generalize statistically about deficits and outcomes may not be productive.

Finally, the LD follow-up literature contributed relatively little to understanding either the etiology or prevalence of learning disabilities. It appears that it will be impossible to obtain definitive and reliable information concerning LD's natural history until a consensus definition can be achieved. All too often, the term learning disability was defined loosely and without operational specification. Consequently, there was an ambiguity surrounding the nature of the sample under study. The variety of terminology used, such as dyslexia, minimal brain dysfunction, hyperactivity, attention deficit disorder, and the like, sometimes referred to different children but, at other times, referred to the same children. There was no consistency, which makes generalization difficult.

Besides definitional issues, other methodological considerations should be incorporated into future research. The ideal follow-up study of LD children should use a longitudinal design, beginning with children selected prior to the onset of LD (i.e., probably during the preschool period). This procedure has proven valuable in the study of schizophrenia (e.g., Garmerzy, 1974) and would be a good model for the LD field. The advantages would include the absence of bias in the target sample, the availability of a valid comparison group, and the availability of current (not exclusively retrospective) information. Such a methodology would provide data for cross-lagged panel designs (Campbell & Stanley, 1969) that would allow for the teasing out of cause and effect relationships between the LD child's symptoms and environmental events (e.g., does school failure lead to behavioral disorders or do behavioral disorders lead to school failure and learning disabilities?). Any future research should also use a wide array of outcome measures to examine the prognosis of LD in a variety of areas (e.g., academic, occupational, social, emotional, neuropsychological). These outcomes should be studied both separately and in interaction to determine the relationships, if any, among areas. These outcomes must also be more tightly controlled for IQ and socioeconomic status. Currently, outcome differences cannot always be related to specific deficits because subjects often differ in general aptitude and family background. Finally, greater specification of treatment variables is necessary so comparisons can be made across studies. The variety of treatments in longitudinal research, even among the same sample, is a serious source of confusion since the interventions vary considerably in length, method, and intensity.

What, then, should we tell the parents of an LD child? Although the data are by no means complete, there is a consistency indicating that the child will possess a high risk of lasting deficits. There is a high risk of repeating one or more grades in school and a somewhat elevated risk of some behavior problems (particularly low self-esteem). Beyond these few generalizations, outcomes appear to depend on the nature and extent of the cognitive and behavioral manifestations of the learning disability, the child's IQ level, and, to some extent, family's socioeconomic level. If the LD child is fortunate enough to possess a high IQ, to have professional parents, and to have been exposed to intensive and long-term treatment, then the prognosis for academic and vocational success is generally good. However, reading and spelling will probably always be difficult for the child. On the other hand, if the child has a low IQ, a lower socioeconomic status, associated behavioral disorders, and is subject to average intervention efforts, then the prognosis is poor, especially with regard to academic failure. However, prognosis for vocational and life adjustment, even with extensive school failure, is not totally gloomy. Although risks for lowered socioeconomic status and psychiatric contact are increased, the total social and occupational outcomes are, as a rule, not entirely negative. For the child in the middle, the "average" LD child, any of the possible outcomes may occur. Parents should be advised that there is a high probability of some noticeable improvement but not enough to allay totally their concerns about their child's future.

References

Aaron, P. G., Baker, C., & Hickox, G. L. (1982). In search of the third dyslexia. *Neuropsychologia, 20,* 203–208.

Abbott, R. C., & Frank, B. E. (1975). A follow-up of LD children in a private special school. *Academic Therapy, 10,* 291–298.

Abrams, J. C., & Kaslow, F. W. (1976). Learning disability and family dynamics: A mutual interaction. *Journal of Clinical Child Psychology, 5,* 35–40.

Abrams, J. C., & Kaslow, F. W. (1977). Family systems and the learning-disabled child: Intervention and treatment. *Journal of Learning Disabilities, 10,* 86–90.

Ackerman, P. T., & Dykman, R. A. (1982). Automatic and effortful information-processing deficits in children with learning and attention disorders. *Topics in Learning and Learning Disabilities, 2,* 12–22.

Ackerman, P. T., Dykman, R. A., & Peters, J. E. (1977). Learning-disabled boys as adolescents: Cognitive factors and achievement. *Journal of the American Academy of Child Psychiatry, 16,* 296–313.

Ackerman, P. T., Elardo, P. T., & Dykman, R. A. (1979). A psychosocial study of hyperactive and learning disabled boys. *Journal of Abnormal Child Psychology, 7,* 91–99.

Adams, M. (1960). *The mentally subnormal.* London: Heineman.

Adamson, W. C. (1972). Helping parents of children with learning disabilities. *Journal of Learning Disabilities, 5,* 327–330.

Adamson, W. C. (1979). Individual psychotherapy: An illustrative case study. In W. C. Adamson & K. K. Adamson (Eds.), *A handbook for specific learning disabilities* (pp. 193–236). New York: Gardner Press.

Adelman, H. S., & Taylor, L. (1982). Enhancing the motivation and skills needed to overcome interpersonal problems. *Learning Disability Quarterly, 5,* 438–446.

Adelman, H. S. & Taylor, L. (1985). The future of the LD field. *Journal of Learning Disabilities, 18,* 422–427.

Alberman, E. (1973). The early prediction of learning disorders. *Developmental Medicine and Child Neurology, 15,* 202–204.

Algozzine, B., & Korinek, J. (1985). Where is special education for students with high prevalence handicaps going? *Exceptional Children, 51,* 388–394.

Algozzine, B., & Ysseldyke, J. (1981). Special education for normal children: Better safe than sorry? *Exceptional Children, 48,* 238–243.

Allen, R. V., & Allen, P. (1970). *Language experience in reading.* Chicago: Encyclopaedia Brittanica.

Alley, G., & Deshler, D. (1979). *Teaching the learning-disabled adolescent: Strategies and methods.* Denver: Love

Alley, G., Deshler, D., Clark, F., Schumaker, J., & Warner, M. (1983). Learning disabilities in adolescent and adult populations: Part II: Research Implications. *Focus on Exceptional Children, 15*(9), 1–14.

Allington, R. L., & Flemming, J. T. (1978). The misreading of high-frequency words. *Journal of Special Education, 12,* 417–421.

Altwerger, B., & Bird, L. (1982). The learner or the curriculum? *Topics in Learning and Learning Disabilities, 1,* 69–78.

Aman, M. G. (1978). Drugs, learning, and the psychotherapies. In J. S. Werry (Ed.), *Pediatric psychopharmacology: The use of behavior modifying drugs in children* (pp. 79–108). New York: Brunner/Mazel.

Aman, M. G. (1980). Psychotropic drugs and learning problems — A selective review. *Journal of Learning Disabilities, 13,* 87–97.

Aman, M. G. (1982). Psychotropic drugs in the treatment of reading disorders. In R. N. Malatesha & P. G. Aaron (Eds.), *Reading disorders: Varieties and treatments.* New York: Academic Press.

Aman, M. G., & Werry, J. S. (1982). Methylphenidate and diazepam in severe reading retardation. *Journal of the American Academy of Child Psychiatry, 1,* 31–37.

Ambrose, A. (1974). Personality. In R. Sears & S. Feldman (Eds.), *The seven ages of man* (pp. 10–14). Los Altos, CA: Kaufmann.

Americaner, M. H., & Omizo, M. M. (1984). Family interaction and learning disability. *Journal of Learning Disabilities, 17*(9), 540–543.

Anderson, C. A., & Jennings, D. L. (1980). When experiences of failure promote expectations of success. The impact of attributing failure to ineffective strategies. *Journal of Personality, 48,* 393–407.

Anderson, D. (1976). Pruning the fuzziness and flab from learning disabilities research. *Journal of Special Education, 10,* 157–161.

Anderson, J. R. (1975). *Cognitive psychology and its implications.* San Francisco: Freeman.

Anderson, R. C. (1977). The notion of schemata and the educational enterprise. In R. Anderson, R. Spiro, & W. Montague (Eds.), *Schooling and the acquisition of knowledge* (pp. 415–531). Hillsdale, NJ: Lawrence Erlbaum.

Anderson, T. H. (1980). Study strategies and adjunct aids. In R. J. Spiro, B. B. Bruce, & W. F. Brewer (Eds.), *Theoretical issues in reading comprehension* (pp. 484–502). Hillsdale, NJ: Lawrence Erlbaum.

André, M. E. D. A., & Anderson, T. H. (1978-1979). The development and evaluation of a self-questioning study technique. *Reading Research Quarterly, 14,* 605–623.

Andrews, N., & Shaw, J. E. (1986). *Child Care, Health and Development, 12*(1), 53–62.

Applebee, A. N. (1971). Research in reading retardation: Two critical problems. *Journal of Child Psychology and Psychiatry, 12,* 91–113.

Application for admission Ben D. Caudle Special Learning Center. (Undated). Clarksville, AR: The College of the Ozarks.

Arkowitz, H. (1981). Assessment of social skills. In M. Hersen & A. S. Bellack (Eds.), *Behavioral assessment* (pp. 296–327). New York: Pergamon Press.

Armstrong, J. (1973). A generalized model for the evaluation of instructional materials and media. In J. Armstrong (Ed.), *A sourcebook for the evaluation of instructional materials and media.* Madison: University of Wisconsin, Special Education Instructional Materials Center.

Arter, J. A., & Jenkins, J. R. (1977). Examining the benefits and prevalence of modality considerations in special education. *Journal of Special Education, 11,* 281–298.

Arter, J. A., & Jenkins, J. R. (1979). Differential diagnosis — prescriptiive teaching: A critical appraisal. *Review of Educational Research, 49,* 517–555.

Asher, S., & Hymel, S. (1981). Children's social competence in peer relations: Sociometric and behavioral assessment. In J. D. Wine & M. D. Syme (Eds.), *Social competence.* New York: Guilford Press.

Ashlock, R. B. (1976). *Error patterns in computation: A semi-programmed approach.* Columbus, OH: Merrill.

Ashlock, R. B. (1986). *Error patterns in computation: A semi-programmed approach* (4th ed.). Columbus, OH: Merrill.

Ashlock, R. B., & Washbon, C. A. (1978). Games: Practice activities for the basic facts. In M. N. Suydam & R. E. Reys (Eds.), *Developing computational skills: 1978 yearbook* (pp. 39–50). Reston, VA: National Council of Teachers of Mathematics.

Averch, H. A., Carroll, S. J., Donaldson, T. S., Kiesling, H. J., & Pincus, J. (1984). *How effective is schooling? A critical review and synthesis of the research.* Englewood Cliffs, NJ: Educational Technology Publications.

Axelrod, L. (1982). Social perception in learning disabled adolescents. *Journal of Learning Disabilities, 15,* 610–613.

Ayllon, T., Layman, D., & Kandel, H. J. (1975). A behavioral-educational alternative to drug control of hyperactive children. *Journal of Applied Behavior Analysis, 8,* 137–146.

Ayllon, T., & Roberts, M. D. (1974). Eliminating discipline problems by strengthening academic performance. *Journal of Applied Behavior Analysis, 7,* 71–76.

Ayres, L. P. (1917). *Ayres scales for measuring handwriting.* Princeton, NJ: Educational Testing Service.

Bachara, G. (1976). Empathy in learning disabled children. *Perceptual and Motor Skills, 43,* 541–542.

Badian, N. A. (1983). Dyscalculia and nonverbal disorders of learning. In H. R. Myklebust (Ed.), *Progress in learning disabilities* (Vol. V, pp. 235–264). New York: Grune & Stratton.

Bailey, J., & Bostow, D. (1979). *Research methods in applied behavioral analysis.* Tallahassee: Behavior Management Consultants.

Bain, A. M. (1980). *Handwriting survey.* Unpublished paper, Loyola College, Baltimore.

Baker, H. J., & Leland, B. (1967). *Detroit Tests of Learning Aptitude* (rev. ed.). Indianapolis: Bobbs-Merrill.

Baker, L. (1979, July). *Do I understand or do I not understand: That is the question.* (Reading Education Report No. 10). Urbana: University of Illinois, Center for the Study of Reading.

Baker, L., & Brown, A. (1984a). Metacognitive skills and reading. In P. D. Pearson (Ed.), *Handbook of reading research* (pp. 353–394). New York: Longman.

Baker, L., & Brown, A. L. (1984b). Cognitive monitoring in reading. In J. Flood (Ed.). *Understanding reading comprehension* (pp. 21–44). Newark, DE: International Reading Association.

Balkwell, C., & Halverson, C. F., Jr. (1980). The hyperactive child as a source of stress in the family: Consequences and suggestions for intervention. *Family Relations, 29,* 550–557.

Balow, B. (1965). The long-term effects of remedial reading. *The Reading Teacher, 18,* 581–586.

Banikowski, A. L. (1981). *The verbal cognitive-socialization and strategies used by learning disabled and non-learning disabled junior high school adolescents in a peer-to-peer interaction activity.* Unpublished doctoral dissertation, University of Kansas, Lawrence.

Bannatyne, A. (1974). Diagnosis: A note on recategorization of the WISC scaled scores. *Journal of Learning Disabilities, 7,* 272–273.

Barat College Learning Opportunities Program case history. (1982, April). Lake Forest, IL: Barat College.

Barbaro, F. (1982). The learning disabled college student: Some considerations in setting objectives. *Journal of Learning Disabilities, 15,* 559–603.

Barkley, R. A. (1981a). *Hyperactive children: A handbook for diagnosis and treatment.* New York: Guilford Press.

Barkley, R. A. (1981b). Learning disabilities. In E. J. Mash & L. G. Terdal (Eds.), *Behavioral assessment of childhood disorders.* New York: Guilford Press.

Barkley, R. A., & Cunningham, C. E. (1978). Do stimulant drugs improve the academic performance of hyperkinetic children? *Clinical Pediatrics, 17,* 85–92.

Barkley, R. A., Cunningham, C. E., & Karlsson, J. (1983). The speech of hyperactive children and their mothers: Comparison with normal children and stimulant drug effects. *Journal of Learning Disabilities, 16,* 105–110.

Barsch, R. W. (1961). Counseling the parent of the brain-injured child. *Journal of Rehabilitation, 37,* 26–27, 40–42.

Barsch, R. (1967). *Achieving perceptual-motor efficiency.* Seattle: Special Child Publication.

Bateman, B. (1964). Learning disabilities — Yesterday, today, and tomorrow. *Exceptional Children, 31,* 167–177.

Bateman, R. J. (1966). Learning disorders. *Review of Educational Research, 36,* 93–119.

Battle, J. (1979). Self-esteem of students in regular and special classes. *Psychological Reports, 44,* 212–214.

Beattie, I. D., & Scheer, J. K. (1982). *Using the diagnostic stamp kit.* Port Roberts, WA: Janian Educational Materials.

Beck, R. J. (1977). *Remediation of learning deficits through precision teaching: A follow-up study.* Unpublished doctoral dissertation, University of Montana.

Becker, H. (1983). How schools use microcomputers. *Computer Room Learning,* 41–144.

Becker, W. C. (1977). Teaching reading and language to the disadvantaged — what we have learned from field research. *Harvard Educational Review, 47,* 518–543.

Becker, W. C., & Carnine, D. W. (1981). Direct instruction: A behavior theory model for comprehensive educational intervention with the disadvantaged. In S. W. Bijou & R. Ruis (Eds.), *Behavior modification: Contributions to education.* Hillsdale, NJ: Lawrence Erlbaum.

Becker, W. C., & Engleman, S. (1977). *The Oregon Direct Instruction Model: Comparative results in project Follow Through, a summary of nine years work.* Eugene: University of Oregon.

Beers, C. S. (1980). The relationship of cognitive development to spelling and reading abilities. In E. H. Henderson & J. W. Beers (Eds.), *Developmental and cognitive aspects of learning to spell.* Newark, DE: International Reading Associates.

Beers, J. W. (1980). Developmental strategies of spelling competence in primary school children. In E. H. Henderson & J. W. Beers (Eds.), *Developmental and cognitive aspects of learning to spell.* Newark, DE: International Reading Associates.

Beery, K. E., & Buktenica, N. A. (1967). *Developmental Test of Visual Motor Integration.* Chicago: Follett.

Begle, S. G. (1979). *Critical variables in mathematics education.* Washington, DC: Mathematics Association of America and the National Council of Teachers of Mathematics.

Beland, R. (1980). *An analysis of role perception and needs assessment of selected special edu-*

cators toward leisure education for the handicapped. Unpublished doctoral dissertation, University of Maryland.

Ben D. Caudle Special Learning Center student handbook. (1981, September) Clarkesville, AR: The College of the Ozarks.

Bennett, A. B. (1982). *Decimal squares: Step by step teacher's guide to readiness to advanced levels in decimals.* Fort Collins, CO: Scott Resources.

Bennett, K. (1981). The effects of syntax and verbal mediation on learning disabled students' verbal mathematical problem solving. *Dissertation Abstracts International, 42,* 1093. (University Microfilms No. 04-19, 4209)

Benton, A. L. (1974). *The revised visual retention test.* New York: Psychological Corporation.

Benton, A. L. (1978). Some conclusions about dyslexia. In A. L. Benton & D. Pearl (Eds.), *Dyslexia: An appraisal of current knowledge* (pp. 451–476). New York: Oxford University Press.

Bentovin, A. (1972). Emotional disturbance of handicapped pre-school children and their families: Attitudes to the child. *British Medical Journal, 3,* 579–581.

Berkell, D. E. (1984). Choosing the right software. *Journal of Learning Disabilities, 19*(4), 431–439.

Berler, E. S., Gross, A. M., & Drabman, R. S. (1982). Social skills training with children: Proceed with caution. *Journal of Applied Behavior Analysis, 15,* 41–53.

Bersoff, D. N., Kabler, M., Fiscus, E., & Ankney, R. (1972). Effectiveness of special class placement for children labeled neurologically handicapped. *Journal of School Psychology, 10,* 157–163.

Bickel, W. E., & Bickel, D. D. (1986). Effective schools, classrooms, and instruction: Implications for special education. *Exceptional Children, 52*(6), 489–500.

Bijou, D. W., Birnbrauer, J. S., Kidder, J. D., & Tague, C. (1966). Programmed instruction as an approach to teaching of reading, writing, and arithmetic to retarded children. *Psychological Record, 16,* 505–522.

Bingham, A. (1981). Exploratory process in career development: Implications for learning disabled students. *Career Development for Exceptional Individuals, 4*(2), 77–80.

Bingham, G. (1978). Career attitudes among boys with and without specific learning disabilities. *Exceptional Children, 44,* 341–342.

Bireley, M., & Manley, E. (1980). The learning disabled student in a college environment: A report of Wright State University's program. *Journal of Learning Disabilities, 13,* 12–15.

Birenbaum, A. (1970). On managing courtesy stigma. *Journal of Health and Social Behavior, 11,* 196–206.

Blackwell, P. M., Engen, E., Fischgrund, J. E., & Zarcadoolas, C. (1978). *Sentences and other systems: A language and learning curriculum for hearing impaired children.* Washington, DC: The Alexander Graham Bell Association for the Deaf.

Blair, J. R. (1972). The effects of differential reinforcement on the discrimination learning of normal and low-achieving middle class boys. *Child Development, 43,* 251–255.

Blalock, J. (1982a). Residual learning disabilities in young adults: Implications for rehabilitation. *Journal of Applied Rehabilitation Counseling, 13*(2), 9–13.

Blalock, J. (1982b). Persistent auditory language deficits in adults with learning disabilities. *Journal of Learning Disabilities, 15,* 604–609.

Blankenship, C., & Lilly, M. S. (1981). *Mainstreaming students with learning and behavioral problems: Techniques for the classroom teacher.* New York: Holt, Rinehart & Winston.

Blankenship, C. S. (1985). Linking assessment to curriculum assessment. In J. F. Cawley (Ed.), *Mathematics appraisal of the learning disabled.* Rockville, MD: Aspen Publications.

Blatt, B. (1958). The physical, personality, and academic status of children who are mentally retarded attending special classes as compared with children who are mentally retarded attending regular classes. *American Journal of Mental Deficiency, 62,* 810–818.

Blatt, B. (1980). Why educational research fails. *Journal of Learning Disabilities, 13,* 3–4.

Blau, H., & Loveless, E. (1982). Specific hemispheric routing — TAK/V to teach spelling to dyslexics: VAK and VAKT challenged. *Journal of Learning Disabilities, 15,* 461–466.

Bley, N. S., & Thornton, C. A. (1981). *Teaching mathematics to the learning disabled.* Rockville, MD: Aspen Publications.

Bloom, B. (1976). *Human characteristics and school learning.* New York: McGraw-Hill.

Bloomer, C. H. (1978). *A six year follow-up study on learning disabled children in a resource room program.* Unpublished doctoral dissertation, Columbia University, New York.

Blouin, A., Bornstein, R., & Trites, R. (1978). Teenage alcohol use among hyperactive children: A 5-year follow-up study. *Journal of Pediatric Psychology, 3,* 188–194.

Boder, E. (1971). Developmental dyslexia: A diagnostic screening procedure based on three characteristic patterns of reading and spelling. In B. Bateman (Ed.), *Learning disorders* (Vol. 4). Seattle: Special Child Publications.

Boersma, F. J., & Chapman, J. W. (1981). Academic self-concept, achievement expectations, and locus of control in elementary learning-disabled children. *Canadian Journal of Behavioural Science, 13,* 349–358.

Boggs, E. (1979). Economic factors in family care. In R.H. Bruininks & G. C. Krantz (Eds.), *Family care of developmentally disabled members: Conference proceedings.* Minneapolis: University of Minnesota.

Bognar, C., & Martin, W. R. W. (1982). A sociological perspective on diagnosing learning difficulties. *Journal of Learning Disabilities, 15,* 347–351.

Bork, A., & Franklin, S. (1979). Personal computers in learning. *Educational Technology, 19,* 7–12.

Borkowski, J. G., & Cavanaugh, J. C. (1979). Maintenance and generalization of skills and strategies by the retarded. In N. R. Ellis (Ed.), *Handbook of mental deficiency: Psychological theory and research* (2nd ed., pp. 569–618). Hillsdale, NJ: Lawrence Erlbaum.

Borkowski, J. G., Johnston, M. B., & Reid, M. K. (in press). Metacognition, motivation, and the transfer of control processes. In S. J. Ceci (Ed.), *Handbook of cognition, social and neuropsychological aspects of learning disabilities.* Hillsdale, NJ: Lawrence Erlbaum.

Borkowski, J. G., & Konarski, E. A. (1981). Educational implications of efforts to train intelligence. *Journal of Special Education, 15*(2), 289–305.

Borland, B. L., & Heckman, H. K. (1976). Hyperactive boys and their brothers: A 25-year follow-up study. *Archives of General Psychiatry, 33,* 669–675.

Bose, A. (1970). *Information system design methodology based on PERT/CPN networking.* (ERIC Document Reproduction Service No. AR 711 670).

Bracht, G. H. (1970). Experimental factors related to aptitude-treatment interactions. *Review of Educational Research, 40,* 627–645.

Bradley, C. (1937). The behavior of children receiving benzedrine. *American Journal of Psychiatry, 94,* 577–585.

Bradley, C. (1957). Characteristics and management of children with behavior problems associated with organic brain damage. *Pediatric Clinics of North America, 4,* 1049–1060.

Bradley, C., & Bowen, M. (1940). School performance of children receiving amphetamine (Benzedrine) sulfate. *American Journal of Orthopsychiatry, 10,* 782–788.

Brannan, R., & Schaaf, O. (1983). An instructional approach to problem solving. In G. Schfelt (Ed.), *The agenda in action.* Reston, VA: National Council of Teachers of Mathematics.

Brannan, S. A. (1977). A special education viewpoint: Consultation in the public schools. In J. Goldstein (Ed.), *Consultation: Enhancing leisure service delivery to handicapped children and youth* (pp. 51–79). Arlington, VA: National Recreation and Park Association.

Brannan, S., Chinn, K., & Verhoven, P. (1981). *What is leisure education? ... A primer for persons working with handicapped children and youth.* Washington, DC: Hawkins and Associates.

Braun, C. (1976). Teacher expectations: Socio-psychological dynamics. *Review of Educational Research, 46,* 185–213.

Brewer, G., & Kakalik, J. (1979). *Handicapped children: Strategies for improving services.* New York: McGraw-Hill.

Briard, F. K. (1976). Counseling parents of children with learning disabilities. *Social Casework, 57,* 581–585.

Brightbill, C. (1961). *Man and leisure: A philosophy of recreation.* Englewood Cliffs, NJ: Prentice-Hall.

Broden, M., Hall, R. V., Dunlap, A., & Clark, R. (1970). Effects of teacher attention and a token reinforcement system in a junior high school special education class. *Exceptional Children, 36,* 341–349.

Broden, M., Hall, R. V., & Mitts, B. (1971). The effect of self-recording on the classroom behavior of two eighth-grade students. *Journal of Applied Behavioral Analysis, 4,* 191–199.

Brolin, D. E. (Ed.). (1978, 1983). *Life-centered career education: A competency based approach.* Reston, VA: Council for Exceptional Children.

Brolin, D. E. (1982). Life-centered career education for exceptional children. *Focus on Exceptional Children, 14*(7), 1–15.

Brolin, D. E. (1983). Career education: Where do we go from here? *Career Development for Exceptional Individuals, 6*(1), 3–14.

Brolin, D. E. (1985). Preparing handicapped students to be productive adults. [Special issue: Transition from school to the world of work]. *Technique, 1*(6), 447–454.

Brolin, D. E., & Carver, J. T. (1982). Lifelong career development for adults with handicaps: A new model. *Journal of Career Education, 8*(4), 280–282.

Brolin, D. E., & Kokaska, C. (1979). *Career education for handicapped children and youth.* Columbus, OH: Merrill.

Brolin, D. E., McKay, D., & West, L. (1978). *Trainer's guide for life-centered career education.* Reston, VA: Council for Exceptional Children.

Broughton, S. F., & Lahey, B. B. (1978). Direct and collateral effects of positive reinforcement, response cost, and mixed contingencies for academic performance. *Journal of School Psychology, 16,* 126–136.

Brown, A. L. (1978). Knowing when, where, and how to remember. A problem of metacognition. In R. Glaser (Ed.), *Advances in instructional psychology.* Hillsdale, NJ: Lawrence Erlbaum.

Brown, A. L. (1980). Metacognitive development and reading. In R. J. Spiro, B. B. Bruce, & W. F. Brewer (Eds.), *Theoretical issues in reading comprehension* (pp. 453–481). Hillsdale, NJ: Lawrence Erlbaum.

Brown, A. L., Campione, J. C., & Barclay, C. R. (1979). Training self-checking routines for estimating test readiness: Generalization from list learning to prose recall. *Child Development, 50,* 501–512.

Brown, D. (1982). *Counseling and accommodating the student with learning disabilities.* Washington, DC: President's Committee on Employment of the Handicapped. (ERIC Document Reproduction Service No. ED 214 338).

Brown, J. S., & Burton, R. R. (1978). Diagnostic models for procedural bugs in basic mathematical skills. *Cognitive Science, 2,* 155–192.

Brown, L. & Perlmutter, L. (1971). Teaching functional reading to trainable level retarded students. *Education and Training of the Mentally Retarded, 6,* 74–84.

Bruck, M., & Hebert, M. (1982). Correlates of learning disabled students' peer-interaction patterns. *Learning Disability Quarterly, 5,* 353–362.

Bruininks, V. L. (1978a). Actual and perceived peer status of learning disabled students in mainstream programs. *Journal of Special Education, 12,* 51–58.

Bruininks, V. L. (1978b). Peer status and personality characteristics of learning disabled and non-disabled students. *Journal of Learning Disabilities, 11,* 29–34.

Bruno, R. M. (1981). Interpretation of pictorially presented social situations by learning disabled and normal children. *Journal of Learning Disabilities, 14,* 350–352.

Bryan, J. H., & Perlmutter, B. (1979). Immediate impressions of LD children by female adults. *Learning Disability Quarterly, 2*(1), 80–88.

Bryan, J. H., & Sherman, R. (1981). Immediate impressions of nonverbal ingratiation attempts by learning disabled boys. *Learning Disability Quarterly, 3*(2), 19–28.

Bryan, J. H., Sherman, R., & Fisher, A. (1980). Learning disabled boys' nonverbal behaviors within a dyadic interview. *Learning Disability Quarterly, 3*(1), 65–72.

Bryan, J. H., & Sonnefeld, J. J. (1981). Children's social desirability ratings of ingratiation tactics. *Learning Disability Quarterly, 4,* 287–293.

Bryan, J. H., Sonnefeld, L. J., & Greenberg, F. Z. (1981). Children's and parents' views on ingratiation tactics. *Learning Disability Quarterly, 4,* 170–179.

Bryan, T. (1982). Social skills of learning disabled children and youth: An overview. *Learning Disability Quarterly, 5,* 332–333.

Bryan, T., Pearl, R., Donahue, M., Bryan, J., & Pflaum, S. (1983). The Chicago Institute for the study of learning disabilities. *Exceptional Education Quarterly, 4*(1), 1–22.

Bryan, T. H. (1974a). An observational study of classroom behaviors of children with learning disabilities. *Journal of Learning Disabilities, 7,* 26–34.

Bryan, T. H. (1974b). Peer popularity of learning disabled children. *Journal of Learning Disabilities, 7,* 621–625.

Bryan, T. H. (1976). Peer popularity of learning disabled children: A replication. *Journal of Learning Disabilities, 9,* 307–311.

Bryan, T. H. (1977). Learning disabled children's comprehension of nonverbal communication. *Journal of Learning Disabilities, 10,* 501–506.

Bryan, T. H., & Bryan, J. H. (1977). Research: The perpetual revolution. In R. D. Kneedler & S. G. Tarver (Eds.), *Changing perspectives in special education* (pp. 273–294). Columbus, OH: Merrill.

Bryan, T. H., & Bryan, J. H. (1978). Social interactions of learning disabled children. *Learning Disability Quarterly, 1*(1), 33–38.

Bryan, T. H., Cosden, M., & Pearl, R. (1982). The effects of cooperative models on LD and NLD students. *Learning Disability Quarterly, 5,* 415–421.

Bryan, T. H., Donahue, M., & Pearl, R. (1981). Learning disabled children's peer interactions during a small-group problem solving task. *Learning Disability Quarterly, 4,* 13–22.

Bryan, T. H., Donahue, M., Pearl, R., & Sturm, C. (1981). Learning disabled children's conversational skills — the "T.V. talk show." *Learning Disability Quarterly, 4,* 250–259.

Bryan, T. H., & Pflaum, S. (1978). Social interactions of learning disabled children: A linguistic, social, and cognitive analysis. *Learning Disability Quarterly, 1*(3), 70–79.

Bryan, T. H., Werner, M., & Pearl, R. (1982). Learning disabled students' conformity responses to prosocial and antisocial situations. *Learning Disability Quarterly, 5,* 344–352.

Bryan, T. H., & Wheeler, R. (1972). Perception of children with learning disabilities: The eye of the observer. *Journal of Learning Disabilities, 5,* 484–488.

Bryan, T. H., Wheeler, R., Felcan, J., & Henek, T. (1976). "Come on Dummy" An observational study of children's communications. *Journal of Learning Disabilities, 9,* 661–669.

Budoff, M., & Gottlieb, J. (1976). Special-class EMR children mainstreamed: A study of an aptitude (learning potential) x treatment interaction. *American Journal of Mental Deficiency, 81,* 1–11.

Burstein, L., & Guiton, G. W. (1984). Methodological perspectives on documenting program impact. In B. K. Keogh (Ed.), *Advances in Special Education* (Vol. 4, pp. 21–42). Greenwich, CT: JAI Press.

Burton, L., & Bero, F. (1984). Is career education really being taught? *Academic Therapy, 19*(4), 389–395.

Bush, W. J., & Giles, M. T. (1969). *Aids to psycholinguistic teaching.* Columbus, OH: Merrill.

Butkowsky, I. S., & Willows, D. M. (1980). Cognitive-motivational characteristics of children varying in reading ability: Evidence for learned helplessness in poor readers. *Journal of Educational Psychology, 72,* 408–422.

Calfee, R., & Drum, P. (1978). Learning to read: Theory, research and practice. *Curriculum Inquiry, 8,* 183–249.

Calfee, R., Venezky, R., & Chapman, R. (1969). *Pronunciation of synthetic words with predictable and unpredictable letter-sound correspondences* (Tech. Rep. 71). Madison: Wisconsin Research and Development Center for Cognitive Learning.

Campbell, D. T. (1969). Reforms as experiments. *American Psychologist, 24,* 409–429.

Campbell, D. T., & Stanley, J. C. (1969). *Experimental and quasi-experimental designs for research.* Chicago: Rand McNally.

Campbell, L. (1968). *Study of curriculum planning.* Sacramento: California Department of Education.

Canney, G., & Winograd, P. (1979). *Schemata for reading and reading comprehension performance* (Tech. Rep. No. 120). Urbana: University of Illinois, Center for the Study of Reading.

Cantwell, D. P., & Carlson, G. R. (1978). Stimulants. In J. S. Werry (Ed.), *Pediatric psychopharmacology: The use of behavior modifying drugs in children* (pp. 171–207). New York: Brunner/Mazel.

Cantwell, D. P., & Satterfield, J. H. (1978). The prevalence of academic underachievement in hyperactive children. *Journal of Pediatric Psychology, 3,* 161–168.

Carlberg, C., & Kavale, K. (1980). The efficacy of special versus regular class placement for exceptional children: A meta-analysis. *Journal of Special Education, 14,* 295–309.

Carnine, D. (1983). Direct instruction: In search of instructional solutions for educational problems. In *Interdisciplinary voices in learning disabilities and remedial education* (pp. 1–66). Austin, TX: Pro-Ed.

Carnine, D. A. (1987). A response to "False standards, a distorting and disintegrating effect on education, turning away from useful purposes, being inevitably unfulfilled, and remaining unrealistic and irrelevant." *Remedial and Special Education, 8*(1), 42–43.

Caroll, A. W. (1967). The effects of segregated and partially integrated school programs on self-concept and academic achievement of educable mentally retarded. *Exceptional Children, 34,* 93–99.

Carpenter, T. P., Corbitt, M. K., Keprer, H. S., Lindquist, M. M., & Reys, R. E. (1981). Decimals: Results and implications from national assessment. *Arithmetic Teacher, 28,* 34–37.

Carpenter, T. P., Hiebert, J., & Moser, J. (1981). The effect of problem structure on first grader's initial solution procedures for simple addition and subtraction problems. *Journal for Research in Mathematics Education, 12,* 27–39.

Carr, T. H. (1982). What's in a model: Reading theory and reading instruction. In M. Singer (Ed.), *Competent reader, disabled reader: Research and application* (pp. 119–140). Hillsdale, NJ: Lawrence Erlbaum.

Carroll, J. A. (1984). Process into product: Teacher awareness of the writing process affects students' written products. In R. Beach & L. S. Bridwell (Eds.), *New directions in composition research.* New York: Guilford Press.

Carver, R. P. (1978). The case against statistical significance testing. *Harvard Educational Review, 48,* 378–399.

Case, R. (1982). General developmental influences on the acquisition of elementary concepts and algorithms in arithmetic. In T. P. Carpenter, J. M. Moser, & T. A. Romberg (Eds.), *Addition and subtraction: A cognitive perspective.* Hillsdale, NJ: Lawrence Erlbaum.

Cawley, J. F. (1981). Commentary. *Topics in Learning and Learning Disabilities, 1,* 3.

Cawley, J. R. (1984). *Developmental teaching of mathematics for the learning disabled.* Rockville, MD: Aspen Publications.

Cegelka, W. J. (1978). Educational materials: Curriculum guides for the mentally retarded: An analysis and recommendations. *Education and Training of the Mentally Retarded, 13,* 187–188.

Cegelka, W. J., & Tyler, J. L. (1970). The efficacy of special class placement for the mentally retarded in proper perspective. *Training School Bulletin, 67,* 33–68.

Chadwick, B. A., & Day, R. C. (1971). Systematic reinforcement: Academic performance of underachieving students. *Journal of Applied Behavior Analysis, 4,* 311–319.

Chalfant, J., & Scheffelin, M. (1969). *Central processing dysfunctions in children* (NINDS Monograph No. 9). Washington, DC: U.S. Government Printing Office.

Chall, J. S. (1979). The great debate: Ten years later with a modest proposal for reading stage. In L. Resnick & P. Weaver (Eds.), *Theory and practice of early reading* (Vol. 1, pp. 29–55). Hillsdale, NJ: Lawrence Erlbaum.

Charles, L., & Schain, R. (1981). A four-year follow-up study of the effects of methylphenidate on the behavior and academic achievement of hyperactive children. *Child Psychology, 9,* 495–505.

Chassan, J. B. (1979). *Research design in clinical psychology and psychiatry* (2nd ed.). New York: Irvington.

Chesler, B. M. (1980). *A talking mouth speaks about learning disabled college students.* Sacramento: Author.

Chi, M. T. H. (1985). Interactive roles of knowledge and strategies in development. In S. Chipman, J. Segal, & R. Glaser (Eds.), *Thinking and learning skills: Current research and open questions* (Vol. 2, pp. 457–483). Hillsdale, NJ: Lawrence Erlbaum.

Childs, R. E. (1979). A drastic change in curriculum for the educable mentally retarded child. *Mental Retardation, 17,* 299–301.

Chomsky, C. (1970). Reading, writing, and phonology. *Harvard Educational Review, 40*(2), 287–309.

Chomsky, N. (1965). *Aspects of the theory of syntax.* Cambridge, MA: MIT Press.

Christopolos, F., & Renz, P. (1969). A critical examination of special education programs. *Journal of Special Education, 3,* 371–379.

Church, G., & Bender, M. (1984). A pilot survey on computer awareness. Unpublished manuscript, Johns Hopkins University, Baltimore.

Clark, C. A., & Walberg, H. J. (1979). The use of secondary reinforcement in teaching inner-city school children. *Journal of Special Education, 3,* 177–185.

Clark, G. M. (1979). *Career education for the handicapped child in the elementary classroom.* Denver: Love Publishing.

Clark, L. (1980). *Instructions for implementing and maintaining the exceptional education management and information system (EEMIS).* Jacksonville, FL: Duval County Schools.

Clift, J., Edwards, M., Reese, S., & Vincent, R. (1977). Therapeutic recreation with hyperactive children. *Therapeutic Recreation Journal, 11,* 165-171.

Cobb, R. M., & Crump, W. D. (1984). *Post-school status of young adults identified as learning disabled while enrolled in public schools: A comparison of those enrolled and not enrolled in learning disabilities programs.* Washington, DC: U.S. Department of Education, Research Projects Section.

Cohen, A. (1969). Studies in visual perception and reading in disadvantaged children. *Journal of Learning Disabilities, 2,* 298-303.

Cohen, S. (1976). The last word. *Journal of Special Education, 10,* 167-170.

Cohen, S. A. (1976). The fuzziness and the flab: Some solutions to research problems in learning disabilities. *Journal of Special Education, 10,* 129-139.

Cohn, R. (1971). Arithmetic and learning disabilities. In H. R. Myklebust (Ed.), *Progress in learning disabilities* (Vol. 2, pp. 322-389). New York: Grune & Stratton.

Colarusso, R., & Hammill, D. (1972). *Motor-Free Visual Perception Test.* San Rafael, CA: Academic Therapy.

Coleman, N., & Harmer, W. (1982). A comparison of standardized reading tests and informal placement procedures. *Journal of Learning Disabilities, 19,* 396-398.

Coles, G. S. (1978). The learning-disabilities test battery: Empirical and social issues. *Harvard Educational Review, 48,* 313-340.

Coles, R. E., & Goodman, Y. (1980). Do we really need those oversized pencils to write with? *Theory into Practice, 19*(3), 194-196.

Collard, K. (1981). Leisure education in the schools: Why, who, and the need for advocacy. *Therapeutic Recreation Journal, 15,* 8-16.

Collins, A., & Smith, E. E. (1980, Sept.) *Teaching the process of reading comprehension* (Tech. Rep. No. 182). Urbana: University of Illinois, Center for the Study of Reading.

Conners, C. K. (1970). Symptom patterns in hyperkinetic, neurotic, and normal children. *Child Development, 41,* 667-682.

Cooke, T. P., & Apolloni, L. (1976). Developing positive social emotional behaviors: A study of training and generalization effects. *Journal of Applied Behavior Analysis, 9,* 65-78.

Cooper, C. R. (1977). Holistic evaluation of writing. In C. R. Cooper & L. Odell (Eds.), *Evaluating writing* (pp. 3-31). Urbana, IL: NCTE.

Cordoni, B. K. (1979). Assisting dyslexic college students: An experimental program design at a university. *Bulletin of the Orton Society, 29,* 261-268.

Cordoni, B. K. (1980). College options for the learning disabled. *Learning Disabilities, 4*(11).

Cordoni, B. K. (1982a). Services for college dyslexics. In R. M. Malatesha & P. G. Aaron (Eds.), *Neuropsychology of developmental dyslexia and acquired alexia and treatment. Perspectives in neurolinguistics* (Vol. 21). New York: Academic Press.

Cordoni, B. K. (1982b). Personal adjustment: The psycho-social aspects of learning disabilities. In M. R. Schmidt & H. Z. Sprandel (Eds.), *New directions for student services: Helping the learning disabled student* (No. 18). San Francisco: Jossey-Bass.

Cordoni, B. K., O'Donnell, J. P., Ramaniah, N. V., Kurtz, J., & Rosenshein, K. (1981). Wechsler Adult Intelligence score patterns for learning disabled young adults. *Journal of Learning Disabilities, 14,* 404-407.

Cornfort, R. L. (1985). Social work with unconventional children and their families. *Social Work, 30*(4), 367-368, 384.

Corno, L., & Mandinach, E. B. (1983). The role of cognition engagement in classroom learning and motivation. *Educational Psychologist, 18*(2), 88-108.

Council for Exceptional Children Ad Hoc Committee. (1984). Reply to "A Nation at Risk." *Exceptional Children, 50,* 484-494.

Coval, T., Gilhool, T., & Laski, F. (1977). Rules and tactics in institutionalization proceedings for mentally retarded persons: The role of the courts in assuring access to services in the community. *Education and Training of the Mentally Retarded, 12,* 177–185.

Cowen, E. L., Pederson, A., Babigian, H., Izzo, L. D., & Trost, M. A. (1973). Long-term follow-up of early detected vulnerable children. *Journal of Consulting and Clinical Psychology, 41,* 438–446.

Coyne, P. (1981). The status of recreation as a related service in P.L. 94-142. *Therapeutic Recreation Journal, 14,* 4–15.

Cratty, B. (1969). *Perceptual motor behavior and educational process.* Springfield, IL: Thomas.

Cratty, B. (1970). *Motor activities, motor ability, and the education of children.* Springfield, IL: Thomas.

Creager, R., & Van Riper, C. (1967). The effect of methylphenidate on the verbal productivity of children with cerebral dysfunction. *Journal of Speech and Hearing Research, 10,* 623–628.

Crimando, W., & Nichols, B. (1982). A model for vocational explanation and selective placement of the learning disabled. *Vocational Evaluation and Work Adjustment Bulletin, 15*(3), 98–102.

Crnic, K. A., Friedrich, W. N., & Greenberg, M. T. (1983). Adaptation of families with mentally retarded children: A model of stress, coping and family ecology. *American Journal of Mental Deficiency, 88,* 125–138.

Cromer, R. F. (1980). Spontaneous spelling of language-disordered children. In Ute Frith (Ed.), *Cognitive processes in spelling.* London: Academic Press.

Cronin, M. E., & Gerber, P. J. (1982). Preparing the learning disabled adolescent for adulthood. *Topics in Learning and Learning Disabilities, 2,* 55–68.

Cruickshank, W. (1967). *The brain-injured child in the home, school, and community.* Syracuse, NY: Syracuse University Press.

Cruickshank, W., Morse, W., & Johns, J. (1980). *Learning disabilities: The struggle from adolescence toward adulthood.* Syracuse, NY: Syracuse University Press.

Cullinan, D., Gadow, K. D., & Epstein, M. H. (in press). Psychotropic drug treatment among learning disabled, educable mentally retarded, and seriously emotionally disturbed students. *Journal of Abnormal Child Psychology.*

Cullinan, D., Lloyd, J, & Epstein, M. H. (1981). Strategy training: A structured approach to arithmetic instruction. *Exceptional Education Quarterly, 2,* 41–49.

Cunningham, C., & Barkley, R. (1979). The interactions of normal and hyperactive children with their mothers in free play and structured tasks. *Child Development, 50,* 217–224.

Daiute, C. (1985). *Writing and computers.* Reading, MA: Addison-Wesley.

Delacatto, C. (1959). *Treatment and prevention of reading problems.* Springfield, IL: Thomas.

Dembinski, R. J. (1977). What parents of the learning disabled really want from professionals. *Journal of Learning Disabilities, 10,* 578.

Denckla, M. B. (1977). Minimal brain dysfunction and dyslexia: Beyond diagnosis and exclusion. In M. E. Blaw, I. Rapin, & M. Kinsbourne (Eds.), *Topics in child neurology.* New York: Spectrum Publications.

Denckla, M. B., & Rudel, R. C. (1976). Rapid "automized" naming (R.A.N.): Dyslexia differentiated from other learning disabilities. *Neuropsychologia, 14,* 471–479.

Denham, C., & Lieberman, A. (1980). *Time to learn.* Washington, DC: National Institute of Education.

Deno, E. (1970). Special education as developmental capital. *Exceptional Children, 37,* 229–237.

Deno, S., Mirkin, P., & Chiang, B. (1982). Identifying valid measures of reading. *Exceptional Children, 49,* 36–45.

Department of Education. (1982). Independent study sheds light on employment statistics. *Programs for the Handicapped, July/August*(4), 13(b).

Deshler, D. D. (1978). Issues related to the education of learning disabled adolescents. *Learning Disability Quarterly, 1,* 2–10.

Deshler, D. D., Alley, G. R., Warner, M. M., & Schumaker, J. B. (1981). Instructional practices for promoting skill acquisition and generalization in severely learning disabled adolescents. *Learning Disability Quarterly, 4,* 415–421.

Deshler, D. D., & Schumaker, J. B. (1983). Social skills of learning disabled adolescents: Characteristics and intervention. *Topics in Learning and Learning Disabilities, 3*(2), 15–23.

Deshler, D., Schumaker, J., Alley, G., Warner, M., & Clark, F. (1982). Learning disabilities in adolescent and young adult populations: Research implications. *Focus on Exceptional Children, 15*(1), 1–12.

Deschler, D. D., Schumaker, J. B., & Lenz, B. K. (1984). Academic and cognitive interventions for LD adolescents: Part I. *Journal of Learning Disabilities, 17,* 108–117.

Dickstein, E. B., & Warren, D. R. (1980). Role-taking deficits in learning disabled children. *Journal of Learning Disabilities, 13,* 378–382.

Dil, N. (1983). Affective curricula: Theory, models and implementation. *Topics in Early Childhood Special Education, 2,* 25–33.

Dinsmore, J. A., & Isacson, D. K. (1986). Tactics for teaching dyslexic students. *Academic Therapy, 21*(3), 293–300.

Disimoni, F. (1978). *The Token Test for Children.* New York: Teaching Resources.

Dobbert, D. (1973). Procedures for the selection of instructional material at various stages of the evaluative process. In J. Armstrong (Ed.), *A sourcebook for the evaluation of instructional materials and media* (pp. 453–462). Madison: University of Wisconsin, Special Education Instructional Materials Center.

Dobbins, D. A. (1985). A classification of poor readers. *Early Child Development and Care, 19*(3), 183–198.

Doehring, D. G., & Hoshko, I. M. (1977). Classification of reading problems by the Q-technique of factor analysis. *Cortex, 13,* 281–292, 284.

Doehring, D. G., Hoshko, I. M., & Bryans. (1979). Statistical classification of children with reading problems. *Journal of Clinical Neuropsychology, 1,* 5–16.

Doehring, D. G., Trites, R. L., Patel, P. G., & Fiedorowicz, C. A. M. (1981). *Reading disabilities: The interaction of reading, language, and neuropsychological deficits.* New York: Academic Press.

Donahue, M., & Bryan, T. (1983). Conversational skills and modeling in learning disabled boys. *Applied Psycholinguistics, 4,* 251–278.

Donahue, M., Pearl, R., & Bryan, T. (1980). Learning disabled children's conversational competence: Responses to inadequate messages. *Applied Psycholinguistics, 1,* 387–403.

Donahue, M., Pearl, R., & Bryan, T. (1982). Learning disabled children's syntactic proficiency during a communicative task. *Journal of Speech and Hearing Disorders, 47,* 397–403.

Donahue, M. L. (1981). Requesting strategies of learning disabled children. *Applied Psycholinguistics, 2,* 213–234.

Donmoyer, R. (1985). The rescue from relativism: Two failed attempts and an alternative strategy. *Educational Researcher, 14,* 13–20.

Douglas, V. I. (1972). Stop, look, and listen: The problem of sustained attention and impulse control in hyperactive and normal children. *Canadian Journal of Behavioural Science, 4,* 259–282.

Downing, J. (1970). Children's concepts of language in learning to read. *Educational Research, 12,* 106–112.

Downing, J. (1972). Children's developing concepts of spoken and written language.

Journal of Reading Behavior, 4, 1-19.

Downing, J. (1978). Linguistic awareness. English orthography and reading instruction. *Journal of Reading Behavior, 10,* 103-114.

Downing, J. (1979). *Reading and reasoning.* New York: Springer-Verlag.

Downing, J., & Oliver, P. (1974). The child's concept of 'a word.' *Reading Research Quarterly, 9,* 568-582.

Drabman, R. S., Spitalnik, R., & O'Leary, K. D. (1973). Teaching self-control to disruptive children. *Journal of Abnormal Psychology, 82,* 10-16.

Duffy, F. H., Denckla, M. B., Bartels, P. H., & Sandini, G. (1980). Dyslexia: Automated diagnosis by computerized classification of brain electrical activity. *Annals of Neurology,* 421-428.

Duffy, J. (1974). *Type it.* Cambridge, MA: Educators Publishing Service.

Dunkin, M. J., & Biddle, B. J. (1974). *The study of teaching.* New York: Holt, Rinehart & Winston.

Dunn, L. M. (1968). Special education for the mildly retarded — is much of it justifiable? *Exceptional Children, 35,* 5-22.

Dunn, L. M., & Markwardt, F. C. (1970). *Peabody Individual Achievement Test.* Circle Pines, NM: American Guidance Service.

Dweck, C. S. (1975). Achievement. In M. E. Lamb (Ed.), *Social and personality development* (pp. 114-130). New York: Holt, Rinehart & Winston.

Dykman, R. A., Ackerman, P. T., & McCray, D. S. (1980). Effects of methylphenidate on selective and sustained attention in hyperactive, reading-disabled and presumably attention-disordered boys. *Journal of Nervous and Mental Diseases, 168,* 745-752.

Edgington, R. E. (1975). SLD children: A ten-year follow-up. *Academic Therapy, 11,* 53-64.

Egelman, C. D. (1981). Career workshops for the disabled. *Journal of College Student Personnel, 22*(6), 567-568.

Ehri, L. C. (1979). Linguistic insight: Threshold of reading acquisition. In T. G. Waller & G. E. MacKinnon (Eds.), *Reading research: Advances in theory and practice* (Vol. 1). New York: Academic Press.

Elenbogen, M. L. (1957). A comparative study of some aspects of academic and social adjustment of two groups of mentally retarded children in special classes and in regular classes (Doctoral dissertation, Northwestern University, 1957). *Dissertation Abstracts, 17,* 2496.

Elkind, D. (1983). Viewpoint: The curriculum disabled child. *Topics in Learning and Learning Disabilities, 3,* 71-78.

Ellington, C., & Winskoff, L. (1982). Low cost implementation of a career education program for elementary school children with handicaps. *Journal of Career Education, 8,* 246-255.

Engelmann, S. (1969). *Preventing failure in the primary grades.* Chicago: SRA.

Englert, C. S. (1983). Measuring special education teacher effectiveness. *Exceptional Children, 50*(3), 247-254.

Entwisle, D. R. (1976). Young children's expectations for reading. In J. Guthrie (Ed.), *Aspects of reading acquisition* (pp. 37-38). Baltimore: Johns Hopkins University Press.

Epps, S., Ysseldyke, J. E., & Algozzine, B. (1983). Impact of different definitions of learning disabilities on the number of students identified. *Journal of Psychoeducational Assessment, 1,* 341-352.

Epps, S., Ysseldyke, J. E., & Algozzine, B. (1985). An analysis of the conceptual framework underlying definitions of learning disabilities. *Journal of School Psychology, 23,* 133-144.

Erikson, E. H. (1963). *Child and society* (2nd ed.). New York: Norton.

Evans, G. W., & Oswalt, G. L. (1968). Acceleration of academic progress through the manipulation of peer influence. *Behavior Research and Therapy, 6,* 189–195.

Evenson, T. L., & Evenson, M. L. (1983). An innovative approach to career development of disabled college students. *Journal of Rehabilitation, 49*(2), 64–67.

Faerstein, L. M. (1981). Stress and coping in families of learning disabled children: A literature review. *Journal of Learning Disabilities, 14,* 420–423.

Fafard, M. B., & Haubrich, P. A. (1981). Vocational and social adjustment of learning disabled young adults: A follow-up study. *Learning Disability Quarterly, 4,* 122–130.

Farber, B. (1960). Family organization and crisis: Maintenance of integration in families with a severely retarded child. *Monographs of the Society for Research in Child Development, 25,* 1–25.

Farber, B. (1979). Sociological ambivalence and family care. In R. H. Bruininks & G. C. Krantz (Eds.), *Family care of developmentally disabled members: Conference proceedings.* Minneapolis: University of Minnesota.

Farber, B., & Jenne, W. (1963). Interaction with retarded siblings and life goals of children. *Marriage and Family Living, 25,* 96–98.

Farber, B., & Jenne, W. (1979). Sociological ambivalence and family care. In R. H. Bruininks & G. C. Krantz (Eds.), *Family care of developmentally disabled members: Conference proceedings.* Minneapolis: University of Minnesota.

Farnham–Diggory, S. (1972). The development of an equivalence system. In S. Farnham–Diggory (Ed.), *Information processing in children.* New York: Academic Press.

Farnham–Diggory, S., & Nelson, B. (1984). Cognitive analyses of basic school tests. *Applied Developmental Psychology, 1,* 21–74.

Favell, J. (1973). Reduction of stereotypes by reinforcement of toy play. *Mental Retardation, 11,* 21–23.

Fayne, H., & Bryant, N. D. (1981). Relative effects of various word synthesis strategies on phonics achievement of the learning disabled. *Journal of Educational Psychology, 73,* 616–623.

Feagans, L. (1983). Discourse processes in learning disabled children. In J. D. McKinney & L. Feagans (Eds.), *Current topics in learning disabilities* (Vol. 1, pp. 87–115). Norwood, NJ: Ablex.

Feagans, L., & Applebaum, M. I. (1986). Language subtypes and their validation in learning disabled children. *Journal of Educational Psychology, 78*(5), 358–364.

Feagans, L., & McKinney, J. D. (1981). The pattern of exceptionality across domains in learning disabled children. *Journal of Applied Developmental Psychology, 1,* 313–328.

Federal Register. (1977, Wednesday, May 4). Nondiscrimination on basis of handicap. Washington, DC, pp. 22676–22702.

Federal Register. (1977, December 29). Washington, DC, pp. 65082–65085.

Feingold, B. F. (1976). Hyperkinesis and learning disabilities linked to the ingestion of artificial food colors and flavors. *Journal of Learning Disabilities, 9,* 551–559.

Feldman, K. A. (1971). Using the work of others: Some observations of reviewing and integrating. *Sociology of Education, 44,* 86–102.

Ferhold, J. B., & Solnit, A. J. (1978). Counseling parents of mentally retarded and learning disabled children. In L. E. Arnold (Ed.), *Helping parents help their children.* New York: Brunner/Mazel.

Fernald, G. (1943). Remedial techniques in basic school subjects. New York: McGraw-Hill.

Ferritor, D. E., Buckholdt, D., Hamblin, R. L., & Smith, L. (1972). The non-effects of contingent reinforcement for attending behavior on work accomplished. *Journal of Applied Behavior Analysis, 5,* 7–17.

Fincham, F. (1977). A comparison of moral judgment in learning disabled and normal-achieving boys. *Journal of Psychology, 96*, 153–160.

Fisher, C. W., & Berliner, D. C. (1985). *Perspectives on instructional time.* White Plaines, NY: Longman.

Fisk, J., & Rourke, B. (1979). Identification of subtypes of learning disabled children at three age levels: A multivariate approach. *Journal of Clinical Neuropsychology, 1*, 289–310.

Fitzgerald, E. (1966). *Straight language for the deaf.* Washington, DC: Volta Bureau.

Fitzmaurice-Hayes, A. M. (1984). Curriculum and instructional activities grade 2 through grade 4. In J. F. Cawley (Ed.), *Developmental teaching of mathematics for the learning disabled.* Rockville, MD: Aspen Publications.

Fitzmaurice-Hayes, A. M. (1985). Whole numbers: Concepts and skills. In J. F. Cawley (Ed.), *Secondary school mathematics for the learning disabled.* Rockville, MD: Aspen Publications.

Flack, V. (1973). Application of management principles to instructional methods. *Exceptional Children, 39*(5), 401–407.

Flavell, J. H. (1976). Metacognitive aspects of problem solving. In L. B. Resnick (Ed.), *The nature of intelligence* (pp. 231–235). Hillsdale, NJ: Lawrence Erlbaum.

Fleischner, J. E. (1983). *Arithmetic Task Force progress report.* Unpublished manuscript, Columbia University, Teacher's College, Institute for the Study of Learning Disabilities, New York.

Fleischner, J. E. (1985). Arithmetic instruction for handicapped children in elementary grades. *Focus on Learning Problems in Mathematics, 7*, 23–24.

Fleischner, J. E., & Garnett, K. (1983). Arithmetic difficulties among learning-disabled children: Background and current directions. *Learning Disabilities, 2*, 111–124.

Fleischner, J. E., Garnett, K., & Preddy, D. (1982). *Mastery of basic number facts by learning disabled students: An intervention study* (Tech. Rep. No. 17). New York: Columbia University, Teachers College.

Fleischner, J. E., Garnett, K., & Shepherd, M. J. (1982). Proficiency in arithmetic basic fact computation of learning disabled and nondisabled children. *Focus on Learning problems in Mathematics, 4*, 47–55.

Fleischner, J. E., Nuzum, M. B., & Marzola, E. S. (1987). Devising an instructional program to teach arithmetic problem solving skills to students with learning disabilities. *Journal of Learning Disabilities, 20*, 214–217.

Fleischner, J. E., & Shepherd, M. J. (1980). *Improving the performance of children with learning disabilities: Instruction matters* (Tech. Rep. No. 27). New York: Columbia University, Teachers College, The Research Institute for the Study of Learning Disabilities.

Fleisher, L. A., & Jenkins, J. R. (1983). The effect of word- and comprehension-emphasis instruction on reading performance. *Learning Disability Quarterly, 6*(2), 146–154.

Fleisher, L. S., Jenkins, J. R., & Pany, D. (1979). Effects on poor readers' comprehension of training in rapid decoding. *Reading Research Quarterly, 15*, 30–48.

Flower, L. (1985). *Problem-solving strategies for writing* (2nd ed.). San Diego: Harcourt Brace Jovanovich.

Flynn, P. A. (1985). Adapting computer software to accommodate the learning disabled student. *Journal of Reading, Writing, and Learning Disabilities International, 1*(4), 93–97.

Fokes, J. (1976). *Fokes sentence builder.* New York: Teacher Resources.

Ford, A., Brown, L., Pumpian, I., Baumgart, D., Nisbet, J., Schroeder, J., & Loomis, R. (1980). *Strategies for developing individualized recreation/leisure plans for adolescent and young adult severely handicapped students.* Madison: University of Wisconsin.

Forness, S. (1981). Concepts of school learning and behavior disorders: Implications for research and practice. *Exceptional Children, 48*, 56–64.

Forness, S. R. (1982). Diagnosing dyslexia: A note on the need for ecologic assessment. *American Journal of Diseases of Children, 134,* 237–242.

Forness, S. R. (1983). Diagnostic schooling for children or adolescents with behavior disorders. *Behavior Disorders, 8,* 176–190.

Forness, S. R., & Esveldt, K. C. (1975). Prediction of high-risk kindergarten children through observation. *Journal of Special Education, 9,* 375–388.

Forness, S. R., Guthrie, D., & Hall, R. J. (1976). Follow-up of high-risk children identified in kindergarten through direct classroom observation. *Psychology in the Schools, 13,* 45–49.

Forness, S. R., Hall, R. J., & Guthrie, D. (1977). Eventual school placement of kindergartners observed as high risk in the classroom. *Psychology in the Schools, 14,* 315–317.

Forness, S. R., & Kavale, K. A. (1984). Education of the mentally retarded: A note on policy. *Education and Training of the Mentally Retarded, 19,* 239–245.

Forness, S. R., & Kavale, K. A. (1987). Holistic inquiry and the scientific challenge in special education: A reply to Iano. *Remedial and Special Education, 8*(1), 47–51.

Forrest, D. L., & Waleer, T. G. (1980). *What do children know about their reading and study skills?* Paper presented at the annual meeting of the American Educational Resource Association, Boston.

Foster, G. E. (1972). *A short-term follow-up study of the academic, social, and vocational adjustment and achievement of children five to ten years following placement in a perceptual development program.* Unpublished doctoral dissertation, Wayne State University, Detroit.

Fox, B., & Routh, D. K. (1975). Analyzing spoken language into words, syllables and phonemes: A developmental study. *Journal of Psycholinguistic Research, 4,* 331–342.

Francis–Williams, J. (1976). Early identification of children likely to have specific learning difficulties. Report of a follow-up. *Developmental Medicine and Child Neurology, 18,* 71–77.

Franklin, G. S., & Sparkman, W. E. (1978). The cost effectiveness of two program delivery systems for exceptional children. *Journal of Educational Finance, 3,* 305–314.

Frauenheim, J. G. (1978). Academic achievement characteristics of adult males who were diagnosed as dyslexic in childhood. *Journal of Learning Disabilities, 11,* 476–483.

Frederickson, C. H. (1979). Discourse comprehension and early reading. In L. Resnick & P. Weaver (Eds.), *Theory and practice of early reading* (Vol. 1). Hillsdale, NJ: Lawrence Erlbaum.

Freeman, D. J., Kuhs, T. M., Knappen, L. B., & Porter, A. C. (1982). A closer look at standardized tests. *The Arithmetic Teacher, 29,* 50–54.

Friars, E., & Gelmann, N. (1981). *Special education management by information: A design handbook.* Washington, DC: National Association of State Directors of Special Education.

Frostig, M., & Horn, D. (1964). *The Frostig program for the development of visual perception.* Chicago: Follett Education Corporation.

Fuchs, L. S., & Fuchs, D. (1986). Effects of systematic formative evaluation: A meta-analysis. *Exceptional Children, 53*(3), 199–208.

Gable, R., Hendrickson, J., Young, C., Shores, R., & Stowitschek, J. (1983). A comparison of teacher approved statements across categories of exceptionality. *Journal of Special Education Technology, 6,* 15–22.

Gadow, K. D. (1981). Prevalence of drug treatment for hyperactivity and other childhood behavior disorders. In K. D. Gadow & J. Loney (Eds.), *Psychosocial aspects of drug treatment for hyperactivity.* Boulder, CO: Westview Press.

Gadow, K. D. (1983). Effects of stimulant drugs on academic performance in hyperactive and learning disabled children. *Journal of Learning Disabilities, 16,* 290–299.

Gadow, K. D. (1985). Relative efficacy of pharmacological, behavioral, and combination treatments for enhancing academic performance. *Clinical Psychology Review, 5,* 513–533.

Gadow, K. D. (1986). *Children on medication: I. Hyperactivity, learning disabilities, and mental retardation.* San Diego: College-Hill Press.

Gadow, K. D., & Sprague, R. L. (1980, September). *An anterospective followup of hyperactive children into adolescence: Licit and illicit drug use.* Paper presented at the meeting of the American Psychological Association, Montreal.

Gadow, K. D., & Swanson, H. L. (1985). Assessing drug effects on academic performance. *Psychopharmacology Bulletin, 21,* 877–886.

Gadow, K. D., Torgeson, J., Greenstein, J., & Schell, R. (1985). Learning disabilities. In M. Hersen (Ed.), *Pharmacological and behavioral treatment: An integrated approach.* New York: Wiley & Sons.

Gage, N. L. (Ed.). (1976). *The psychology of teaching methods: The 75th yearbook of the National Society for the Study of Education, Part I.* Chicago: University of Chicago Press.

Gagne, R. (1965). *The conditions of learning.* New York: Holt, Rinehart & Winston.

Gagne, R. (1968). Instructional variables and learning outcomes. CSE Report No. 16.

Garmezy, N. (1974). Children at risk — the search for antecedents of schizophrenia: I. Conceptual models and research methods. *Schizophrenia Bulletin, 1,* 14–90.

Garner, R. (1980). Monitoring of understanding: An investigation of good and poor readers' awareness of induced miscomprehension of text. *Journal of Reading Behavior, 12,* 55–63.

Garner, R. (1981). Monitoring of passage inconsistency among poor comprehenders: A preliminary text of the "Piecemeal Processing" explanation. *Journal of Educational Research, 74,* 159–162.

Garner, R., & Kraus, C. (1982). Good and poor comprehender differences in knowing and regulating reading behaviors. *Educational Research Quarterly, 6,* 5–12.

Garner, R., & Reis, R. (1981). Monitoring and resolving comprehension obstacles: An investigation of spontaneous text lookbacks among upper-grade good and poor comprehenders. *Reading Research Quarterly, 14,* 569–582.

Garner, R., & Taylor, N. (1982). Monitoring of understanding: An investigation of attentional assistance needs at different grade and reading proficiency levels. *Reading Psychology, 3,* 1–6.

Garnett, K., & Fleischner, J. E. (1987). Mathematical disabilities. *Pediatric Annals, 16,* 159–176.

Garnett, K., Frank, B., & Fleischner, J. A. (1983a). *A strategies generalization approach to basic fact learning (Addition and subtraction lessons)* (Manual No. 3). New York: Columbia University, Teachers College, Research Institute for the Study of Learning Disabilities.

Garnett, K., Frank, B., & Fleischner, J. (1983b). *A mastery/motivation approach to basic fact learning (Addition and subtraction lessons)* (Manual No. 4). New York: Columbia University, Teachers College, Research Institute for the Study of Learning Disabilities.

Garnett, K., Frank, B., & Fleischner, J. (1983c). *A strategies generalization approach to basic fact learning (Multiplication lessons).* New York: Columbia University, Teachers College, Research Institute for the Study of Learning Disabilities.

Garnett, K., Frank, B., & Fleischner, J. (1983d). *A mastery/motivation approach to basic fact learning* (Multiplication lessons). New York: Columbia University, Teachers College, Research Institute for the Study of Learning Disabilities.

Garrett, M. K., & Crump, W. D. (1980). Peer acceptance, teacher preferences, and self-appraisal of social status among learning disabled students. *Learning Disability Quarterly, 3,* 42–48.

Gath, A. (1973). The school age siblings of Mongol children. *British Journal of Psychiatry, 123,* 161–167.

Geiger, W. L., Brownsmith, K., & Forgnone, C. (1978). Differential importance of skills for TMR students as perceived by teachers. *Education and Training of the Mentally Retarded, 13,* 259–264.

Geist, C. S., & McGrath, C. (1983). Psychosocial aspects of the adult learning disabled person in the world of work: A vocational rehabilitation perspective. *Rehabilitation Literature, 44*(7–8), 210–213.

Gelman, R., & Gallistel, C. R. (1978). *The child's understanding of numbers.* Cambridge, MA: Harvard University Press.

Gerber, M. M. (1984). The Department of Education's Sixth Annual Report to Congress on PL 94-142: Is Congress getting the full story? *Exceptional Children, 51,* 209–224.

Gerber, M. M. (1983). Learning disabilities and cognitive strategies: A case for training or constraining problem solving? *Journal of Learning Disabilities 16*(5), 255–260.

Gerber, M. M., & Semmel, M. I. (1984). Teacher as imperfect test: Reconceptualizing the referral process. *Educational Psychologist, 19,* 137–148.

Gerber, P. J., & Zinkgraf, S. A. (1982). A comparative study of social-perceptual ability in learning disabled and non-handicapped students. *Learning Disability Quarterly, 5,* 374–378.

Gershman, J. (1976). *A follow-up study of graduates of the perceptual and behavioral special classes* (Research Report No. 143). Toronto, Canada: Board of Education. (ERIC Document Reproduction Service No. ED 135 169)

Gibson, E. (1972). Reading for some purpose. In J. Kavanaugh & I. Mattingly (Eds.), *Language by ear and by eye: The relationship between speech and reading* (pp. 3–19). Cambridge, MA: MIT Press.

Gibson, E. J., & Levin, H. (1975). *The psychology of reading.* Cambridge, MA: MIT Press.

Gilhool, T. (1976). Changing public policies in the individualization of instruction: Roots and force. *Education and Training of the Mentally Retarded, 11,* 180–188.

Gillet, P. (1978). *Career education for children with learning disabilities.* San Rafael, CA: Academic Therapy Publications.

Gillet, P. (1980). Career education and the learning disabled student. *Career Development for Exceptional Individuals, 3,*(2) 67–73.

Gillet, P. (1981). *Of work and worth: Career education for the handicapped.* Salt Lake City: Olympus Publishing.

Gillingham, A., & Stillman, B. W. (1960). *Remedial training for children with specific disability in reading, spelling, and penmanship.* Cambridge, MA: Educators Publishing Service.

Ginsburg, H. P. (Ed.). (1983). *The development of mathematical thinking.* New York: Academic Press.

Giordano, G. (1978). Convergent research on language and teaching reading. *Exceptional Children, 44,* 604–611.

Gittelman, R. (1985). Controlled trials of remedial approaches to reading disability. *Journal of Child Psychology and Psychiatry and Applied Disciplines, 26*(6), 843–846.

Gittelman, R., Klein, D. F., & Feingold, I. (1983). Children with reading disorders — II. Effects of methylphenidate in combination with reading remediation. *Journal of Child Psychology and Psychiatry, 24,* 193–212.

Gittelman–Klein, R., & Klein, D. F. (1976). Methylphenidate effects in learning disabilities. *Archives of General Psychiatry, 33,* 655–664.

Glaser, R. (1972). Individuals and learning: The new aptitudes. *Educational Researcher, 6,* 5–13.

Glass, G. (1973). *Teaching decoding as separate from reading.* Garden City, NY: Adelphi

University Press.

Glass, G. V. (1979). Policy for the unpredictable (uncertainty research and policy). *Educational Researcher, 8,* 12-14.

Glass, G. V., McGaw, B., & Smith, M. L. (1981). *Meta-analysis in social research.* Beverly Hills, CA: Sage.

Glass, G. V., & Robbins, M. P. (1967). A critique of experiments of the role of neurological organization in reading performance. *Reading Research Quarterly, 3,* 5-52.

Glavin, J. P. (1974). Behaviorally oriented resource rooms: A follow-up. *The Journal of Special Education, 8,* 337-347.

Glavin, J. P., Quay, H. C., Annesley, R. F., & Werry, J. S. (1971). An experimental resource room for behavior problem children. *Exceptional Children, 38,* 131-137.

Glazzard, P. (1982). Long-range kindergarten prediction of reading achievement in first through sixth grades. *Learning Disability Quarterly, 5,* 85-88.

Gleason, G. (1981). Microcomputers in education: The state of the art. *Educational Technology, 2*(1), 7-18.

Gleitman, L., & Rozin, P. (1977). The structure and acquisition of reading. I: Relations between orthographics and the structure of reading. In A. Reber & D. Scarborough (Eds.), *Toward a psychology of reading* (pp. 1-54). Hillsdale, NJ: Lawrence Erlbaum.

Glenwick, D. S., & Barocas, R. (1979). Training impulsive children in verbal self-control by the use of natural change agents. *Journal of Special Education, 13,* 387-398.

Glusker, P. (1968). An integrational approach to spelling. In J. Arens (Ed.), *Building spelling skills in dyslexic children.* San Rafael, CA: Academic Therapy Press.

Goldman, R., & Hardin, V. (1982). The social perception of learning disabled and non-learning disabled children. *The Exceptional Child, 29*(1), 57-63.

Goldstein, H. (1975). *The social learning curriculum.* Columbus, OH: Merrill.

Goldstein, H., Moss, J. W., & Jordan, L. J. (1965). *The efficacy of special class training on the development of mentally retarded children* (Cooperative Research Progress Report No. 619). Urbana: University of Illinois, Institute for Research on Exceptional Children. (ERIC Document Reproduction Service No. ED 002 907)

Goldstein, H., & Siegle, D. (1958). *A curriculum guide for teachers of the educable mentally handicapped.* Springfield, IL: Department of Public Instruction.

Golick, M. (1973). *Deal me in! The use of playing cards in teaching learning.* New York: Jeffrey Norton.

Gollub, W. L. (1977). Family communication rituals to aid children's learning. *Langauge Arts, 54,* 655-660.

Good, T. L. (1983). Classroom research: A decade of progress. *Educational Psychologist, 18,* 127-144.

Goodlad, J. I., & Klein, M. F. (1970). *Behind the classroom door.* Worthington, OH: Jones.

Goodman, K., & Goodman, Y. (1979). Learning to read is natural. In L. Resnick & P. Weaver (Eds.), *Theory and practice in early reading* (Vol. 1). Hillsdale, NJ: Lawrence Erlbaum.

Goodman, K. S. (1967). Reading: A psycholinguistic guessing game. *Journal of the Reading Specialist, 6,* 126-133.

Goodman, L., & Hammill, D. (1973). The effectiveness of Kephart-Getman activities in developing perceptual-motor and cognitive skills. *Focus on Exceptional Children, 4,* 1-9.

Goodstein, H. A. (1984). Measurement and assessment group and individual techniques. In J. F. Cawley (Ed.), *Secondary school mathematics for the learning disabled.* Rockville, MD: Aspen Publications.

Goodstein, H. A., & Kahn, H. (1974). Pattern of achievement among children with learning difficulties. *Exceptional Children, 5,* 47-49.

Gorman, R. (1974). *The psychology of classroom learning: An inductive approach.* Columbus, OH: Merrill.

Gorney–Krupsaw, B., Atwater, J., Powell, L., & Morris, E. K. (1981). *Improving social interactions between learning disabled adolescents and teachers: A child effects approach* (Research Report No. 45). Lawrence: University of Kansas, Institute for Research in Learning Disabilities.

Gottesman, R. L. (1978). *Follow-up study of reading achievement in learning disabled children* (Final Report). Washington, DC: Department of Health, Education, and Welfare. (ERIC Document Reproduction Service No. ED 155 833)

Gottesman, R. L. (1979). Follow-up of learning disabled children. *Learning Disability Quarterly, 2,* 60–69.

Gough, P. (1972). One second of reading. In J. Kavanaugh & I. Mattingly (Eds.), *Language by ear and by eye: The relationship between speech and reading.* Cambridge, MA: MIT Press.

Gough, P., & Hillinger, M. (1980). Learning to read: An unnatural act. *Bulletin of the Orton Society, 30,* 179–196.

Gough, P. B., & Turner, W. E. (1986). Decoding, reading, and reading disability. *Remedial and Special Education, 7*(1).

Graham, F. K., & Kendall, B. S. (1960). Memory-For-Designs Test: Revised General Manual. *Perceptual and Motor Skills Monograph* (Suppl. 2), 6, 147–188.

Gralicker, B., Fishler, K., & Koch, R. (1962). Teenage reaction to a mentally retarded sibling. *American Journal of Mental Deficiency, 66,* 838–843.

Graves, D. H. (1985). All children can write. *Learning Disabilities Focus, 1*(1), 36–43.

Gray, W. S. (1952). *The twenty-fourth yearbook of the National Society for the Study of Education: Part I.* Bloomington, IL: Public School Publishing.

Green, T. (1968). *Work, leisure, and the American Schools.* New York: Random House.

Greenan, J. R. (1982). Problems and issues in delivering vocational education instruction and support services to students with learning disabilities. *Journal of Learning Disabilities, 15,* 231–235.

Greene, V. E., & Enfield, M. (1979). *Framing your thoughts.* Bloomington, MN: Winston Press.

Gregg, L. W., & Farnham–Diggory, S. (1979). How to study reading: An information processing analysis. In L. Resnick & P. Weaver (Eds.), *Theory and practice of early reading* (Vol. 3, pp. 53–70). Hillsdale, NJ: Lawrence Erlbaum.

Gresham, F. M. (1981). Social skills training with handicapped children: A review. *Review of Educational Research, 51,* 139–176.

Groen, G., & Parkman, L. A. (1972). Chronometric analysis of simple addition. *Psychological Review, 79,* 329–343.

Grossman, F. (1972). *Brothers and sisters of retarded children: An exploratory study.* Syracuse, NY: Syracuse University Press.

Gunn, S., & Peterson, C. (1978). *Therapeutic recreation program design: Principles and practices.* Englewood Cliffs, NJ: Prentice-Hall.

Guskin, S., & Spicker, H. (1968). Educational research in mental retardation. In N. O. Ellis (Ed.), *International review of mental retardation* (Vol. 3, pp. 217–278). New York: Academic Press.

Guthrie, J. T. (1973). Models of reading and reading disability. *Journal of Educational Psychology, 65,* 9–18.

Guthrie, J. T. (1978). Principles of instruction: A critique of Johnson's "Remedial Approaches to Dyslexia." In A. L. Benton & D. Pearl (Eds.), *An appraisal of current knowledge* (pp. 423–433). New York: Oxford University Press.

Guthrie, J. T., Martuza, V., & Seifert, M. (1979). Impacts of instructional time in reading. In L. Resnick & P. Weaver (Eds.), *Theory and practice of early reading* (Vol. 3, pp. 153–

178). Hillsdale, NJ: Lawrence Erlbaum.

Guthrie, J. T., & Seifert, M. (1978). Education for children with reading disabilities. In H. Myklebust (Ed.), *Progress in learning disabilities* (Vol. 4, pp. 223–225). New York: Grune & Stratton.

Hakes, D., Evans, J., & Tunmer, W. (1980). *The development of metalinguistic abilities in children*. New York: Springer-Verlag.

Hall, R. J. (1980). An information processing approach to the study of exceptional children. In B. Keogh (Ed.), *Advances in special education* (Vol. 2, pp. 79–110). Greenwich, CT: JAI.

Hall, R. J., & Humphreys, M. (1982). Research on specific learning disabilities: Deficits and remediation. *Topics in Learning and Learning Disabilities, 2,* 68–78.

Hallahan, D. P. (Ed.). (1980). Teaching exceptional children to use cognitive strategies. *Exceptional Education Quarterly, 1.*

Hallahan, D. P., & Cruickshank, W. M. (1973). *Psychoeducational foundations of learning disabilities*. Englewood Cliffs, NJ: Prentice-Hall.

Hallahan, D. P., Hall, R. J., Ianna, S. O., Kneedler, R. D., Lloyd, J. W., Loper, A. B., & Reeve, R. E. (1983). Summary of the research findings at the University of Virginia Learning Disabilities Research Institute. *Exceptional Education Quarterly, 4*(1), 95–114.

Hallahan, D. P., & Kauffman, J. (1976). *Introduction to learning disabilities: A psychobehavioral approach*. Englewood Cliffs, NJ: Prentice-Hall.

Hallahan, D. P., Lloyd, J. W., Kauffman, J. M., & Loper, A. B. (1983). Academic problems. In R. J. Morris & T. R. Kratochiwill (Eds.), *The practice of child therapy*. New York: Pergamon.

Hallahan, D. P., Lloyd, J., Kosiewicz, M. M., Kauffman, J. M., & Graves, A. W. (1979). Self-monitoring of attention as a treatment for a learning-disabled boy's off-task behavior. *Learning Disability Quarterly, 2,* 24–34.

Hallahan, D. P., & Reeve, R. C. (1980). Selective attention and distractability. In B. K. Keogh (Ed.), *Advances in special education* (Vol. 1, pp. 141–181). Greenwich, CT: JAI Press.

Halpern, N. (1984). Artificial intelligence and the education of the learning disabled. *Journal of Learning Disabilities, 17*(2), 118–120.

Hambleton, R. A. (1973). A review of testing and decision-making procedures for selected instructional programs. *ACT Technical Bulletin, No. 15.*

Hammil, D., & Bartel, N. R. (1975). *Teaching students with learning and behavioral problems*. Boston: Allyn and Bacon.

Hammill, D. D., Brown, V. I., Larsen, S. C., & Wiederholt, J. L. (1980). *Test of adolescent language*. Austin, TX: Pro-Ed.

Hammill, D. D., & Larsen, S. (1974). The effectiveness of psycholinguistic training. *Exceptional Children, 41,* 5–15.

Hammill, D. D., & Larsen, S. C. (1978). The effectiveness of psycholinguistic training: A reaffirmation of position. *Exceptional Children, 44,* 402–414.

Hammill, D. D., & Larsen, S. C. (1983). *Test of written language*. Austin, TX: Pro-Ed.

Hanna, P. R., Hodges, R. F., & Hanna, J. S. (1971). *Spelling: Structures and strategies*. Boston: Houghton Mifflin.

Hannaford, A., & Sloane, E. (1981). Microcomputers: Powerful learning tool with proper programming. *Teaching Exceptional Children, 14*(2), 54–56.

Hardin, V. (1978). Ecological assessment and interaction for learning disabled students. *Learning Disability Quarterly, 1,* 15–20.

Hargis, C. H. (1982). Word recognition development. *Focus on Exceptional Children, 14*(9), 1–8.

Haring, N. G., & Hauck, M. A. (1969). Improved learning conditions in the establishment of reading skills with disabled readers. *Exceptional Children, 35,* 34–352.

Harris, A., & Sarver, B. (1966). The CRAFT project: Instructional time in reading research. *Reading Research Quarterly, 2,* 27–57.

Harris, A. J. (1982). How many kinds of reading disability are there? *Journal of Learning Disabilities, 19,* 456–460.

Harris, F. C., & Lahey, B. B. (1978). A method for combining occurrence and nonoccurrence interobserver agreement scores. *Journal of Behavior Analysis, 11,* 523–527.

Harris, K. R. (1985). Conceptual, methodological, and clinical issues in cognitive-behavioral assessment. *Journal of Abnormal Child Psychology, 13,* 373–390.

Harris, L. A., & Sherman, J. A. (1972). Effects of homework assignments and consequences on performance in social studies and mathematics. *Journal of Applied Behavior Analysis, 7,* 505–519.

Harris, L. A., Sherman, J. A., Henderson, D. G., & Harris, M. S. (1973). *Effects of peer tutoring on the spelling performance of elementary classroom students. A new direction for education: Behavior analysis.* Lawrence: University of Kansas, Support and Development Center for Follow Through.

Hart, B. M., & Risley, T. R. (1968). Establishing use of descriptive adjectives in the spontaneous speech of disadvantaged preschool children. *Journal of Applied Behavior Analysis, 1,* 109–120.

Hartman, D. P. (1977). Considerations in the choice of interobserver reliability estimates. *Journal of Applied Behavioral Analysis, 10,* 103–116.

Harvey, B. (1983). Stop saying "computer literacy." One man's controversial opinion. *Classroom Computer News, 3*(6), 56–57.

Haworth, M. (1971). The effects of rhythmic-motor training and gross-motor training on the reading and writing abilities of educable mentally retarded children. *Dissertation Abstracts International, 31,* 3391-A.

Hayden, D. A., Vance, H. B., & Irwin, J. J. (1982). A special education management system. *Journal of Learning Disabilities, 15*(7), 428–429.

Hayden, D. L. (1972). *NRRC/P Diagnostic prescriptive instructional data bank for teachers of handicapped children.* Harrisburg, PA: The National Regional Resource Center of Pennsylvania.

Hazel, J. S., Schumaker, J. B., & Sheldon, J. (1984). *Evaluation of a training program for court service officers for the treatment of learning disabled and other social skill deficient adolescents* (Research Report #62). Lawrence: The University of Kansas, Research Institute for Research in Learning Disabilities.

Hazel, J. S., Schumaker, J. B., Sherman, J. A., & Sheldon, J. (1982). Application of a group training program in social skills and problem solving skills to learning disabled and non-learning disabled youth. *Learning Disability Quarterly, 5,* 398–408.

Hazel, J. S., Schumaker, J. B., Sherman, J. A., & Sheldon-Wildgen, J. (1981). The development and evaluation of a group training program for teaching social and problem solving skills to court-adjudicated youth. In D. Upper & S. M. Ross (Eds.), *Behavioral group therapy.* Champaign, IL: Research Press.

Hazel, J. S., Smalter, M. C., & Schumaker, J. B. (1983, October). *A learner-managed social skills curriculum for mildly handicapped young adults.* Presentation at the International Conference on Learning Disabilities, San Francisco.

Hechtman, L., Weiss, G., & Perlman, T. (1984). Young adult outcome of hyperactive children who received long-term stimulant treatment. *Journal of the American Academy of Child Psychiatry, 23,* 261–269.

Hechtman, L., Weiss, G., Perlman, T., Hopkins, J., & Wener, A. (1979). Hyperactive children in young adulthood: A controlled prospective ten-year follow-up. *International Journal of Mental Health, 8,* 52–66.

Hedges, L. V., & Olkin, I. (1980). Vote-counting methods in research synthesis. *Psy-*

chological Bulletin, 88, 359-369.

Hegge, T. G., Kirk, S., & Kirk, W. (1936). *Remedial reading drills.* Ann Arbor, MI: Wahr.

Heller, K. A., Holtzman, W. H., & Messick, S. (1982). *Placing children in special education: A strategy for equity.* Washington, DC: National Academy Press.

Helms, H. B. (1970). Big chalkboard for big movement. In J. Arena (Ed.), *Building handwriting skills in dyslexic children.* San Rafael, CA: Academic Therapy.

Helwig, J. (1976). Measurement of visual-verbal feedback on changes in manuscript letter formation. *Dissertation Abstracts International, 36,* 5196-A.

Hemry, F. P. (1973). Effect of reinforcement conditions on a discrimination learning task for impulsive versus reflective children. *Child Development, 44,* 657-660.

Henderson, E. H. (1980). Word knowledge and reading disability. In E. J. Henderson & J. W. Beers (Eds.), *Developmental aspects of learning to spell.* Newark, DE: International Reading Associates.

Heron, T. E., & Heward, N. (1982). Ecologic assessment: Implications for teachers of learning disabled students. *Learning Disability Quarterly, 5,* 117-125.

Herr, C. M. (1976). Mainstreaming — Is it effective: A follow-up study of learning disabled children. *Division for Children with Learning Disabilities Newsletter, 2,* 22-29.

Hersen, M., & Barlow, D. (1976). *Strategies for studying behavioral change.* New York: Pergamon Press.

Heshusius, L. (1982). At the heart of the advocacy dilemma: A mechanistic word view. *Exceptional Children, 49,* 6-13.

Heshusius, L. (1986). Paradigm shifts and special education: A response to Ulman and Rosenberg. *Exceptional Children, 52,* 461-465.

Hewett, F. M., Taylor, F., & Artuso, A. (1968). The Madison plan really swings. *Today's Education, 59,* 15-17.

Hiebert, B., Wong, B. Y. L., & Hunter, M. (1982). Affective influences on learning-disabled adolescents. *Learning Disability Quarterly, 5*(4), 334-343.

Hillman, H. H., & Snowdon, R. L. (1960). Part-time classes for young backward readers. *British Journal of Educational Psychology, 30,* 168-172.

Hines, C. W., & Bruno, G. (1985). LD career success after high school. *Academic Therapy, 21*(2), 171-176.

Hines, C. W., & Hohenshil, T. A. (1985). Career development and career education for handicapped students: A reexamination. *Vocational Guidance Quarterly, 34*(1), 31-40.

Hinton, G. G., & Knights, R. M. (1971). Children with learning problems: Academic prediction and adjustment three years after assessment. *Exceptional Children, 37,* 513-519.

Hodges, R. E. (1977). *Learning to spell — Theory and research into practice.* Urbana, IL: NCTE.

Hofmeister, A., & Thorkildsen, R. (1981). Videodisc technology and the preparation of special education teachers. *Teacher Education and Special Education, 4*(3), 34-39.

Holt, M., Kocsis, J., & Reisman, K. (1980). *Special education data base information retrieval system.* Dallas, TX: Central Dallas Independent School District, Research and Evaluation Department.

Holyoak, K. J., & Gordon, P. C. (1984). Information processing and social cognition. In R. S. Wyer, Jr., & T. K. Srull (Eds.), *Handbook of social cognition* (pp. 39-70). Hillsdale, NJ: Lawrence Erlbaum.

Holznagel, D. (1981). Which courseware is right for you? *Microcomputing, 5*(10), 38-40.

Hopps, H. (1981). Behavioral assessment of exceptional children's development. *Exceptional Education Quarterly, 4,* 31-43.

Horn, W. F., O'Donnell, J. P., & Vitulano, L. A. (1983). Long-term follow-up studies of learning disabled persons. *Journal of Learning Disabilities, 16,* 542-555.

Horowitz, E. C. (1981). Popularity, decentering ability and role-taking skills in learning disabled and normal children. *Learning Disability Quarterly, 4,* 23–30.

Howe, C. (1981). From leisure ethic to reindustrialization. *Leisure Today, 12,* 23–39.

Hoyt, K. B. (1980, June 24). *Career education for persons with visual handicaps.* Paper presented at the Helen Keller Centennial Conference, Boston.

Huessy, H. R., Metoyer, M., & Townsend, M. (1974). 8-10 year follow-up of 84 children treated for behavioral disorder in rural Vermont. *Acta Paedopsychiatrica, 40,* 230–235.

Huey, E. B. (1968). *The psychology and pedagogy of reading.* Cambridge, MA: MIT Press.

Humes, C. W., & Bronner, G. (1985). LD career success after high school. *Academic Therapy, 21*(2), 171–176.

Hummel, J. W., & Balcom, F. W. (1984). Microcomputers: Not just a place for a practice. *Journal of Learning Disabilities, 17*(7), 432–434.

Hummel, J. W., & Farr, S. D. (1985). Options for creating and modifying CAI software for the handicapped. *Journal of Learning Disabilities, 18*(3), 166–168.

Hunt, K. W. (1977). Early blooming and late blooming syntactic structures. In C. R. Cooper & L. Odell (Eds.), *Evaluating writing.* Urbana, IL: NCTE.

Iano, R. P. (1986). The study of development of teaching: With implications for the advancement of special education. *Remedial and Special Education, 7*(5), 50–61.

Ingram, C. P. (1935). *Education of the slow-learning child.* Yonkers: World Book Co.

Ingram, T. T. S. (1969). Developmental disorders of speech. In P. Vinken & G. Bruyn (Eds.), *Handbook of clinical neurology* (Vol. 4). Amsterdam: North Holland.

Institute for Career and Leisure Development. (1979). *Special education for leisure fulfillment — A facilitator's instructional guide.* Washington, DC.

Ito, H. R. (1980). Long-term effects of resource room programs on learning disabled children's reading. *Journal of Learning Disabilities, 13,* 322–326.

Ito, H. R. (1981). After the resource room — then what? *Academic Therapy, 16,* 283–287.

Iwata, B. A., & Bailey, J. S. (1974). Reward versus cost token systems: An analysis of the effects on students and teacher. *Journal of Applied Behavior Analysis, 7,* 564–576.

Jackson, G. B. (1980). Methods for integrative reviews. *Review of Educational Research, 50,* 438–460.

Jastak, J. F., & Jastak, S. R. (1978). *The Wide Range Achievement Test* (Rev. Ed.). Wilmington, DE: Guidance Associates.

Jastak, S., & Wilkinson, G. (1984). *The Wide Range Achievement Test—Revised: Administration manual.* Wilmington, DE: Jastak Associates.

Jenkins, J. R., & Pany, D. (1978). Standardized achievement tests: How useful for special education? *Exceptional Children, 44,* 448–453.

Jennings, D. L. (1981). *The effects of attributions in social settings: Changes in strategy use, expectations, and performance quality following failure.* Unpublished manuscript.

Johnson, D. J. (1978). Remedial approaches to dyslexia. In A. L. Benton & D. Pearl (Eds.), *Dyslexia: An appraisal of current knowledge* (pp. 397–421). New York: Oxford University Press.

Johnson, D. J., & Myklebust, H. (1967). *Learning disabilities: Educational principles and practices.* New York: Grune & Stratton.

Johnson, G. O. (1962). Special education for the mentally handicapped — A paradox. *Exceptional Children, 29,* 62–69.

Johnson, W. T. (1977). *The Johnson handwriting program.* Cambridge, MA: Educators Publishing Service.

Jones, J. C., Trap, J., & Cooper, J. (1977). Technical report: Students self-recording of manuscript letter strokes. *Journal of Applied Behavior Analysis, 10,* 509–514.

Jones, R. L. (1974). Student views of special placement and their own special classes: A clarification. *Exceptional Children, 41,* 22–29.

Jongsma, E. (1971). *The cloze procedure as a teaching technique.* Newark, DE: International Reading Association.

Joyce, B., & Weil, M. (1972). *Models of teaching*. Englewood Cliffs, NJ: Prentice-Hall.

Kagan, J. (1966). Reflection-impulsivity: The generality and dynamics of conceptual tempo. *Journal of Abnormal Psychology, 71,* 17-24.

Kaliski, L., & Iohga, R. (1970). A musical approach to handwriting. In J. Arena (Ed.), *Building handwriting skills in dyslexic children.* San Rafael, CA: Academic Therapy.

Kaplan, ___. (1964). *The conduct of inquiry.* San Francisco: Chandler.

Kaslow, F. W. (1979). Therapy within the family constellation. In W. Adamson & K. K. Adamson (Eds.), *A handbook for specific learning disabilities* (pp. 313-332). New York: Gardner Press.

Katz, J. (1986). *Arithmetic problem solving strategies of kindergarten children.* Unpublished doctoral dissertation, Teachers College, Columbia University, New York.

Kaufman, K. F., & O'Leary, K. D. (1972). Reward, cost, and self-evaluation procedures for disruptive adolescents in a psychiatric hospital school. *Journal of Applied Behavior Analysis, 5,* 293-309.

Kaufman, M. E., & Alberto, P. A. (1976). Research on efficacy of special education for the mentally retarded. In N. R. Ellis (Ed.), *International review of research in mental retardation* (Vol. 8, pp. 225-255). New York: Academic Press.

Kaufman, M. J., Gottlieb, J., Agard, J. A., & Kukic, M. B. (1975). Mainstreaming: Toward an explication of the construct. In E. Meyen, G. Vergason, & R. Whelan (Eds.), *Alternatives for teaching exceptional children* (pp. 35-54). Denver: Love.

Kavale, K., & Schreiner, R. (1978). Psycholinguistic implications for beginning reading instruction. *Language Arts, 55,* 34-40.

Kavale, K. A. (1981a). Functions of the Illinois Test of Psycholinguistic Abilities (ITPA): Are they trainable? *Exceptional Children, 47,* 496-510.

Kavale, K. A. (1981b). The relationship between auditory perceptual skills and reading ability: A meta-analysis. *Journal of Learning Disabilities, 14,* 539-546.

Kavale, K. A. (1982a). The efficacy of stimulant drug treatment for hyperactivity: A meta-analysis. *Journal of Learning Disabilities, 15,* 280-289.

Kavale, K. A. (1982b). Meta-analysis of the relationship between visual perceptual skills and reading achievement. *Journal of Learning Disablities, 15,* 42-51.

Kavale, K. A. (1982c). Psycholinguistic training programs: Are there differential treatment effects? *The Exceptional Child, 29,* 21-30.

Kavale, K. A., & Andreassen, E. (1984). Factors in diagnosing the learning disabled: Analysis of judgmental policies. *Journal of Learning Disabilities, 17,* 273-278.

Kavale, K. A., & Forness, S. R. (1983). Hyperactivity and diet treatment: A meta-analysis of the Feingold hypothesis. *Journal of Learning Disabilities, 16,* 324-330.

Kavale, K. A., & Forness, S. R. (1984). A meta-analysis assessing the validity of Wechsler scale profiles and recategorizations: Patterns or parodies? *Learning Disability Quarterly, 7,* 136-156.

Kavale, K. A., & Forness, S. R. (1985). *The science of learning disabilities.* San Diego: College-Hill Press.

Kavale, K. A., & Forness, S. R. (1987). The far side of heterogeneity: A critical analysis of empirical subtyping research in learning disabilities. *Journal of Learning Disabilities, 20,* 274-382.

Kavale, K. A., & Forness, S. R. (1987). Substance over style: A quantitative synthesis assessing the efficacy of modality testing and teaching. *Exceptional Children, 54,* 228-234.

Kavale, K. A., & Glass, G. V. (1981). Meta-analysis and the integration of research in special education. *Journal of Learning Disabilities, 14,* 531-538.

Kavale, K. A., & Matson, P. D. (1983). One jumped off the balance beam: Meta-analysis of perceptual-motor training. *Journal of Learning Disabilities, 16,* 165-173.

Kazdin, A., & Erickson, B. (1975). Developing responsiveness to instructions in severely and profoundly retarded residents. *Journal of Behavior Therapy and Experimental Psychiatry, 6,* 17–21.

Keeney, A. H., & Keeney, M. T. (1968). *Dyslexia: Diagnosis and treatment of reading disorders.* St. Louis: Mosby.

Kendall, C. R., Borkowski, J. G., & Cavanaugh, J. C. (1980). Maintenance and generalization of an interrogative strategy by EMR children. *Intelligence, 4,* 270.

Kendall, J. R., & Mason, J. M. (1982). Metacognition from the historical context of teaching reading. *Topics in Learning and Learning Disabilities, 2,* 82–89.

Kent, R. M., & O'Leary, K. D. (1976). A controlled evaluation of behavior modification with conduct problem children. *Journal of Consulting and Clinical Psychology, 44,* 586–596.

Keogh, B. K., Major–Kingsley, S., Omori–Gordon, H., & Reid, H. (1982). *A system of marker variables for the field of learning disabilities.* Syracuse, NY: Syracuse University Press.

Kephart, N. C. (1971). *The slow learner in the classroom.* Columbus, OH: Merrill.

Kerns, K., & Decker, S. (1985). Multifactorial assessment of reading disability: Identifying the best predictors. *Perceptual and Motor Skills 60*(3), 747–753.

Kew, S. (1975). *Handicap and family crisis: A study of siblings of handicapped children.* London: Longman.

Kimmel, G. M. (1968). Teaching spelling in a splash of color. In J. Arena (Ed.), *Building spelling skills in dyslexic children.* San Rafael, CA: Academic Therapy.

Kimmel, G. M. (1970). Handwriting readiness: Motor-coordinative practices. In J. Arena (Ed.), *Building handwriting skills in dyslexic children.* San Rafael, CA: Academic Therapy.

King, D. (1985). *Writing skills for the adolescent.* Cambridge, MA: Educators Publishing Service.

Kirby, F. D., & Shields, F. (1972). Modification of arithmetic response rate and attending behavior in a seventh grade student. *Journal of Applied Behavior Analysis, 5,* 78–84.

Kirk, S. A. (1964). Research in education. In H. A. Stevens & R. Heber (Eds.), *Mental retardation: A review of research* (pp. 57–99). Chicago: University of Chicago Press.

Kirk, S. A., & Elkins, J. (1975). Characteristics of children enrolled in child service demonstration centers. *Journal of Learning Disabilities, 8,* 630–637.

Kirk, S. A., & Kirk, W. D. (1971). *Psycholinguistic learning disabilities: Diagnosis and remediation.* Urbana: University of Illinois Press.

Kirk, S. A., McCarthy, J. J., & Kirk, W. D. (1968). *Illinois Test of Psycholinguistic Abilities.*(Rev. ed.). Urbana: University of Illinois Press.

Kirk, U. (1978). Rule-based instruction: A cognitive approach to beginning handwriting instruction. *Dissertation Abstracts International, 39,* 113-A.

Klein, N. K., Pasch, M., & Frew, T. W. (1979). *Curriculum analysis and design for retarded learners.* Columbus, OH: Merrill.

Knapczyk, D., & Yoppi, J. (1975). Development of cooperative and competitive play responses in developmentally disabled children. *American Journal on Mental Deficiency, 80,* 245–255.

Knight, E. (1975). *KISP: Knight Individualized Spelling Program.* Cambridge, MA: Educators Publishing Service.

Kohn, M. (1977). *Social competence, symptoms and underachievement in childhood: A longitudinal perspective.* Washington, DC: Winston.

Kohn, M., & Rosman, B. L. (1972). Relationship of preschool social–emotional functioning to later intellectual development. *Developmental Psychology, 6,* 445–452.

Kolich, E. (1985). Microcomputer technology with the learning disabled: A review of the literature. *Journal of Learning Disability, 18*(7), 428–431.

Koppell, S. (1979). Testing the attentional deficit notion. *Journal of Learning Disablities, 12,* 43–48.

Koppitz, E. M. (1971). *Children with learning disabilities: A five year follow-up study.* New York: Grune & Stratton.

Kornblum, H. (1982). A social worker's role with mothers of language disordered preschool children. *Journal of Learning Disabilities, 15,* 406–408.

Kornetsky, C. (1975). Minimal brain dysfunction and drugs. In W. Cruickshank & D. Hallahan (Eds.), *Perceptual learning disabilities in children: Research and theory* (Vol. 2, pp. 447–481). Syracuse, NY: Syracuse University Press.

Kosc, L. (1974). Developmental dyscalculia. *Journal of Learning Disabilities, 7,* 164–177.

Kottmeyer, W. (1959). *Teacher's guide for remedial reading.* St. Louis: Webster Publishing.

Kozloff, M. A. (1979). *A program for families of children with learning and behavioral problems.* New York: Wiley.

Kraus, R. (1978). *Recreation and leisure in a modern society.* Santa Monica, CA: Goodyear Publishing.

Kubie, L. S. (1964). Research on protecting preconscious functions in education. In A. H. Passow (Ed.), *Nurturing individual potential.* Washington, DC: Association for Supervision and Curriculum Development.

Kubler–Ross, E. (1969). *On death and dying.* New York: Macmillan.

LaBerge, D., & Samuels, S. J. (1974). Toward a theory of automatic information processing in reading. *Cognitive Psychology, 6,* 293–323.

Labouvie, E. W. (1975). The dialectical nature of measurement activities in the behavioral sciences. *Human Development, 18,* 205–222.

LaGreca, A. M., & Mesibov, G. B. (1981). Facilitating interpersonal functioning with peers in learning disabled children. *Journal of Learning Disabilities, 14,* 197–199, 238.

Lahey, B. B. (1976). Behavior modification with learning disabilities and related problems. In M. Hersen, R. Eisler, & P. Miller (Eds.), *Progress in behavior modification* (Vol. 3, pp. 173–206). New York: Academic Press.

Lahey, B. B. (1977). Research on the role of reinforcement in reading instruction: Some measurement and methodological difficulties. *Corrective and Social Psychiatry, 23,* 27–32.

Lahey, B. B. (1979). *Behavior therapy with hyperactive and learning disabled children.* New York: Oxford University Press.

Lahey, B. B., Busemeyer, M., O'Hara, C., & Beggs, V. E. (1977). Treatment of severe perceptual-motor disorders in children diagnosed as learning disabled. *Behavior Modification, 1,* 123–140.

Lahey, B. B., Delameter, A., Kupfer, D. L., & Hobbs, S. A. (1978). Behavioral aspects of learning disabilities and hyperactivity. *Education and Urban Society, 10,* 447–499.

Lahey, B. B., & Drabman, R. S. (1974). Facilitation of the acquisition and retention of sight-word vocabulary through token reinforcement. *Journal of Applied Behavior Analysis, 7,* 307–312.

Lahey, B. B., Kupfer, D. L., Beggs, V. E., & Landon, D. (1982). Do learning-disabled children exhibit peripheral deficits in selective attention?: Analysis of eye movements during reading. *Journal of Abnormal Child Psychology, 10,* 1–10.

Lahey, B. B., McNees, M. P., & Brown, S. C. (1973). Modification of deficits in reading for comprehension. *Journal of Applied Behavior Analysis, 6,* 475–480.

Lahey, B. B., McNees, M. P., & Schnelle, J. F. (1977). The functional independence of three reading behaviors: A behavior systems analysis. *Corrective and Social Psychiatry, 23,* 44–47.

Lahey, B. B., Vosk, B. N., & Habif, V. L. (1981). Behavioral assessment of learning disabled children: A rationale and strategy. *Behavioral Assessment, 3,* 3–14.

Lahey, B. B., Weller, D. R., & Brown, W. R. (1973). The behavior analysis approach to reading: Phonics discriminations. *Journal of Reading Behavior, 5,* 200–206.

Lambert, N., & Sandoval, J. (1980). The prevalence of learning disabilities in a sample of children considered hyperactive. *Journal of Abnormal Child Psychology, 8,* 33–50.

Lamkin, J. S. (1980). *Getting started: Career education activities for exceptional students (K–9).* Reston, VA: The Council for Exceptional Children.

Landers, S. (1987). Researchers struggling to understand learning disabilities. *APA Monitor, 18*(3), 28–29.

Larsen, S. C., & Hammill, D. D. (1976). *Test of written spelling.* Austin, TX: Pro-Ed.

Larson, C. H. (1981, January). *EBCE State of Iowa dissemination model for MD and LD students.* Ft. Dodge: Iowa Central Community College.

Larson, S. C. (1976). The learning disabilities specialist: Roles and responsibilities. *Journal of Learning Disabilities, 9,* 37–47.

Lasagna, L. (1974). A plea for the "naturalistic" study of medicine (Editorial). *European Journal of Clinical Pharmacology, 7,* 153.

Lee, L. (1974). *Developmental sentence analysis.* Evanston, IL: Northwestern University Press.

Lee, L. (1975). *Interactive language developmental teaching.* Evanston, IL: Northwestern University Press.

Lefton, L. A., Nagle, R. J., Johnson, G., & Fisher, D. G. (1979). Eye movement dynamics of good and poor readers: Then and now. *Journal of Reading Behavior, 11,* 319–328.

Leggett, C. L. (1978). Special education and career education: A call for a new partnership. *Education and Training of the Mentally Retarded, 13,* 430–431.

Lehtinen–Rogan, L., & Hartman, L. D. (1976). *A follow-up study of learning disabled children as adolescents* (Final Report). Washington, DC: Department of Health, Education, and Welfare, Bureau of Education of the Handicapped. (ERIC Document Reproduction Service No. ED 163 728)

Leinhardt, G., & Pallay, A. (1982). Restrictive educational settings. *Review of Educational Research, 52,* 557–578.

Leinhardt, G., Zigmond, N., & Cooley, W. (1981). Reading instruction and its effects. *American Educational Research Journal, 18,* 343–361.

Leisure Information Service (1976). *A systems model for developing a leisure education program for handicapped children and youth (K–12).* Washington, DC: Hawkins and Associates.

Leone, P., Lovitt, T., & Hansen, C. (1981). A descriptive followup study of learning disabled boys. *Learning Disability Quarterly, 4,* 152–162.

Lerer, R. M., Lerer, M. P., & Artner, J. (1977). The effects of methylphenidate on the handwriting of children with minimal brain dysfunction. *Journal of Pediatrics, 91,* 127–132.

Lesgold, A. M., & Perfetti, C. A. (1981). *Interactive processes in reading.* Hillsdale, NJ: Lawrence Erlbaum.

Levin, E. K., Zigmond, N., & Birch, J. W. (1985). A follow-up study of 52 learning disabled adolescents. *Journal of Learning Disabilities, 18,* 2–7.

Levin, J. R. (1973). Inducing comprehension in poor readers: A test of a recent model. *Journal of Educational Psychology, 65,* 19–24.

Levy, B. A. (1978). Speech processing during reading. In A. Lesgold, J. Pellegrino, S. Fokkema, & R. Glaser (Eds.), *Cognitive psychology and instruction.* New York: Plenum.

Levy, B. A. (1980). Interactive processes during reading. In A. Lesgold & C. Perfetti (Eds.), *Interactive processes in reading* (pp. 1–35). Hillsdale, NJ: Lawrence Erlbaum.

Levy, H. B. (1973). *Square pegs, round holes: The learning-disabled child in the classroom and the home.* Boston: Little, Brown.

Levy, J. (1982). Behavioral observation techniques in assessing change in therapeutic recreation/play settings. *Therapeutic Recreation Journal, 5,* 170–173.

Lew, F. (1977). The Feingold diet, experienced [letter]. *Medical Journal of Australia, 1,* 190.

Liberman, I., & Shankweiler, D. (1979). Speech, the alphabet, and teaching to read. In L. Resnick & P. Weaver (Eds.), *Theory and practice of early reading* (Vol. 2, pp. 109–132). Hillsdale, NJ: Lawrence Erlbaum.

Liberman, I., Shankweiler, D., Liberman, A., Fowler, C., & Fischer, F. (1977). Phonetic segmentation and recording in the beginning reader. In A. Reber & D. Scarborough (Eds.), *Toward a psychology of reading* (pp. 207–225). Hillsdale, NJ: Lawrence Erlbaum.

Liberman, I. Y. (1973). Segmentation of the spoken word and reading acquisition. *Bulletin of the Orton Society, 23,* 65–77.

Liberman, I. Y. (1982). A language-oriented view of reading and its disabilities. In H. Myklebust (Ed.), *Progress in learning disabilities* (Vol. 5, pp. 81–101). New York: Grune & Stratton.

Libet, J. M., & Lewinsohn, P. M. (1973). Concept of social skills with special reference to the behavior of depressed persons. *Journal of Consulting and Clinical Psychology, 40,* 304–312.

Licht, B. G. (1983). Cognitive-motivational factors that contribute to the achievement of learning-disabled children. *Journal of Learning Disabilities, 16,* 483–490.

Lieber, J., & Semmel, M. (1985). Effectiveness of computer application to instruction with mildly handicapped learners: A review. *Remedial and Special Education, 6*(5), 5–12.

Lieby, J. (1981). *Automatization, cognitive style, and the selection of an instructional method for teaching basic facts to learning disabled and compensatory education students.* Unpublished doctoral dissertation, Teachers College, Columbia University, New York.

Light, R. J., & Smith, P. V. (1971). Accumulating evidence: procedures for resolving contradictions among different research studies. *Harvard Educational Review, 41,* 429–471.

Lincoln, A. L. (1949). *Diagnostic Spelling Test, Form 3.* New York: Educational Records Bureau.

Lincoln, A. L. (1959). *Lincoln Intermediate Spelling Test, Form A for grades 4–8.* New York: Educational Records Bureau.

Lindquist, M. M., Carpenter, T. P., Silver, E. A., & Matthews, W. (1983). The third national mathematics assessment: Results and implications for elementary and middle schools. *Arithmetic Teacher, 31,* 14–19.

Lindsey, J. D., & Kerlin, M. A. (1979). Learning disabilities and reading disorders: A brief review of the secondary level literature. *Journal of Learning Disabilities, 12,* 408–415.

Lindvall, C., & Cox, R. (1970). The IPI evaluation program. AERA monograph series on *Curriculum Evaluation.* Chicago: Rand McNally.

Litman, T. (1974). The family as a basic unit in health and medical care: A social-behavioral overview. *Social Science and Medicine, 8,* 495–519.

Lloyd, J. (1975). The pedagogical orientation: An argument for improving instruction. *Journal of Learning Disabilities, 8*(2), 74–78.

Lloyd, J. (1980). Academic instruction and cognitive behavior modification: The need for attack strategy training. *Exceptional Education Quarterly, 1*(1), 53–63.

Lloyd, J., Cullinan, D., Heins, E. D., & Epstein, M. H. (1980). Direct instruction: Effects on oral and written language comprehension. *Learning Disability Quarterly, 3*(4), 70–76.

Lloyd, J., Saltzman, N. J., & Kauffman, J. M. (1981). Predictable generalization in academic learning as a result of preskills and strategy training. *Learning Disablity Quarterly, 4,* 203–216.

Lloyd, J. W. (1984). How shall we individualize instruction — Or should we? *Remedial and Special Education, 5*(1), 7–15.

Lloyd, J. W. (1987). The art and science of research on teaching. *Remedial and Special Education, 8*(1), 44–46.

Lloyd-Jones, R. (1977). Primary trait scoring. In C. R. Cooper & L. Odell (Eds.), *Evaluation writing.* Urbana, IL: NCTE.

Loney, J., Kramer, J., & Kosier, T. (1981, August). *Medicated vs. unmedicated hyperactive adolescents: Academic, delinquent and symptomatological outcome.* Paper presented at the meeting of the American Psychological Association, Los Angeles.

Loney, J., Kramer, J., & Milich, R. (1981). The hyperactive child grows up: Predictors of symptoms, delinquency, and achievement at followup. In K. D. Gadow & J. Loney (Eds.), *Psychosocial aspects of drug treatment for hyperactivity.* Boulder, CO: Westview Press.

Lopez, M., & Clyde-Snyder, M. (1983). Higher education for learning disabled students. *NASPA Journal, 20*(4), 34–39.

Lovitt, T. C., & Smith, D. D. (1974). Using withdrawal of positive reinforcement to alter subtraction performance. *Exceptional Children, 40,* 357–358.

Ludlow, C., Rapoport, J., Bessich, S., & Mikkelsen, E. (1980). The differential effects dextroamphetamine on the language and performance in hyperactive and normal children. In R. Knights & D. Bakker (Eds.), *Treatment of hyperactive and learning disordered children: Current research* (pp. 185–206). Baltimore: University Park Press.

Lund, K. A., Foster, G. E., & McCall-Perez, F. C. (1978). The effectiveness of psycholinguistic training: A reevaluation. *Exceptional Children, 44,* 310–319.

Lyon, G. R., (1983). Learning disabled readers: Identification of subgroups. In H. Myklebust (Ed.), *Progress in learning disabilities* (Vol. 5, pp. 103–134). New York: Grune & Stratton.

Lyon, G. R. (1985a). Educational validation of learning disability subtypes. In B. Rourke (Ed.), *The neuropsychology of learning disabilities: Essentials of subtype analysis* (pp. 228–253). New York: Guilford Press.

Lyon, G. R. (1985b). Neuropsychology and learning disabilities. *Neurology and Neurosurgery Update, 5,* 2–8.

Lyon, G. R., & Risucci, D. (in press). Classification issues in learning disabilities. In K. Kavale (Ed.), *Learning disabilities: State of the art and practice.* San Diego: College-Hill Press.

Lyon, G. R., Rietta, S., Watson, B., Porch, B., & Rhodes, J. (1981). Selected linguistic and perceptual abilities of empirically derived subgroups of learning disabled readers. *Journal of School Psychology, 19,* 152–166.

Lyon, G. R., Stewart, N., & Freedman, D. (1982) Neuropsychological characteristics of empirically derived subgroups of learning disabled readers. *Journal of Clinical Neuropsychology, 4,* 343–365.

Lyon, R., & Watson, B. (1981). Empirically derived subgroups of learning-disabled readers: Diagnostic characteristics. *Journal of Learning Disabilities, 14,* 256–261.

Mackenzie, D. E. (1983). Research for school improvement: An appraisal of some recent trends. *Educational Researcher, 12*(4), 5–17.

Mackworth, J., & Mackworth, N. (1974). How children read: Matching by sight and sound. *Journal of Reading Behavior, 6,* 295–305.

MacMillan, D. L. (1971). Special education for the mildly retarded: Servant or savant? *Focus on Exceptional Children, 2,* 1–11.

MacMillan, D. L., & Semmel, M. I. (1977). Evaluation of mainstreaming programs. *Focus on Exceptional Children, 9,* 1–14.

Madden, N. A., & Slavin, R. E. (1983). Mainstreaming students with mild handicaps: Academic and social outcomes. *Review of Educational Research, 53*(4), 519–569.

Madison, B. D. (1970). A kinesthetic technique for handwriting development. In J. Arena (Ed.), *Building handwriting skills in dyslexic children.* San Rafael, CA: Academic Therapy.

Madsen, C. H., Becker, W. C., & Thomas, D. R. (1968). Rules, praise, and ignoring: Elements of elementary classroom control. *Journal of Applied Behavior Analysis, 1,* 139–150.

Mager, R. (1962). *Preparing instructional objectives.* San Francisco: Fearon.

Maheady, L., & Maitland, G. E. (1982). Assessing social perception abilities in learning disabled students. *Learning Disability Quarterly, 5,* 363–370.

Major-Kinglsey, S. (1982). *Learning disabled boys as young adults: Achievement, adjustment, and aspirations.* Unpublished doctoral dissertation, University of California, Los Angeles.

Mandler, G. (1981, August). *What's cognitive psychology? What isn't?* Invitational address, Division of Philosophical Psychology, American Psychological Association convention, Los Angeles.

Mangrum, C. T., & Strichart, S. S. (1984). *College and the learning disabled student.* Orlando, FL: Grune & Stratton

Mangrum, C. T., & Strichart, S. S. (1985). *Peterson's guide to colleges with programs for learning-disabled students.* Princeton, NJ: Peterson's Guides.

Margalit, M. (1982). Learning disabled children and their families: Strategies of extension and adaptation of family therapy. *Journal of Learning Disabilities, 15,* 594–595.

Marholin, D., & Steinman, W. M. (1977). Stimulus control in the classroom as a function of the behavior reinforced. *Journal of Applied Behavior Analysis, 10,* 465–478.

Markman, E. M. (1977). Realizing that you don't understand: A preliminary investigation. *Child Development, 43,* 986–992.

Markman, E. M. (1979). Realizing that you don't understand: Elementary school children's awareness of inconsistencies. *Child Development, 50,* 643–655.

Marland, S. P., Jr. (1971). Career education now. Speech presented before the annual convention of the National Association of Secondary School Principals, Houston.

Martin, F. (1971). TRIC — A computer-based information storage and retrieval for the field of therapeutic recreation service. *Therapeutic Recreation Journal, 5,* 170–173.

Martin, F. (1977). Therapeutic recreation research: An analysis of research content area, methodology and setting. In G. Fain & G. Hitzhusen (Eds.), *Therapeutic recreation: State of the art* (pp. 83–91). Arlington, VA: National Recreation and Park Association.

Martino, L., & Johnson, D. W. (1979). Cooperative and individualistic experiences among disabled and normal children. *Journal of Social Psychology, 107,* 177–183.

Marzola, E. S. (1985). *An arithmetic problem solving model based on a plan for steps to solution, mastery learning, and calculator use in a resource room for learning disabled students.* Unpublished doctoral dissertation, Teachers College, Columbia University, New York

Massari, D. J., & Schack, M. L. (1972). Discrimination learning by reflective and impulsive children as a funciton of reinforcement schedule. *Developmental Psychology, 6,* 183.

Massaro, D. W. (Ed.). (1975). *An information-processing analysis of speech perception, reading, and psycholinguistics.* New York: Academic Press.

Masson, M. A. (1982). A framework of cognitive and metacognitive determinants of reading skill. *Topics in Learning and Learning Disabilities, 2,* 37–43.

Mathews, R., Whang, P., & Fawcett, S. B. (1982). Behavioral assessment of occupational skills of learning disabled adolescents. *Journal of Learning Disabilities, 15,* 41–83.

Mathews, R. M., Whang, P., & Fawcett, S. B. (1980). *Behavioral assessment of job-related skills: Implications for learning disabled young adults* (Research Report No. 6). Lawrence: The University of Kansas, Institute for Research in Learning Disabilities.

Mattingly, I. G. (1972). Reading, the linguistic process, and linguistic awareness. In J. Kavanaugh & I. Mattingly (Eds.), *Language by ear and by eye: The relationship between speech and reading* (pp. 133–148). Cambridge, MA: MIT Press.

Mattis, S. (1978). Dyslexia syndromes: A working hypothesis that works. In A. L. Benton & D. Pearl (Eds.), *Dyslexia: An appraisal of current knowledge* (pp. 43–58). New York: Oxford University Press.

Mattis, S. (1981). Dyslexia syndromes in children: Toward the development of syndrome-specific treatment patterns. In F. J. Pirozzolo & M. C. Wittrock (Eds.), *Neuropsychological and cognitive processes in reading* (pp. 93–107). New York: Academic Press.

Mattis, S., French, J. H., & Rapin, I. (1975). Dyslexia in children and adults: Three independent neuropsychological syndromes. *Developmental Medicine and Child Neurology, 17,* 150–163.

Mayer, W. V. (1982). Curriculum development: A process and a legacy. *Focus on Exceptional Children, 14,* 1–12.

McCormick, S., & Moe, A. J. (1982). The language of instructional materials: A source of reading problems. *Exceptional Children, 49,* 48–53.

McDowell, R. L., & Brown, G. B. (1978). The emotionally disturbed adolescent: Development of program alternatives in secondary education. *Focus on Exceptional Children, 10,* 1–16.

McIntyre, R. B., & Nelson, C. C. (1969). Empirical evaluation of instructional materials. *Educational Technology, 9*(2), 24–27.

McKinney, J. D., & Feagans, L. (1980). *Learning disabilities in the classroom* (Final Project Report). Chapel Hill: University of North Carolina, Frank Porter Graham Child Development Center.

McKinney, J. D., & Feagans, L. (1984). Academic and behavioral characteristics of learning disabled children and average achievers: Longitudinal studies. *Learning Disability Quarterly, 7,* 251–265.

McKinney, J. D., & Kreuger, M. (1974). *Models for educating the learning disabled (MELD): Project period 1971–1974: Final evaluation report.* Washington, DC: Bureau of Elementary and Secondary Education (DHEW/OE). (ERIC Document Reproduction Service No. ED 108 402)

McKinney, J. D., Mason, J., Perkerson, K., & Clifford, M. (1975). Relationship between classroom behavior and academic achievement. *Journal of Educational Psychology, 67,* 198–203.

McKinney, J. D., McClure, S., & Feagans, L. (1982). Classroom behavior of learning disabled children. *Learning Disability Quarterly, 5,* 45–52.

McKinney, J. D., Short, E. J., & Feagans, L. (1985). Academic consequences of perceptual-linguistic subtypes of learning disabled children. *Learning Disability Quarterly, 1*(1), 6–17.

McKinney, J. D., & Speece, D. L. (1983). Classroom behavior and the academic progress of learning disabled students. *Journal of Applied Developmental Psychology, 4,* 149–161.

McLeod, T. M., & Armstrong, S. W. (1982). Learning disabilities in mathematics skill deficits and remedial approaches at the intermediate and secondary level. *Learning*

Disability Quarterly, 5, 303–311.

McNeil, J. D. (1976). *Designing curriculum of self-instructional modules.* Boston: Little, Brown.

Meichenbaum, D. (1977). *Cognitive-behavior modification: An integrative approach.* New York: Plenum.

Meichenbaum, D., & Asarnow, J. (1978). Cognitive-behavioral modification and meta-cognitive development: Implications for the classroom. In P. Kendall & S. Hollon (Eds.), *Cognitive-behavioral interventions: Theory, research and procedure.* New York: Academic Press.

Meichenbaum, D., & Goodman, J. (1971). Training impulsive children to talk to themselves: A means of developing self-control. *Journal of Abnormal Psychology, 77,* 115–126.

Mendelson, W. B., Johnson, N. E., & Stewart, M. A. (1971). Hyperactive children as teenagers: A follow-up study. *Journal of Nervous and Mental Disease, 153,* 273–279.

Mercer, C. D., & Mercer, A. R. (1981). *Teaching students with learning problems.* Columbus, OH: Merrill.

Meyen, E. L. (1972). *Developing units of instruction: For the mentally retarded and other children with learning problems.* Dubuque, IA: Brown.

Meyen, E. L., & Horner, R. D. (1976). Curriculum development. In J. Wortis (Ed.), *Mental retardation and developmental disabilities.* New York: Grune & Stratton.

Meyen, E. L., & Schumaker, J. B. (1981). *A learner-managed social skills curriculum development project.* Washington, DC: U.S. Office of Education (Contract No. 300-81-0349).

Meyen, E. L., & White, W. J. (1980). Career education and PL 94-142: Some views. In G. M. Clark & W. J. White (Eds.), *Career education for the handicapped: Current perspectives for teachers.* Boothwyn, PA: Educational Resources Center.

Meyers, C. E., MacMillan, D. L., & Yoshida, R. K. (1980). Regular class education of EMR students, from efficacy to mainstreaming: A review of issues and research. In J. Gottlieb (Ed.), *Educating mentally retarded persons in the mainstream* (pp. 176–206). Baltimore: University Park Press.

Miccinati, J. (1979). The Fernald technique: Modifications increase the probability of success. *Journal of Learning Disabilities, 12,* 139–142.

Michelson, L., Foster, S., & Ritchey, W. (1981). Behavioral assessment of children's social skills. In B. B. Lahey & A. E. Kazdin (Eds.), *Advances in clinical child psychology* (Vol. 3). New York: Plenum.

Milazzo, T. C. (1970). *Special class placement or how to destroy in the name of help.* Paper presented at the 49th annual international convention of the Council for Exceptional Children, Chicago. (ERIC Document Reproduction Service No. ED 039 383)

Miller, C. D., McKinley, D. L., & Ryan, M. (1979). College students: Learning disabilities and services. *The Personnel and Guidance Journal, 58,* 154–158.

Miller, G. A., Galanter, E., & Pribram, K. H. (1960). *Plans and the structure of behavior.* New York: Holt, Rinehart & Winston.

Miller, L. G. (1968). Toward a greater understanding of the parents of the mentally retarded child. *Pediatrics, 73,* 699–705.

Miller, L. K., & Schneider, R. (1970). The use of a token system in project Head Start. *Journal of Applied Behavior Analysis, 3,* 213–220.

Millman, J. (1973). Passing scores and test lengths for domain-referenced measures. *Review of Educational Research, 43*(2), 205–215.

Minde, K., Lewin, D., Weiss, G., Lavigueur, H., Douglas, V., & Sykes, E. (1971). The hyperactive child in elementary school: A 5 year, controlled followup. *Exceptional Children, 38,* 215–221.

Minde, K. K., Weiss, G., & Mendelson, N. A. (1972). A 5-year follow-up study of 91 hyperactive school children. *Journal of the American Academy of Child Psychiatry, 11,* 595–610.

Mineo, B., & Cavalier, A. R. (1985). From idea to implementation: Cognitive software for students with learning disabilities. *Journal of Learning Disabilities, 18*(10), 613–618.

Minskoff, E. (1975). Research on psycholinguistic training: Critique and guidelines. *Exceptional Children, 42,* 136–144.

Mitchell, G. D. (1981). *School related achievement of high risk learning disabled students: A follow-up study.* Unpublished doctoral dissertation, Duke University, Durham, NC.

Miyake, N., & Norman, D. A. (1979). To ask a question, one must know enough to know what is not known. *Journal of Verbal Learning and Verbal Behavior, 18,* 357–364.

Molitch, M., & Sullivan, J. P. (1937). Effect of benzedrine sulfate on children taking New Stanford Achievement Test. *American Journal of Orthopsychiatry, 7,* 519–522.

Moore, S. R., & Simpson, R. L. (1984). Reciprocity in the teacher–pupil and peer verbal interactions of learning disabled, behavior-disordered and regular education students. *Learning Disability Quarterly, 7,* 30–38.

Mori, A. A. (1980). Career education for the learning disabled — where are we now? *Learning Disability Quarterly, 1*(3), 91–101.

Mori, A. A. (1982a). Career attitudes and job knowledge among junior high school regular, special, and academically talented students. *Career Development for Exceptional Individuals, 5*(1), 62–69.

Mori, A. A. (1982b). School-based career assessment programs: Where are we now and where are we going? *Exceptional Education Quarterly, 3,* 41–48.

Mori, A. A., & Neisworth, J. T. (1983). Curricula in early childhood education: Some generic and special condsiderations. *Topics in Early Childhood Special Education, 2,* 1–8.

Morrison, G. M., Lieber, J., & Morrison, R. L. (in press). A multi-dimensional view of teacher perceptions of special education episodes. *Remedial and Special Education.*

Morrison, G. M., & MacMillan, D. L. (1983). Defining, describing, and explaining the social status of mildly handicapped children: A discussion of methodological problems. In J. M Berg (Ed.), *Prospectives and progress in mental retardation: I. Social, psychological, and educational aspects* (pp. 43–52). Baltimore: University Park Press.

Morrison, G. M., MacMillan, D. L., & Kavale, K. (1985). System identification of learning disabled children: Implications for research sampling. *Learning Disability Quarterly, 8,* 1–10.

Morsink, C. V., Soar, R. S., Soar, R. M., & Thomas, R. (1986). Research on teaching: Opening the door to special education classrooms. *Exceptional Children, 53*(1), 32–40.

Moulton, J. R., & Bader, M. S. (1985). The writing process: A powerful approach for the language-disabled student. *Annals of Dyslexia, 35,* 161–173.

Muenster, G. E. (1982). The career development process at the elementary level. *Journal of Career Development, 8,* 238–245.

Mullen, F., & Itkin, W. (1961). The value of special classes for the mentally handicapped. *Chicago Schools Journal, 42,* 353–363.

Mullins, J., Joseph, F., Turner, C., Zawadyski, R., & Saltzman, L. (1972). A handwriting model for children with learning disabilities. *Journal of Learning Disabilities, 5,* 306–311.

Mullis, I. (1980). *The primary trait system for scoring writing tasks* (NAEP Report No. 05-W-50). Denver, CO: Education Commission of the United States.

Mundy, J. (1975). *Systems approach to leisure education.* Tallahassee: Florida State University.

Munester, G. E. (1982). The career development process at the elementary level. *Journal of Career Development, 8,* 238–245.

Muraski, J. A. (1982). Designing career education programs that work. *Academic Therapy, 18,* 65–71.

Myers, A. C., & Thornton, C. A. (1977). The learning disabled child: Learning the basic facts. *Arithmetic Teacher, 24,* 46–50.

Myers, J. K. (1976). The efficacy of the special day school for EMR pupils. *Mental Retardation, 14,* 3–11.

Myers, P. I., & Hammill, D. (1982). *Learning disabilities: Basic concepts, assessment practices, and instructional strategies.* Austin, TX: Pro-Ed.

Myklebust, H. (1965). *Development and disorders of written language: Picture story language test* (Vol. 1). New York: Grune & Stratton.

Myklebust, H. R., & Johnson, D. J. (1962). Dyslexia in children. *Exceptional Children, 29,* 14–25.

Nagle, R. J., & Thwaite, B. C. (1979). Modeling effects of impulsivity with learning disabled children. *Journal of Learning Disabilities, 12,* 331–336.

Nash, K., & Geyer, C. (1983). *Touch to type.* North Billerica, ME: Curriculum Associates.

National Assessment of Educational Progress. (1977). *Write/rewrite: An assessment of revision skills* (Writing Report No. 05-W-04). Washington, DC: U. S. Government Printing Office.

National Council of Teachers of Mathematics. (1980). *An agenda for action: Recommendations for school mathematics of the 1980's.* Reston, VA: Author.

National Joint Committee for Learning Disabilities. (1981). *Learning disabilities: Issues on definition.* Unpublished position paper. (Available from NJCLD Committee Chairperson, c/o Orton Society, 8419 Bellona Lange, Touson, MD 21204).

Neal, L. (1970). *Recreation's role in the rehabilitation of the mentally retarded.* Eugene: University of Oregon Rehabilitation and Training Center in Mental Retardation.

Neeley, M. D., & Lindsley, O. R. (1978). Phonetic, linguistic, and sight readers produce similar learning with exceptional children. *Journal of Special Education, 12,* 423–441.

Nelson, H. E. (1980). Analysis of spelling errors in normal dyslexic children. In U. Frith (Ed.), *Cognitive processes in spelling.* London: Academic Press.

Newcombe, F., & Marshall, J. (1981). On psycholinguistic classification of the acquired dyslexias. *Bulletin of the Orton Society, 31,* 29–46.

Newcomer, P., Larsen, S., & Hammill, D. (1975). A response. *Exceptional Children, 42,* 144–148.

Nichols, P. L., & Chen, T. C. (1981). *Minimal brain dysfunction: A prospective study.* Hillsdale, NJ: Lawrence Erlbaum.

Noel, M. M. (1980). Referential communication abilities of learning disabled children. *Learning Disability Quarterly, 3,* 70–75.

Novak, A., & Heal, L. (Eds.). (1980). *Integration of developmentally disabled individuals into the community.* Baltimore: Paul H. Brookes.

Novy, P., Burnett, J., Powers, M., & Sulzer-Azaroff, B. (1973). Modifying attending-to-work behavior of a learning disabled child. *Journal of Learning Disabilities, 6,* 217, 221.

Nuzum, M. (1982). *The effects of a curriculum based on the information processing paradigm on the arithmetic problem solving performance of four learning disabled students.* Unpublished doctoral dissertation, Teachers College, Columbia University, New York.

Oakland, T. (Ed.). (1981). *Psychological assessment of minority children.* New York: Bruner/ Mazel.

Oden, S., & Asher, S. R. (1977). Coaching children in social skills for friendship making. *Child Development, 48,* 459–506.

O'Hara, D. M., Chaiklin, H., & Mosher, B. M. (1980). A family life cycle plan for delivery services for the developmentally disabled. *Child Welfare, 59,* 80–90.

Ohrenstein, D. F. (1979). Parent counseling. In W. C. Adamson (Ed.), *A handbook for specific learning disabilities.* New York: Gardner Press.

Oldesen, C. F. (1974). Instructional materials. In *Thesaurus for special education* (2nd ed.). Education IMC/RMC Network. (ERIC Reproduction Document Service No. EC 070 639.

O'Leary, K. D. (1980). Pills or skills for hyperactive children. *Journal of Applied Behavior Analysis, 13,* 191–204.

O'Leary, K. D., & Becker, W. C. (1967). Behavior modification of an adjustment class: A token reinforcement program. *Exceptional Children, 9,* 637–642.

Olsen, J., & Midgett, J. (1984). Alternative placements: Does a difference exist in the LD population? *Journal of Learning Disabilities, 17*(2), 101–103.

Olsen, K. (1973). *SER-LARS-I. Users manual.* Harrisburg, PA: National Regional Resource Center of Pennsylvania.

Olshansky, S. (1962). Chronic sorrow: A response to having a mentally defective child. *Social Casework, 43,* 190–193.

O'Morrow, G. (1976). *Therapeutic recreation: A helping profession.* Reston, VA: Reston Publishing.

O'Neill, D. R., & Jensen, R. S. (1981). Some aids for teaching place value. *Arithmetic Teacher, 28,* 6–9.

Orton, S. (1937). *Reading, writing, and speech problems in children.* New York: Norton.

Osburn, W. (1953). Handwriting. In O. Buros (Ed.), *Fourth mental measurement yearbook.* Highland Park, NJ: The Gryphon Press.

Osman, B. (1982). *No one to play with: The social side of learning disabilities.* New York: Random House.

Otto, W., McMenemy, R. A., & Smith, P. J. (1973). *Corrective and remedial teaching* (2nd ed.). Boston: Houghton Mifflin.

Otto, W., & Smith, R. J. (1983). Skill-centered and meaning-centered conceptions of remedial instruction: Striking a balance. *Topics in Learning and Learning Disabilities, 2,* 20–26.

Palincsar, A. S. (1982). Improving the reading comprehension of junior high students through reciprocal teaching of comprehension-monitoring strategies. Unpublished doctoral dissertation, University of Illinois, Urbana.

Palmer, D. J. (1980). Factors to consider in placing handicapped children in regular education classes. *Journal of School Psychology, 18,* 163–171.

Palmer, D. J. (1985). The microcomputer and the learning disabled: A useful tool. *Journal of Reading, Writing, and Learning Disabilities International, 1*(1), 24–40.

Palmer, D. J., Drummond, F., Tollison, P., & Zinkgraff, S. (1982). An attributional investigation of performance outcomes for learning disabled and normal-achieving pupils. *Journal of Special Education, 16,* 207–216.

Palmer, D. J., & Goetz, E. T. (1985). Selection and the use of study strategies: The role of the studier's beliefs about self and strategies. Unpublished manuscript, Texas A & M University, College Station.

Palmer, J. T. (1985). The microcomputer and the learning disabled: A useful tool. *Journal of Reading, Writing, and Learning Disabilities, 1*(1), 24–40.

Paloutzian, R., Hasazi, J., Streitel, R., & Edgar, C. (1971). Promotion of positive social interaction in severely retarded young children. *American Journal on Mental Defi-*

ciency, 75, 519–524.

Pany, D., Jenkins, J., & Schreck, J. (1982). Vocabulary instruction: Effects of word knowledge and reading comprehension. *Learning Disability Quarterly, 5,* 203–215.

Parker, J. (1975). A photo-electric pen for producing action feedback to aid development in handicapped children of fine visual-motor skills: Tracing and writing. *Slow Learning Child, 22,* 13–22.

Parker, S., Friars, E., Gelman, N., & Kowacki, W. (1980). *Special education: Management information.* Washington, DC: National Association of State Directors of Special Education.

Parten, M. (1932). Social play among school children. *Journal of Abnormal Psychology, 28,* 136–147.

Parten, M., & Newhall, S. (1943). Social behavior of preschool children. In R. Barker, J. Kounin, & H. Wright (Eds.), *Child behavior and development.* New York: McGraw-Hill.

Pearl, R. (1982). Learning-disabled children's attributions for success and failure: A replication with a labeled learning-disabled sample. *Learning Disability Quarterly, 5,* 173–176.

Pearl, R. (1985). Cognitive behavioral interventions for increasing motivation. *Journal of Abnormal Child Psychology, 13,* 443–454.

Pearl, R., Bryan, T., & Donahue, M. (1980). Learning-disabled children's attributions for success and failure. *Learning Disability Quarterly, 3,* 3–9.

Pearl, R., Bryan, T., & Donahue, M. (1983). Social behaviors of learning disabled children: A review. *Topics in Learning and Learning Disabilities, 3*(2), 1–14.

Pearl, R., Bryan, T., & Herzog, A. (1983). Learning-disabled and nondisabled children's strategy analyses under high and low success conditions. *Learning Disability Quarterly, 6,* 67–74.

Pearl, R., & Cosden, M. (1982). Sizing up a situation: LD children's understanding of social interactions. *Learning Disability Quarterly, 5,* 371–373.

Pearl, R., Donahue, M., & Bryan, T. (1983). The development of tact: Children's strategies for delivering bad news. Unpublished manuscript. University of Illinois at Chicago.

Pearson, P. D. (1978). Some practical applications of psycholinguistic models of reading. In S. J. Samuels (Ed.), *What research has to say about reading instruction* (pp. 84–95). Newark, DL: International Reading Association.

Peck, D. M., & Jencks, S. M. (1981). Conceptual issues in the teaching and learning of fractions. *Journal of Research in Mathematics Education, 12,* 339–348.

Peck, M., & Fairchild, S. H. (1980). Another decade of research in handwriting: Progress and prospect in the 1970s. *Journal of Educational Research, 73*(5), 283–298.

Pelham, W. E. (1983). The effects of psychostimulants on academic achievement in hyperactive and learning-disabled children. *Thalamus, 3,* 1–49.

Pelham, W. E. (1985). The effects of psychostimulant drugs on learning and academic achievement in children with attention deficit disorders and learning disabilities. In J. K. Torgeson & B. Wong (Eds.), *Psychological and educational perspectives on learning disabilities* (pp. 259–295). Orlando, FL: Academic Press.

Pelham, W. E., Bender, M. E., Caddell, J., Booth, S., & Moorer, S. H. (1985). Methylphenidate and children with attention deficit disorder: Dose effects on classroom academic and social behavior. *Archives of General Psychiatry, 42,* 948–952.

Pelham, W. E., Milich, R., & Walker, J. L. (1986). The effects of continuous and partial reinforcement and methylphenidate on learning in children with attention deficit disorder. *Journal of Abnormal Psychology, 95,* 319–325.

Pelham, W. E., & Murphy, H. A. (1985). Behavioral and pharmacological treatment of attention deficit and conduct disorders. In M. Hersen (Ed.), *Pharmacological and behavioral treatment: An integrative approach.* New York: Wiley.

Pelham, W. E., Swanson, J., Bender, M., & Wilson, J. (1980, September). *Effects of pemoline on hyperactivity: Laboratory and classroom measures.* Paper presented at the annual meeting of the American Psychological Association, Montreal.

Pennhurst State School and Hospital v. Halderman. (1981). 451 US 1.

Pepe, H. J. (1974). A comparison of the effectiveness of itinerant and resource room model programs designed to serve children with learning disabilities. Doctoral dissertation, University of Kansas. *Dissertation Abstracts International, 1,* 75–92.

Perfetti, C. A., & Lesgold, A. M. (1977). *Coding and comprehension in skilled reading and implications for reading instruction.* Pittsburgh, PA: University of Pittsburgh, Learning Research and Development Center.

Perfetti, C. A., & Lesgold, A. M. (1979). Coding and comprehension in skilled reading and implications for reading instruction. In L. Resnick & P. Weaver (Eds.), *Theory and practice of early reading* (Vol. 1, pp. 57–84). Hillsdale, NJ: Lawrence Erlbaum.

Perlmutter, B. F., Crocker, J., Cordray, D., & Garstecki, D. (1983). Sociometric status and related personality characteristics of mainstreamed learning disabled adolescents. *Learning Disability Quarterly, 6,* 20–30.

Perry, D. C. (1981). The disabled student and college counseling centers. *Journal of College Student Personnel, 22*(6), 533–538.

Peterson, P. L., & Walberg, H. J. (Eds.). *Research on teaching: Concepts, findings, and implications.* Berkeley, CA: McCutchan.

Petrauskas, R., & Rourke, B. (1979). Identification of subgroups of retarded readers: A neuropsychological multivariate approach. *Journal of Clinical Neuropsychology, 1,* 17–37.

Pflaum, S. W., & Pascarella, E. T. (1980). Interactive effects of prior reading achievement and training in context on the reading of learning disabled children. *Reading Research Quarterly, 16,* 138–158.

Phelps, J., Stempel, L., & Speck, G. (1982). *Children's handwriting evaluation scale: A new diagnostic tool.* Unpublished manuscript.

Phelps–Gunn, T., & Phelps–Terasaki, D. (1982). *Written language instruction.* Rockville, MD: Aspen Publications.

Phelps–Terasaki, D., & Phelps, T. (1980). *Teaching written expression: The Phelps sentence guide program.* Novato, CA: Academic Therapy.

Phillips, D. (1983). After the wake: Post positivistic educational thought. *Educational Researcher, 12,* 4–12.

Phillips, D. C. (1980). What do the researcher and the practitioner have to offer each other? *Educational Researcher, 9,* 17–20, 24.

Piaget, J. (1951). *Dreams and imitation in childhood.* New York: Norton.

Piers, M. (1972). *Play and development.* New York: Norton.

Pirozzolo, F. (1979). *The neuropsychology of developmental reading disorders.* New York: Praeger.

Polloway, E. A. (1984). The integration of mildly retarded students in the schools: A historical review. *Remedial and Special Education, 5*(4), 18–19.

Polloway, E. A., Payne, J. S., Patton, J. R., & Payne, R. A. (1985). *Strategies for teaching retarded and special needs learners* (3rd ed.). Columbus, OH: Merrill.

Polsgrove, L. (1979). Self-control: Methods for child training. *Behavioral Disorders, 4,* 116–130.

Popham, W., Eisner, E., Sullivan, H., & Tyler, L. (1969). Instructional objectives. *AERA Monograph Series of Curriculum Evaluation.* Chicago: Rand McNally.

Poplin, M. (1979). The science of curriculum development applied to special education and the IEP. *Focus on Exceptional Children, 12,* 1–16.

Poplin, M., & Gray, R. (1980). A conceptual framework for assessment of curriculum and student progress. *Exceptional Education Quarterly, 1,* 75–86.

Posner, M. I. (1979). Applying theories and theorizing about applications. In L. Resnick & P. Weaver (Eds.), *Theory and practice of early reading* (Vol. 1, pp. 331–342)). Hillsdale, NJ: Lawrence Erlbaum.

Poteet, J. A. (1980). Informal assessment of written expression. *Learning Disability Quarterly, 3,* 88–98.

President's Committee on Mental Retardation. (1974). *America's needs in habilitation and employment of the mentally retarded.* Washington, DC: U.S. Government Printing Office.

Pratt, D. (1980). *Curriculum design and development.* New York: Harcourt Brace Jovanovich.

Prillaman, D. (1981). Acceptance of learning disabled students in the mainstream environment: A failure to replicate. *Journal of Learning Disabilities, 14,* 344–346.

Project Achieve case information. (Undated). Carbondale: Southern Illinois University.

Public Law 94-142. (1977, August 23). Education for All Handicapped Children Act. *Federal Register, 42.*

Purkey, S. C., & Smith, M. S. (1983). Effective schools: A review. *Elementary School Journal, 83,* 427–452.

Quandt, D. F. (1985). *Mathematical problem solving performance of learning disabled, low achieving, and average achieving children.* Unpublished doctoral dissertation, Teachers College, Columbia University, New York.

Quay, H. C., Glavin, J. R., Annesley, F. R., & Werry, J. S. (1972). The modification of problem behavior and academic achievement in a resource room. *Journal of School Psychology, 10,* 187–198.

Quinn, P., & Rapoport, J. (1975). One-year follow-up of hyperactive boys treated with imipramine and methylphenidate. *American Journal of Psychiatry, 132,* 241–245.

Rabinovitch, R. D. (1962). Dyslexia: Psychiatric considerations. In J. Money (Ed.), *Reading disability: Progress and research needs in dyslexia.* Baltimore: Johns Hopkins Press.

Ramming, J. (1970). Using the chalkboard to overcome handwriting difficulties. In J. Arena (Ed.), *Building handwriting skills in dyslexic children.* San Rafael, CA: Academic Therapy Publications.

Rapoport, J. L. (1980). The "real" and "ideal" management of stimulant drug treatment for hyperactive children: Recent findings and a report from clinical practice. In C. K. Whalen & B. Henker (Eds.), *Hyperactive children: The social ecology of identification and treatment.* New York: Academic Press.

Rapoport, J. L., Quinn, P. O., Bradbard, G., Riddle, K. D., & Brooks, E. (1974). Imipramine and methylphenidate treatments of hyperactive boys. *Archives of General Psychiatry, 30,* 789–793.

Rapport, M. .D., Murphy, A., & Bailey, J. S. (1980). The effects of a response cost treatment tactic on hyperactive children. *Journal of School Psychology, 18,* 98–111.

Rapport, M. D., Murphy, H. A., & Bailey, J. S. (1982). Ritalin vs. response cost in the control of hyperactive children.: A within-subject comparison. *Journal of Applied Behavior Analysis, 15,* 205–216.

Rapport, M. D., Stoner, G., DuPaul, G. J., Birmingham, B. K., & Tucker, S. (1985). Methylphenidate in hyperactive children: Differential effects of dose on academic learning and social behavior. *Journal of Abnormal Child Psychology, 13,* 227–244.

Raskind, M. H., Drew, D. E., & Regan, J. O. (1983). Nonverbal communication signals in behavior-disordered and non-disordered LD boys and NLD boys. *Learning Disability Quarterly, 6,* 12–19.

Rasmussen, S. (1980). *Key to fractions.* Berkeley, CA: Key Curriculum Project.

Raven, J. C. (1956). *Standard progresive matrices.* London: H. K. Lewis.

Read, C. (1980). Pre-school children's knowledge of English phonology. In M. Wolf, M.

McQuillan, & E. Radwin (Eds.), Thought & language/language and reading. *Harvard Educational Review* (Reprint Series No. 14, pp. 150–179).

Redden, M. R., Levering, C., & DiQuinzio, D. (1978). *Recruitment, admissions and handicapped students*. Washington, DC: The American Association of College Registrars and Admissions Officers and the American Council on Education.

Reed, J. C. (1968). The ability deficits of good and poor readers. *Journal of Learning Disabilities, 1*, 134–139.

Reeves, R. A., & Brown, A. L. (1985). Metacognition reconsidered: Implications for intervention research. *Journal of Abnormal Child Psychology, 13*, 343–356.

Reid, D. K., & Hresko, W. P. (1981a). *A cognitive approach to learning disabilities*. New York: McGraw-Hill.

Reid, D. K., & Hresko, W. P. (1981b). From the editors. *Topics in Learning and Learning Disabilities, 1*, viii–ix.

Reisman, F. K., & Kauffman, S. H. (1980). *Teaching mathematics to children with special needs*. Columbus, OH: Merrill.

Resnick, L., & Beck, I. (1976). Designing instruction in reading: Interaction of theory and practice. In J. Guthrie (Ed.), *Aspects of reading acquisition* (pp. 180–204). Baltimore: Johns Hopkins University Press.

Resnick, L. B. (1981). Instructional psychology. In M. R. Rosenzweig & L. W. Porter (Eds.), *Annual review of psychology* (Vol. 32, pp. 741–704) Palo Alto, CA: Annual Review.

Reynolds, M. C., & Birch, J. W. (1982). *Teaching exceptional children in all America's schools* (rev. ed.). Reston, VA: The Council for Exceptional Children.

Rhodes, L. K., & Shannon, J. L. (1982). Psycholinguistic principles in operation in a primary learning disabilities classroom. *Topics in Learning and Learning Disabilities, 1*, 1–10.

Rhodes, S. L. (1977). A developmental approach to the life cycle of the family. *Social Casework, 58*, 301–304.

Rhodes, S. S. (1985). Mini-assessment: A practical approach to classroom identification of learning disabled readers. *Reading Horizons, 25*(3), 186–193.

Riddle, D., & Rapoport, J. (1976). A 2-year follow-up of 72 hyperactive boys. *Journal of Nervous and Mental Disease, 162*, 126–134.

Rie, H. E., Rie, E. D., Stewart, S., & Ambuel, J. P. (1976). Effects of methylphenidate on underachieving children. *Journal of Consulting and Clinical Psychology, 44*, 250–260.

Risner, M. T. (1979). *NICSEM special education thesaurus*. Los Angeles: The National Information Center for Special Education Media.

Ritter, D. R. (1978). Surviving in the regular classroom: A follow-up of mainstreamed children with learning disabilities. *Journal of School Psychology, 16*, 253–256.

Roberts, G. H. (1968). The failure strategies of third grade arithmetic pupils. *The Arithmetic Teacher, 15*, 442–446.

Robins, L. N. (1977). Problems in follow-up studies. *American Journal of Psychiatry, 134*, 904–907.

Robins, L. N. (1979). Follow-up studies of behavior disorders in children. In H. C. Quay & J. S. Werry (Eds.), *Psychopathological disorders of childhood* (pp. 483–513). New York: Wiley.

Robinson, S. P. (1974). *Study skills for superior students in secondary schools* (2nd ed.). New York: Macmillan.

Roddy, E. A. (1984). When are resource rooms going to share in the declining enrollment trend? Another look at mainstreaming. *Journal of Learning Disabilities, 17*(5), 279–281.

Roff, M., Sells, S. B., & Golden, M. M. (1972). *Social adjustment and personality develop-*

ment in children. Minneapolis: University of Minnesota Press.

Rose, T., Lessen, E., & Gottlieb, J. (1982). A discussion of transfer of training in mainstreaming progress. *Journal of Learning Disabilities, 15*(3), 162–165.

Rosegrant, T. (1985). Using the microcomputer as a tool for learning to read and write. *Journal of Learning Disabilities, 18*(2), 113–115.

Rosen, L. A., O'Leary, S. G., & Conway, G. (1983). *The withdrawal of stimulant medication for hyperactivity: A case study.* Unpublished manuscript, SUNY, Department of Psychology, Stony Brook, NY.

Rosenshine, B. V., & Berliner, D. C. (1978). Academic engaged time. *British Journal of Teacher Education, 4,* 3–16.

Rosenthal, R., & Jacobson, L. (1968). *Pygmalion in the classroom.* New York: Holt, Rinehart & Winston.

Rosenthal, R., & Rubin, D. B. (1978). Interpersonal expectancy effects: The first 345 studies. *The Behavioral and Brain Sciences, 3,* 377–415.

Rosenthal, R., & Rubin, D. R. (1982). A simple, general purpose display of the magnitude of experimental effect. *Journal of Educational Psychology, 74,* 166–169.

Ross, A. O. (1976). *Psychological aspects of learning disabilities and reading disorders.* New York: McGraw-Hill.

Ross, A. O. (1981). *Child behavior therapy.* New York: Wiley.

Ross, S. K., & O'Brien, M. B. (1981). *504 and admissions: Making the law work for the applicant and the college.* Minneapolis, MN: St Mary's College. (ERIC Document Reproduction Service No. ED 206 335)

Rourke, B. P. (1978). Reading, spelling, arithmetic disabilities: A neuropsychological perspective. In H. R. Myklebust (Ed.), *Progress in learning disabilities* (Vol. 4, pp. 97–120). New York: Grune & Stratton.

Rourke, B. P. (Ed.). (1985). *Neuropsychology of learning disabilities: Advances in subtype analysis.* New York: Guilford Press.

Rourke, B. P., & Finlayson, M. A. (1978). Neuropsychological significance of variations patterns of academic performance: Verbal and visual spatial abilities. *Journal of Abnormal Child Psychology, 6,* 121–133.

Rourke, B. P., & Orr, R. R. (1977). Prediction of the reading and spelling performances of normal and retarded readers: A four-year follow-up. *Journal of Abnormal Child Psychology, 5,* 9–20.

Rubin, L. J. (Ed.). (1977). *Curriculum handbook.* Boston: Allyn and Bacon.

Rumelhart, D. E. (1977). Toward an interactive model of reading. In S. Dornic (Ed.), *Attention and performance* (Vol. 6). New York: Wiley.

Russell, R. L., & Ginsburg, H. P. (1981). *Cognitive analysis of children's mathematics difficulties.* Rochester, NY: University of Rochester.

Rutter, M. (1978). Prevalence and types of dyslexia. In A. L. Benton & D. Pearl (Eds.), *Dyslexia: An appraisal of current knowledge* (pp. 3–28). New York: Oxford University Press.

Rutter, M., & Yule, W. (1975). The concept of specific reading retardation. *Journal of Child Psychology and Psychiatry, 16,* 181–197.

Ryback, D., & Staats, A. W. (1970). Parents as behavior-therapy technicians in treating reading deficits (dyslexia). *Journal of Behavior Therapy and Experimental Psychiatry, 1,* 109–119.

Sabatino, D. A. (1971). An evaluation of resource rooms for children with learning disabilities. *Journal of Learning Disabilities, 4,* 27–35.

Sabatino, D. (1976). *Learning disabilities handbook: A technical guide to program development.* Dekalb: Northern Illinois University.

Safer, D., & Allen, R. (1976). *Hyperactive children: Diagnosis and management.* Baltimore:

University Park Press.

Safer, D. J., & Krager, J. M. (1984). Trends in medication treatment of hyperactive school children. In K. D. Gadow (Ed.), *Advances in learning and behavioral disabilites* (Vol. 3, pp. 125–149). Greenwich, CT: JAI Press.

Salend, S. J. (1984). Factors contributing to the development of successful mainstreaming programs. *Exceptional Children, 50,* 409–416.

Salend, S. J., & Lutz, J. G. (1984). Mainstreaming or maintaining: A competency based approach to mainstreaming. *Journal of Learning Disabilities, 17,* 27–29.

Salend, S. J., & Salend, S. M. (1985). The implications of using microcomputers in classroom testing. *Journal of Learning Disabilities, 18*(1), 51–53.

Salomon, G. (1972). Heuristic models for the generation of aptitude-treatment interaction hypotheses. *Review of Educational Research, 42,* 327–343.

Salvia, J., & Ysseldyke, J. E. (1985). *Assessment in special and remedial education* (3rd ed.). Boston: Houghton Mifflin.

Samaras, M., & Ball, T. (1975). Reinforcement of cooperation between profoundly retarded adults. *American Journal on Mental Deficiency, 80,* 63–71.

Samuels, S. J. (1986). Why children fail to learn and what to do about it. *Exceptional Children, 53*(1), 7–16.

Satterfield, J. H., Cantwell, D. P., & Satterfield, B. T. (1979). Multimodality treatment: A one-year follow-up of 84 hyperactive boys. *Archives of General Psychiatry, 35,* 965–974.

Satterfield, J. H., Satterfield, B. T., & Cantwell, D. P. (1980). Multimodality treatment: A two year evaluation of 61 hyperactive boys. *Archives of General Psychiatry, 37,* 915–918.

Satterfield, J. H., Satterfield, B. T., & Cantwell, D. P. (1981). Three-year multimodality treatment study of 100 hyperactive boys. *Journal of Pediatrics, 98,* 650–655.

Satz, P., & Morris, R. (1981). Learning disability subtypes: A review. In F. J. Pirozzolo & M. C. Wittrock (Eds.), *Neuropsychological and cognitive processes in reading* (pp. 109–141). New York: Academic Press.

Satz, P., Taylor, H. G., Friel, J., & Fletcher, J. (1978). Some developmental and predictive precursors of reading disabilities: A six-year follow-up. In A. L. Benton & D. Pearl (Eds.), *Dyslexia: An appraisal of current knowledge* (pp. 313–348). New York: Oxford University Press.

Savage, J. F., & Mooney, J. F. (1979). *Teaching reading to children with special needs.* Boston: Allyn and Bacon.

Schacht, E. J. (1967). A study of the mathematical errors of low achievers in elementary school mathematics. *Dissertation Abstracts International, 29A,* 920–921.

Schaefer, E. S. (1981). Development of adaptive behavior: Conceptual models and family correlates. In M. Begab, H. Garber, & H. C. Haywood (Eds.), *Prevention of retarded development in psychosocially disadvantaged children.* Baltimore: University Park Press.

Schain, R. J., & Reynard, C. L. (1975). Observations on the effects of central stimulant drug (methylphenidate) in children with hyperactive behavior. *Pediatrics, 55,* 709–716.

Schenck, S. J. (1980). The diagnostic-instructional link in individualized education programs. *Journal of Special Education, 14,* 337–345.

Schleien, S. (1982). *Effects of an individualized leisure education instructional program of cooperative leisure skill activities on severely learning disabled children.* Unpublished doctoral dissertation, University of Maryland.

Schleien, S., Porter, R., & Wehman, P. (1979). An assessment of the leisure skill needs of developmentally disabled individuals. *Therapeutic Recreation Journal, 13,* 16–21.

Schumaker, J., Hovell, M., & Sherman, J. (1977a). An analysis of daily report cards and

parent managed privileges in the improvement of adolescents' classroom performance. *Journal of Applied Behavior Analysis, 10,* 449–464.

Schumaker, J., Hovell, M., & Sherman, J. (1977b). *A home-based achievement system.* Lawrence, KS: Excel Enterprises.

Schumaker, J. B., Deshler, D. D., Alley, G. R., & Warner, M. M. (1983). Toward the
development of an intervention model for learning disabled adolescents: The University of Kansas Institute. *Exceptional Education Quarterly, 4*(1), 45–74.

Schumaker, J. B., & Ellis, E. (1982). Social skills training of LD adolescents: A generalization study. *Learning Disability Quarterly, 5,* 409–414.

Schumaker, J. B., Hazel, J. S., & Pederson, C. (1988). *Social skills for daily living.* Circle
Pines, MN: American Guidance Service.

Schumaker, J. B., Hazel, J. S., Pederson, C. S., & Nolan, S. (in preparation). *Evaluation of a
method for promoting generalization of newly learned social skills* (Research Report). Lawrence: The University of Kansas Institute for Research in Learning Disabilities.

Schumaker, J. B., Hazel, J. S., Sherman, J. A., & Sheldon, J. (1982). Social skill performances of learning disabled and non-learning disabled, and delinquent adolescents.
Learning Disability Quarterly, 5, 409–414.

Schumaker, J. B., Pederson, C. S., Hazel, J. S., & Meyen, E. L. (1983). Social skills
curricula for mildly handicapped adolescents: A review. *Focus on Exceptional
Children, 16*(4), 1–16.

Schumaker, J. B., Sheldon–Wildgen, J., & Sherman, J. A. (1980). *An observational study of
the academic and social behaviors of learning disabled adolscents in the regular classroom*
(Research Report No. 22). Lawrence: The University of Kansas Institute for
Research in Learning Disabilities.

Schwartz, J. S. (1977). *A longitudinal study to determine the effectiveness of a special program
for the learning disabled child.* Unpublished doctoral dissertation, Fordham University, Bronx, NY.

Schworm, R. W. (1979). The effects of selective attention on the decoding skills of
children with learning disabilities. *Journal of Learning Disabilities, 12,* 639–644.

Scranton, T., & Ryckman, D. (1979). Sociometric status of learning disabled children in
an interactive program. *Journal of Learning Disabilities, 12,* 402–407.

Scribner, W. (1953). Evaluation of the Lincoln diagnostic spelling tests. In O. Buros
(Ed.), *The fourth annual mental measurements yearbook.* Highland Park, NJ: Gryphon
Press.

Seabaugh, G. O., & Schumaker, J. B. (1981). *The effects of self-regulation training on the
academic productivity training of LD and NLD adolescents* (Research Report No. 37).
Lawrence: University of Kansas Institute for Research in Learning Disabilities.

Semmel, M. I., Gottlieb, J., & Robinson, N. M. (1979). Mainstreaming: Perspectives on
educating handicapped children in the public school. In D. C. Berliner (Ed.),
Review of research in education (pp. 223–279). Washington, DC: American Educational Research Association.

Senf, G. M. (1972). An information-integration theory and its application to normal
reading acquisition and reading disability. In N. D. Bryant & C. E. Kass (Eds.),
Leadership training institute in learning disabilities (Vol. 2, pp. 305–391, Final Report).
Tucson, AZ: University of Arizona.

Senf, G. M. (1978). Implications of the final procedures for evaluating specific learning
disabilities. *Journal of Learning Disabilities, 11,* 124–126.

Serna, L., Hazel, S., Schumaker, J. B., & Sheldon, J. (1984, May). Training reciprocal
skills to parents of problem adolescents. In L. Serna (Chair), *Parent–adolescent communication programs and family data analysis.* Symposium conducted at the Tenth
Annual Convention of the Association for Behavioral Analysis, Nashville, TN.

Serna, L. A., Schumaker, J. B., Hazel, J. S., & Sheldon, J. B. (1986). Teaching reciprocal social skills to parents and their delinquent adolescents. *Journal of Clinical Psychology, 15,* 64–77.

Seymour, D. (1970). What do you mean "auditory perception"? *Elementary School Journal, 70,* 175–179.

Seymour, P. H., & Porpodas, C. D. (1980). Lexical and non-lexical processing in dyslexia. In U. Frith (Ed.), *Cognitive processes in spelling.* London: Academic Press.

Sharma, M. (1979). Children at risk for disabilities in mathematics. *Focus on Learning Problems, 1,* 63–94.

Shattuck, M. (1946). Segregation versus non-segregation of exceptional children. *Journal of Exceptional Children, 12,* 235–240.

Sheehan, R., & Keogh, B. K. (1984). Approaches to evaluation in special education. In B. K. Keogh (Ed.), *Advances in special education* (Vol. 4, pp. 1–20). Greenwich, CT: JAI Press.

Sheridan, J. J., & Meister, K. A. (1982). *Food additives and hyperactivity.* New York: American Council on Science and Health.

Shulman, R. (1976). Recreation programming for children with specific learning disabilities. *Leisurability, 3,* 13.

Siefferman, L. D. (1983). Vocational education — the post-secondary connection for learning disabled students. *The Journal for Vocational Special Needs Education, 5*(2), 28–29.

Siegel, S. (1956). *Nonparametric statistics for the behavioral sciences.* New York: McGraw–Hill.

Silberberg, N. E., Iverson, I. A., & Goins, J. T. (1973). Which remedial method works best? *Journal of Learning Disabilities, 6,* 547–555.

Silberberg, N. E., & Silberberg, M. C. (1969). Myths in remedial education. *Journal of Learning Disabilities, 2,* 209–217.

Silbert, J., Carnine, D., & Stein, M. (1981). *Direct instruction mathematics.* Columbus, OH: Merrill.

Silver, A. A., & Hagin, R. A. (1976). *SEARCH.* New York: Walker Educational Book Corp.

Silver, A. A., Hagin, R. A., & Beecher, R. (1978). Scanning, diagnosis, and intervention in the prevention of reading disabilities: I. SEARCH: The scanning measure; II. TEACH: Learning tasks for the prevention of learning disabilities. *Journal of Learning Disabilities, 11,* 439–449.

Silver, A. A., Hagin, R. A., & Beecher, R. (1981). A program for secondary prevention of learning disabilities: Results in academic achievement and in emotional adjustment. *Journal of Preventive Psychiatry, 1,* 77–87.

Silver, L. B. (1974). Emotional and social problems of the family with a child who has developmental disabilities. In R. W. Weber (Ed.), *Handbook on learning disabilities: A prognosis for the child, the adolescent, the adult.* Englewood Cliffs, NJ: Prentice–Hall.

Simches, G., & Bohn, R. (1963). Issues in curriculum: Research and responsibility. *Mental Retardation, 1,* 84–87.

Sinclair, A., Jarvella, R., & Levelt, W. (1978). *The child's conception of language.* New York: Springer–Verlag.

Sindelar, P. T., & Deno, S. L. (1978). The effectiveness of resource programming. *The Journal of Special Education, 12,* 17–28.

Singer, M. H. (1982). Reading disability research: A misguided search for difference. In M. Singer (Ed.), *Competent reader, disabled reader: Research and application* (pp. 39–54). Hillsdale, NJ: Lawrence Erlbaum.

Siperstein, G. N., Bopp, M. J., & Bak, J. J. (1978). Social status of learning disabled children. *Journal of Learning Disabilities, 11,* 98–102.

Sleator, E. K. (1985). Measurement of compliance. *Psychopharmacology Bulletin, 21,*

1089-1093.

Sleator, E. K., Ullman, R. K., & von Neumann, A. (1982). How do hyperactive children feel about taking stimulants and will they tell the doctor? *Clinical Pediatrics, 21,* 474–479.

Sleator, E. K., von Neumann, A. W., & Sprague, R. L. (1974). Hyperactive children: A continuous long-term placebo controlled follow-up. *Journal of the American Medical Association, 229,* 316–317.

Slingerland, B. (1970). *Slingerland screening tests for identifying children with specific language disability.* Cambridge, MA: Educators Publishing Service.

Slingerland, B. (1981). *A multi-sensory approach to language arts for specific language disability children.* Cambridge, MA: Educators Publishing Service.

Smiley, A., & Bryan, T. (1983a). *Learning disabled boys' problem solving and visual interactions during raft building.* Chicago: Chicago Institute for the Study of Learning Disabilities.

Smiley, A., & Bryan, T. (1983b). *Learning disabled junior high boys' motor performance and trust during obstacle course activities.* Unpublished manuscript, University of Illinois at Chicago.

Smith, C. R. (1983). *Learning disabilities: The interaction of learner, task, and setting.* Boston: Little, Brown.

Smith, D. D., Lovitt, T. C., & Kidder, J.S. (1972). Using reinforcement contingencies and teaching aids to alter the subtraction performance of children with learning disabilities. In G. Semb (Ed.), *Behavior analysis and education.* Lawrence: University of Kansas Department of Human Development.

Smith, F. (1971). *Understanding reading: A psycholinguistic analysis of reading and learning to read.* New York: Holt, Rinehart & Winston.

Smith, F. (1977). Making sense of reading — And of reading instruction. *Harvard Educational Review, 47,* 386–395.

Smith, F., & Goodman, K. S. (1971). On the psycholinguistic method of teaching reading. *Elementary School Journal, 71,* 177–181.

Smith, G., & Smith, D. (1985). A mainstreaming program that really works. *Journal of Learning Disabilities, 18,* 369–372.

Smith, H. W., & Kennedy, W. A. (1967). Effects of three educational programs on mentally retarded children. *Perceptual and Motor Skills, 24,* 174.

Smith, J. D., & Dexter, B. L. (1980). The basics movement: What does it mean for the education of the mentally retarded students? *Education and Training of the Mentally Retarded, 15,* 72–74.

Smith, M. D., Coleman, J. M., Dokecki, P. R., & Davis, E. E. (1977). Intellectual characteristics of school labeled learning disabled children. *Exceptional Children, 43,* 352–357.

Smith, P. L., & Tomkins, G. E. (1984). Selecting software for your LD students. *Academic Therapy, 20*(2), 221–224.

Smith, T. E. C., Flexter, R. W., & Sigelman, C. K. (1980). Attitudes of secondary principals toward the learning disabled, mentally retarded and workstudy program. *Journal of Learning Disabilities, 13,* 62–64.

Snodgrass, G. (1980). *Computerized IEP and management information system.* Washington, DC: National Association of State Directors of Special Education.

Snowling, M. J. (1980). The development of grapheme-phoneme correspondence in normal and dyslexic readers. *Journal of Experimental Child Psychology, 29,* 294–305.

Soltis, J. (1984). On the nature of educational research. *Educational Researcher, 13,* 5–10.

Søvik, N. (1976). The effects of different principles of instruction in children's copying performance. *Journal of Experimental Education, 45,* 38–45.

Spache, G. D. (1963). *Toward better reading.* Champaign, IL: Garrard.

Spache, G. D. (1976). *Investigating the issue of reading disabilities.* Boston: Allyn and Bacon.

Speece, D. L. (1985). *Information processing and reading in subtypes of learning disabled children.* Unpublished manuscript, University of Maryland, Department of Special Education.

Speece, D. L., McKinney, J. D., & Applebaum, M. I. (1984). Classification and validation of behavior subtypes of learning disabled children. *Journal of Educational Psychology, 77,* 67–77.

Spekman, N. J. (1981). Dyadic verbal communication abilities of learning disabled and normally achieving fourth- and fifth-grade boys. *Learning Disability Quarterly, 4,* 139–151.

Spollen, J. C., & Ballif, B. F. (1971). Effectiveness of individualized instruction for kindergarten children with a developmental lag. *Exceptional Children, 38,* 205–209.

Sprague, R. L., & Berger, B. D. (1980). Drug effects on learning performance: Relevance of animal research to pediatric psychopharmacology. In R. M. Knights & B. J. Bakker (Eds.), *Treatment of hyperactive and learning disordered children: Current research* (pp. 167–184). Baltimore: University Park Press.

Sprague, R. L., & Sleator, E. K. (1973). Effects of psychopharmacologic agents on learning disorders. *Pediatric Clinics of North America, 20,* 719–735.

Sprague, R. L., & Sleator, E. K. (1975). What is the proper dose of stimulant drugs in children? *International Journal of Mental Health, 4,* 75–104.

Sprague, R. L., & Sleator, E. K. (1977). Methylphenidate in hyperactive children: Differences in dose effects on learning and social behavior. *Science, 198,* 1274–1276.

Spuck, D., Junter, S. N., Owen, S. P., & Belt, S. L. (1975). *Computer management of individualized instruction* (Tech. Report 55). Madison: University of Wisconsin, Wisconsin Research and Development Center for Cognitive Learning.

Squires, D. (1983). *Effective schools and classrooms: A research-based perspective.* Alexandria, VA: Association for Supervision and Curriculum Development.

Staats, A. W., & Butterfield, W. H. (1965). Treatment of nonreading in a culturally deprived juvenile delinquent: An application of reinforcement principles. *Child Development, 36,* 925–942.

Stainback, W., Stainback, S., Courtnage, L., & Jaben, T. (1985). Facilitating mainstreaming by modifying the mainstream. *Exceptional Children, 52,* 144–152.

Stanovich, K. E. (1982a). Individual differences in the cognitive processes of reading: I. Word decoding. *Journal of Learning Disabilities, 15,* 485–493.

Stanovich, K. E. (1982b). Individual differences in the cognitive process of reading: II. Text level processes. *Journal of Learning Disabilities, 15,* 549–554.

Stanovich, K. E. (1980). Toward an interactive compensatory model of individual differences in the development of reading fluency. *Reading Research Quarterly, 16,* 32–71.

Stanovich, K. E. (1981). Relationships between word decoding speed, general name-retrieval ability and reading progress in first-grade children. *Journal of Educational Psychology, 73,* 809–815.

Stanovich, K. E. (1985). Explaining variance in reading ability in terms of psychological processes: What have we learned? *Annals of Dyslexia, 35,* 67–69.

Stanton, J. E., & Cassidy, V. M. (1964). Effectiveness of special classes for the educable mentally retarded. *Mental Retardation, 2*(1), 8–13.

Stauffer, R. G. (1975). *Directing the reading-thinking process.* New York: Harper & Row.

Stearns, P. H. (1986). Problem solving and the learning disabled: Looking for answers. *Journal of Learning Disabilities, 19*(2), 116–120.

Stein, R. (1984). Growing up with a physical difference. *Journal of the Association for the Care of Children's Health, 12,* 53–61.

Stein, R. E. K., & Jessup, D. J. (1982). A non-categorical approach to chronic childhood illness. *Public Health Report, 97,* 354–362.

Stephens, R. S., Pelham, W. E., & Skinner, R. (1984). The state-dependent and main effects of methylphenidate and pemoline on paired-associates learning and spelling in hyperactive children. *Journal of Consulting and Clinical Psychology, 523,* 104–113.

Stern, C., & Stern, M. B. (1971). *Children discover arithmetic.* New York: Harper & Row.

Stevens, R., & Rosenshine, B. (1981). Advances in research on teaching. *Exceptional Education Quarterly, 2,* 1–9.

Sticht, T. C. (1979). Applications of the audread model to reading evaluation and instruction. In L. Resnick & P. Weaver (Eds.), *Theory and practice of early reading* (Vol. 1, pp. 209–226). Hillsdale, NJ: Lawrence, Erlbaum.

Stokes, T. F., & Baer, D. M. (1977). An implicit technology of generalization. *Journal of Applied Behavior Analysis, 10,* 349–367.

Stone, M. (1972). Problems with research designs in studies of sensory-response patterns in remedial reading. *Journal of the Association for the Study of Perception, 8,* 8–15.

Strain, P. (1975). Increasing social play of severely retarded preschoolers through sociodramatic activities. *Mental Retardation, 13,* 7–9.

Strain, P. S. (1977). An experimental analysis of peer social initiations on the behavior of withdrawn preschool children: Some training and generalization effects. *Journal of Abnormal Child Psychology, 5,* 445–455.

Strain, P. S., Cooke, T. P., & Apolloni, T. (1976). *Teaching exceptional children: Assessing and modifying social behavior.* New York: Academic Press.

Strain, P. S., Shores, R. E., & Timm, M. A. (1977). Effects of peer social initiations on the behavior of withdrawn preschool children. *Journal of Applied Behavior Analysis, 10,* 289–298.

Strauss, A., & Lehtinen, L. (1947). *Psychopathology and education of the brain-injured child.* New York: Grune & Stratton.

Strickler, E. (1969). Family interaction factors in psychogenic learning disturbance. *Journal of Learning Disabilities, 2,* 31–38.

Stromer, R. (1975). Modifying letter and number reversals in elementary school children. *Journal of Applied Behavior Analysis, 8,* 211.

Stromer, R. (1977). Remediating academic deficiencies in learning disabled children. *Exceptional Children, 43,* 432–440.

Sulzbacher, S. I. (1972). Behavior analysis of drug effects in the classroom. In G. Semb (Ed.). *Behavior analysis and education.* Lawrence, KS: University of Kansas.

Swanson, H. L. (1984a). Semantic and visual memory codes in learning disabled readers. *Journal of Experimental Child Psychology, 37,* 124–140.

Swanson, H. L. (1984b). Does theory guide practice? *Remedial and Special Education, 5*(5), 7–16.

Swanson, J. M., & Kinsbourne, M. (1978). Should you use stimulants to treat the hyperactive child? *Modern Medicine, 46,* 71–80.

Swanson, J. M., & Kinsbourne, M. (1979). The cognitive effects of stimulant drugs on hyperactive children. In G. A. Hale & M. Lewis (Eds.), *Attention and cognitive development.* New York: Plenum Press.

Swanson, J. M., Kinsbourne, M., Roberts, W., & Zucker, K. (1978). Time-response analysis of the effect of stimulant medication on the learning ability of children referred for hyperactivity. *Pediatrics, 61,* 21–29.

Swanson, L. (1982). A multidirectional model for assessing learning disabled students' intelligence: An information processing framework. *Learning Disability Quarterly, 6,* 313–326.

Swift, C., & Lewis, R. (1985). Leisure preferences of elementary aged learning disabled boys. *Remedial and Special Education, 6*(1), 37–42.

Taber, F. (1983). *Microcomputers in special education: Selection and decision making process.* Reston, VA: The Council for Exceptional Children.

Tannenbaum, A. (1970). *The taxonomic instruction process.* New York: Columbia University.

Tarver, S., & Hallahan, D. (1976). Children with learning disabilities: An overview. In J. Kauffman & D. Hallahan (Eds.), *Teaching children with learning disabilities: Personal perspectives* (pp. 2–57). Columbus, OH: Merrill.

Taylor, B. M. (1982). Text structure and children's comprehension and memory for expository material. *Journal of Educational Psychology, 74*, 323–340.

Taylor, B. M., & Beach, R. W. (1984). The effects of text structure on middle-grade students' comprehension and production of expository text. *Reading Research Quarterly, 19*, 134–146.

Taylor, E. (1979). The use of drugs in hyperkinetic states: Clinical issues. *Neuropharmacology, 18*, 951–958.

Tew, B. J., Payne, H., & Lawrence, J. M. (1974). Must a family with a handicapped child be a handicapped family. *Developmental Medicine and Child Neurology, 16*, 95–98.

Texas Department of Mental Health and Mental Retardation. (1976). *Behavioral characteristics progression (BCP).* Fort Worth: Education Service Center, Region XI.

Thomas, S. (1981). Impact of the 1981 rehabilitation regulations on vocatonal evaluation of learning disabled. *Vocational Evaluation and Workshop Bulletin, 14*(1), 28–31.

Thompson, B. J. (1980). Computers in reading. A review of applications and implications. *Educational Technology, 20*, 20–28.

Thorndike, E. L. (1917). Reading as reasoning: A study of mistakes in paragraph reading. *Journal of Educational Psychology, 8*, 323–332.

Thorsell, M. (1961). Organizing experience units for the educable mentally retarded. *Exceptional Children, 27*, 177–185.

Thurlow, M. L., Graden, J., Greener, J. W., & Ysseldyke, J. E. (1982). *Academic responding for learning disabled and non-learning disabled students* (Research Report No. 72). Minneapolis: University of Minnesota, Institute for Research on Learning Disabilities.

Tindal, G. (1985). Investigating the effectiveness of special education: An analysis of methodology. *Journal of Learning Disabilities, 18*, 101–112.

Torgesen, J. K. (1977). The role of nonspecific factors in the task performance of learning-disabled children: A theoretical assessment. *Journal of Learning Disabilities, 10*, 27–34.

Torgesen, J. K. (1979). Factors related to poor performance on memory tasks in reading disabled children. *Learning Disability Quarterly, 2*, 17–23.

Torgesen, J. K. (1980). Implications of the LD child's use of efficient task strategies. *Journal of Learning Disabilities, 13*, 364–371.

Torgesen, J. K. (1981). The study of short-term memory in learning disabled children: Goals, methods, and conclusions. In K. D. Gadow & I. Bialer (Eds.), *Advances in learning and behavior disabilities* (pp. 117–149). Greenwich, CT: JAI Press.

Torgesen J. K. (1982). The learning-disabled child as an inactive learner: educational implications. In B. Y. L. Wong (Ed.), Metacognition and learning disabilities, *Topics in Learning and Learning Disabilities, 2*, 45–52.

Torgesen, J. K., & Licht, B. C. (1983). The learning disabled child as an inactive learner: Retrospect and prospects. In J. D. McKinney, & L. Feagans (Eds.), *Topics in learning disabilities* (pp. 3–31). Norwood, NJ: Ablex.

Torgesen, J. K., Murphy, L. A., & Ivey, C. I. (1979). The influence of an orienting task on the memory performance of children with reading problems. *Journal of Learning Disabilities, 12*, 396–401.

Torgesen, J. K., & Young, K. A. (1983). Priorities for the use of microcomputers with learning disabled children. *Journal of Learning Disabilities, 16*(4), 234–237.

Trammel, C. A. (1974). *A comparison of expressed play interests of children with language and/or learning disabilities and normal children.* Unpublished master's study, Texas Woman's University, Denton.

Traub, N. (1985). *Recipe for math.* North Bergen, NJ: Book Lab.

Traub, M., & Bloom, F. (1975). *Recipe for reading.* Cambridge, MA: Educators Publishing Service.

Treiber, F. A., & Lahey, B. B. (1983). Toward a behavioral model of academic remediation with learning disabled children. *Journal of Learning Disabilities, 16,* 73–136.

Trevino, F. (1979). Siblings of handicapped children: Identifying those at risk. *Social Casework, 60,* 488–492.

Trieber, F., & Lahey, B. (1982). Toward a model of academic remediation with learning disabled children. *Journal of Learning Disabilities, 16,* 111–116.

Trifiletti, J., Frith, G., & Armstrong, S. (1984). Microcomputers versus resource rooms for LD students: A preliminary investigation of the effects on math. *Learning Disability Quarterly, 7,* 69–76.

Trower, P., Bryant, B., & Argyle, M. (1978). *Social skills and mental health.* Pittsburgh: University of Pittsburgh Press.

Tucker, J., Stevens, L., & Ysseldyke, J. (1983). Learning disabilities: The experts speak out. *Journal of Learning Disabilities, 16,* 6–14.

Tucker, J. A. (1980). Ethnic proportions in classes for the learning disabled: Issues in nonbiased assessment. *The Journal of Special Education, 14,* 93–105.

U.S. Department of Education. (1980). *Second annual report to Congress on implementation of the Education of the Handicapped Act.* Washington, DC: U.S. Government Printing Office.

U.S. Department of Health and Human Services. (1979). *Plain talk about children with learning disabilities.* Rockville, MD: Alcohol, Drug Abuse, and Mental Health Administration.

U.S. News & World Report. (1981, August 10). Happiness. *U.S. News & World Report, 58.*

Ulman, J. D., & Rosenberg, M. S. (1986). Science and superstition in special education. *Exceptional Children, 52,* 459–460.

Ullman, C. A. (1957). Teachers, peers, and tests as predictors of adjustment. *Journal of Educational Psychology, 48,* 257–267.

Vacc, N. A. (1968). A study of emotionally disturbed children in regular and special education classes. *Exceptional Children, 35,* 197–204.

Valtin, R. (1974). German studies of dyslexia: Implications for education. *Journal of Research in Reading, 7*(2), 79–109.

Valtin, R. (1978–1979). Dyslexia: Deficit in reading or deficit in research? *Reading Research Quarterly, 14,* 201–221.

Van Hassalt, V. B., Hersen, M., & Bellack, A. S. (1981). The validity of role play tests for assessing social skills in children. *Behavior Therapy, 12,* 202–216.

Van Reusen, A. (1984). *A study of the effects of training learning disabled adolescents in self-advocacy procedures for use in the IEP conference.* Unpublished doctoral dissertation, University of Kansas, Lawrence.

Van Reusen, A., Bos, C., Schumaker, J. B., Deshler, D. D. (1987). *The education planning strategy.* Lawrence, KS: EXCELLENTERPRISES.

Varnen, J. (1983, March). The schoolhouse apple. *Softalk, 4,* 135–136.

Varnen, J. (1983, April). When Rich Hofmann's apple talks, children listen. *Softalk, 3,* 194–199.

Vaughn, S., & Bos, C. S. (1987). Basic knowledge and perception of the resource room: The student's perspective. *Journal of Learning Disabilities, 20*(4), 218–223.

Vellutino, F. R. (1979). *Dyslexia: Theory and research.* Cambridge, MA: MIT Press.

Vellutino, F. R., Steger, B. M., Moyer, G. C., Harding, C. J., & Niles, J. A. (1977). Has the perceptual deficit hypothesis led us astray? *Journal of Learning Disabilities, 10,* 54–64.

Venezky, R. (1970). *The structure of English orthography.* The Hague: Mouton.

Venezky, R., & Massaro, D. (1979). The role of orthographic regularity in word recognition. In L. Resnick & P. Weaver (Eds.), *Theory and practice of early reading* (Vol. 1, pp. 85–108). Hillsdale, NJ: Lawrence Erlbaum.

Verhoven, P., & Goldstein, J. (1976). *Leisure activity participation and handicapped populations.* Arlington, VA: National Recreation and Park Association.

Vetter, A. (1983). *A comparison of the characteristics of learning disabled and non-learning disabled young adults.* Unpublished doctoral dissertation, University of Kansas, Lawrence.

Visonhaler, J., Weinshank, A., Wagner, C., & Polin, R. (1982). Diagnosing children with educational problems: Characteristics of reading and learning disabilities specialists and classroom teachers. *Reading Research Quarterly, 18,* 134–164.

Voeltz, L. M., Evans, I. M., Freedland, K., & Donellon, S. (1982). Teacher decision making in the selection of educational programming priorities for severely handicapped children. *Journal of Special Education, 16,* 179–198.

Vogel, S. A. (1982). On developing LD college programs. *Journal of Learning Disabilities, 15,* 518–528.

Vogel, S. A., & Adelman, P. (1981). Personal development: College and university programs designed for learning disabled adults. *ICEC Quarterly, 1,* 12–18.

Vogel, S. A., & Moran, M. R. (1982). Written language disorders in learning disabled students: A preliminary report. In W. M. Cruickshank & J. W. Lerner (Eds.), *Coming of age: The best of ACLD* (Vol. 3). Syracuse, NY: Syracuse University Press.

Vogel, S. A., & Sattler, J. L. (1981). *The college student with a learning disability: A handbook for college and university admissions officers, faculty, and administration.* Springfield: Illinois Council for Developmental Disabilities.

Voss, J. F. (1982, March). Knowledge and social science problem solving. Paper presented at the AERA meeting, New York.

Voysey, M. (1972). Impression management by parents with disabled children. *Journal of Health and Social Behavior, 13,* 80–89.

Voysey, M. (1975). *A constant burden: The reconstitution of family life.* London: Rutledge and Kegan Paul.

Wadsworth, H. G. (1971). A motivational approach toward the remediation of learning disabled boys. *Exceptional Children, 37,* 33–42.

Walker, V. S. (1974). The efficacy of the resource room for educating retarded children. *Exceptional Children, 40,* 288–289.

Wallace, G., & Larsen, S. C. (1978). *Educational assessment of learning problems: Testing for teaching.* Boston: Allyn and Bacon.

Wallace, G., & McLoughlin, J. A. (1979). *Learning disabilities: Concepts and characteristics.* Columbus, OH: Merrill.

Wallach, M., & Wallach, L. (1976). *Teaching all children to read.* Chicago: University of Chicago Press.

Wallbrown, F. H., Wherry, R. J., Blaha, J., & Counts, D. H. (1974). An empirical test of Myklebust's cognitive structure hypothesis for 70 reading-disabled children. *Journal of Consulting and Clinical Psychology, 42,* 211–218.

Wang, M. C., & Baker, E. T. (1985-1986). Mainstreaming programs design features and effect. *Journal of Special Education, 19,* 503–521.

Wang, M. C., & Birch, J. W. (1984). Comparison of a full-time mainstreaming program and a resource room approach. *Exceptional Children, 51,* 33–40.

Warner, F., Thrapp, R., & Walsh, S. (1973). Attitudes of children toward their special class placement. *Exceptional Children, 40*, 37–38.

Warwick, N. (1968). Notes on spelling tests. In J. Arena (Ed.), *Building spelling skills in dyslexic children.* San Rafael, CA: Academic Therapy Publications.

Webb, G. M. (1974). The neurologically impaired youth goes to college. In R. E. Weber (Ed.), *Handbook on learning disabilities.* Englewood Cliffs, NJ: Prentice–Hall.

Wehman, P. (1977). *Helping the mentally retarded acquire play skills.* Springfield, IL: Thomas.

Wehman, P. (1979). *Recreation programming for developmentally disabled persons.* Baltimore: University Park Press.

Wehman, P., & Schleien, S. (1980). Assessment and selection of leisure skills for severely handicapped individuals. *Education and Training of the Mentally Retarded, 15*, 50–57.

Wehman, P., & Schleien, S. (1981). *Leisure programs for handicapped persons: Adaptations, techniques, and curriculum.* Baltimore: University Park Press.

Weiner, L. H. (1969). An investigation of the effectiveness of resource rooms for children with specific learning disabilities. *Journal of Learning Disabilities, 2*, 223–229.

Weir, S., & Watt, D. (1981). Logo: A computer environment for learning-disabled students. *The Computer Teacher, 8*(5), 11–17.

Weisberg, K. (1984). How consistent is the clinical diagnosis of reading specialists. *Reading Teacher, 38*(2), 205–212.

Weisgerber, R. A., & Rubin, D. P. (1985). Designing and using software for the learning disabled. *Journal of Reading, Writing, and Learning Disabilities International, 1*(2), 133–138.

Weiss, C. (1976). Learning and planning for retirement. *Leisure Today*, 27–28.

Weiss, G. (1979). Controlled studies of efficacy of long-term treatment with stimulants of hyperactive children. In E. Denhoff & L. Stern (Eds.), *Minimal brain dysfunction: A developmental approach.* New York: Masson.

Weiss, G. (1981). Controverial issues of the pharmacotherapy of the hyperactive child. *Canadian Journal of Psychiatry, 26*, 385–392.

Weiss, G., Hechtman, L., Perlman, T., Hopkins, J., & Wener, A. (1979). Hyperactive children as young adults: A controlled prospective 10 year follow-up of the psychiatric status of 75 hyperactive children. *Archives of General Psychiatry, 36*, 675–681.

Weiss, G., Kruger, E., Danielson, U., & Elman, M. (1975). Effects of long-term treatment of hyperactive children with methylphenidate. *Canadian Medical Association Journal, 112*, 159–165.

Wender, E. H. (1977). Food additives and hyperkinesis. *American Journal of Diseases of Children, 131*, 1204–1206.

Wepman, J. M. (1975). *Auditory discrimination test* (rev. 1973). Palm Springs, CA: Research Associates.

Werner, E. E., Blerman, J. M., & French, F. E. (1971). *The children of Kauai: A longitudinal study from the prenatal period to age ten.* Honolulu: University of Hawaii Press.

Werner, E. E., Simonian, K., & Smith, R. S. (1967). Reading achievement, language functioning, and perceptual-motor development of 10 and 11 year olds. *Perceptual and Motor Skills, 25*, 409–420.

Werner, E. E., & Smith, R. S. (1977). *Kauai's children come of age.* Honolulu: University of Hawaii Press.

Werner, E. E., & Smith, R. S. (1979). An epidemiologic perspective on some antecedents and consequences of childhood mental health problems and learning disabilities: A report from the Kauai longitudinal study. *Journal of the American Academy of Child Psychiatry, 18*, 292–306.

Werner, E. E., & Smith, R. S. (1982). *Vulnerable but invincible: A longitudinal study of resilient children and youth*. New York: McGraw–Hill.

Wetter, J. (1972). Parent attitudes toward learning disability. *Exceptional Children, 38,* 490–491.

Whalen, C., Collins, B., Henker, B., Alkus, S., Adams, D., & Stapp, J. (1978). Behavior observations of hyperactive children and methylphenidate effects in systematically structured classroom environments: Now you see them, now you don't. *Journal of Pediatric Psychology, 3,* 177–187.

Whalen, C. K., & Henker, B. (1976). Psychostimulants and children: A review and analysis. *Psychological Bulletin, 83,* 1113–1130.

Whalen, C. K., Henker, B., Collins, B. E., Finck, D., & Dotemoto, S. (1979). A social ecology of hyperactive boys: Medication effects in structured classroom environments. *Journal of Applied Behavior Analysis, 12,* 65–81.

Whalen, C. K., Henker, B., & Finck, D. (1981). Medication effects in the classroom: Three naturalistic indicators. *Canadian Journal of Psychiatry, 26,* 385–392.

Whang, P. L., Fawcett, S. B., & Mathews, R. M. (1981). Teaching job-related social skills to learning disabled adolescents. *Analysis and Intervention in Developmental Disabilities, 4,* 29–38.

White, O. (1971). *A glossary of behavioral terminology*. Champaign, IL: Research Press.

White, O. (1972). *A manual for the calculation and use of the median slope — A technique of progress estimation and prediction in the single case.* Eugene: University of Oregon, Regional Resource Center for Handicapped Children.

White, O. (1974). *The "split middle" — A "quickie" method of trend estimation.* Seattle: University of Washington, Child Development and Mental Retardation Center, Experimental Education Unit.

White, W. J., Alley, G. R., Deshler, D. D., Schumaker, J. B., Warner, M. M., & Clark, F. (1982). Are there learning disabilities after high school? *Exceptional Children, 49,* 273–274.

White, W. J., Deshler, D., Schumaker, J., Warner, M., Alley, G., & Clark, F. (1983). The effects of learning disabilities on postschool adjustment. *Journal of Rehabilitation, 49*(1), 46–50.

White, W. J., Schumaker, J. B., Warner, M. M., Alley, G. R., & Deshler, D. D. (1980). *The current status of young adults identified as learning disabled during their school career* (Research Report No. 21). Lawrence: University of Kansas Institute for Research in Learning Disabilities.

Whitman, T., Mercurio, J., & Caponigri, V. (1970). Development of social responses in two severely retarded children. *Journal of Applied Behavior Analysis, 3,* 133–138.

Wiederholt, J. (1976). Learning disability research in special education. *Journal of Special Education, 10,* 127–128.

Wiener, M., & Cromer, W. (1967). Reading and reading difficulty: A conceptual analysis. *Harvard Educational Review, 37,* 620–643.

Wiig, E. H., & Harris, S. P. (1974). Perception and interpretation of nonverbally expressed emotions by adolescents with learning disabilities. *Perceptual Motor Skills, 38,* 239–245.

Wikler, L. (1980). Chronic stresses of families of mentally retarded children. *Family Relations, 30,* 281–288.

Wikler, L., Wasow, M., & Hatfield, E. (1981). Chronic sorrow revisited: Parent vs. professional depiction of the adjustment of parents of mentally retarded children. *Americal Journal of Orthopsychiatry, 51,* 63–70.

Will, M. C. (1984). Let us pause and reflect — but not too long. *Exceptional Children, 51,* 11–16.

Williams, J. (1979). The ABDs of reading: A program for the learning disabled. In L. Resnick & P. Weaver (Eds.), *Theory and practice of early reading* (Vol. 3, pp. 399–416).

Hillsdale, NJ: Lawrence Erlbaum.

Williams, J. P. (1986). The role of phonemic analysis in reading. In J. K. Torgeson & B. Y. L. Wong (Eds.), *Psychological and educational perspectives in learning diabilities* (pp. 399–416)., New York: Academic Press.

Williams, M., & Lahey, B. B. (1977). The functional independence of response latency and accuracy: Implications for the concept of conceptual tempo. *Journal of Abnormal Child Psychology, 5,* 371–378.

Willner, S. K., & Crane, R. (1979). A parental dilemma: The child with a marginal handicap. *Social Casework, 60,* 30–35.

Willoughby–Herb, S. J. (1983). Selecting relevant curricular objectives. *Topics in Early Childhood Special Education, 2,* 9–14.

Wilson, G. (1969). Status of recreation for the handicapped school centered. *Therapeutic Recreation Journal, 3,* 10–12.

Wilson, K. (1981). Managing the administrative morals of special needs. *Classroom Computer News, 1*(4), 8–9.

Winograd, P. (1984). Strategic difficulties in summarizing texts. *Reading Research Quarterly, 19*(4), 404–425.

Winter, A., & Wright, E. N. (1983). *A follow-up of pupils who entered learning disabilities self-contained classes in 1981-1982* (Research Report No. 171). Toronto, Canada: Board of Education. (ERIC Document Reproduction Service No. ED 238 224)

Wittrock, M. C. (1978). The cognitive movement in instruction. *Educational Psychologist, 13,* 15–30.

Wolf, M. M., Giles, D. K., & Hall, R. V. (1968). Experiments with token reinforcement in a remedial classroom. *Behavior Research and Therapy, 6,* 51–64.

Wolfensberger. W. (1967). Counseling the parents of the retarded. In A. A. Baumeister (Ed.), *Mental retardation: Appraisal, education and rehabilitation* (pp. 329–400). Chicago: Aldine.

Wolraich, M., Drummond, T., Salomon, M. K., O'Brien, M., & Sivage, C. L. (1978). Effects of methylphenidate alone and in combination with behavior modification procedures on the behavior and academic performance of hyperactive children. *Journal of Abnormal Child Psychology, 6,* 149–161.

Wong, B. (1979). The role of theory in learning disabilities research. Part 1. An analysis of problems. *Journal of Learning Disabilities, 12,* 19–28.

Wong, B. (1980). Activating the inactive learner: Use of questions/prompts to enhance comprehension and retention of implied information in learning disabled children. *Learning Disability Quarterly, 3,* 29–37.

Wong, B. Y. (1985). Potential means of enhancing content skill acquisition in learning disabled adolescents. *Focus on Exceptional Children, 17*(5), 1–8.

Wong, B. Y. L. (1985a). Metacognition and learning disabilities. In T. G. Waller, D. Forrest-Pressley, & E. MacKinnon (Eds.), *Metacognition, cognition and human performance* (pp. 137–180). New York: Academic Press.

Wong, B. Y. L. (1985b). Potential means of enhancing content skills acquisition in learning-disabled adolescents. *Focus on Exceptional Children, 17,* 1–8.

Wong, B. Y. L. (1985c). Self-questioning instructional research. *Review of Educational Research, 55*(2), 227–268.

Wong, B. Y. L., & Jones, W. (1982). Increasing metacomprehension in learning-disabled and normally-achieving students through self-questioning training. *Learning Disability Quarterly, 5,* 228–240

Wong, B. Y. L., & Wong, R. (1980). Role-taking skills in normal achieving and learning disabled children. *Learning Disability Quarterly, 3*(2), 11–18.

Wood, M. M., & Hurley, O. L. (1977). Curriculum and instruction. In J. B. Jordan, A. H. Hayden, M. B. Karnes, & M. M. Wood (Eds.), *Early childhood education for excep-*

tional children: A handbook of ideas and exemplary practices. Reston, VA: Council for Exceptional Children.

Woodcock, R. (1973). *Woodcock reading mastery test.* Circle Pines, NM: American Guidance Service.

Woodcock, R., & Johnson, M. (1977). *Woodcock–Johnson psycho-educational battery.* Allen, TX: DLM Teaching Resources.

Worcester, L. H. (1981). *The Canadian Franco-American learning disabled college student at the University of Maine at Orono.* Orono: University of Maine. (ERIC Document Reproduction Service No. ED 204 881)

Wright, L. S., & Stimmel, T. (1984). Perceptions of parents and self among college students reporting learning disabilities. *Exceptional Child, 31*(3), 203–208.

Yates, J. M. (1983). *Research implications for writing in the content areas.* Washington, DC: National Education Association.

Yellin, A. M., Hopwood, J. H., & Greenberg, L. M. (1982). Adults and adolescents with attention deficit disorders: Clinical and behavioral response to psychostimulants. *Journal of Clinical Psychopharmacology, 2,* 133–136.

Yoshida, R. K., Fenton, K. S., Maxwell, J. P., & Kaufman, M. J. (1978). Group decision making in the planning team process: Myth or reality? *Journal of School Psychiatry, 16,* 237–244.

Youngberg v. Romeo. (1982). 102 S.Ct. 2452.

Ysseldyke, J. E. (1983). Current practices in making psychoeducational decisions about learning disabled students. *Journal of Learning Disabilities, 16,* 226–233.

Ysseldyke, J. E., & Algozzine, B. (1982). *Critical issues in special and remedial education.* Boston: Houghton Mifflin.

Ysseldyke, J. E., Algozzine, B., & Richey, L. (1982). Judgment under uncertainty: How many children are handicapped? *Exceptional Children, 48,* 531–534.

Ysseldyke, J. E., Algozzine, B., Richey, L., & Gardner, J. (1982). Declaring students eligible for learning disability services: Why bother with the data? *Learning Disability Quarterly, 5,* 37–44.

Ysseldyke, J. E., & Thurlow, M. L. (1983). *Identification/classifcation research: An integrative summary of findings* (Research Report No. 142). Minneapolis: University of Minnesota, Institute for Research on Learning Disabilities.

Zajonc, R. B. (1980). Feeling and thinking: Preferences need no inferences. *American Psychologist, 35,* 151–175.

Zigmond, N. (1978a). A prototype of comprehensive service for secondary students with learning disabilities: A preliminary report. *Learning Disability Quarterly, 1,* 39–49.

Zigmond, N. (1978b). Remediation of dyslexia: A discussion. In A. L. Benton & D. Pearl (Eds.), *Dyslexia: An appraisal of current knowledge* (pp. 425-448). New York: Oxford University Press.

Zutell, J. (1980). Children's spelling strategies and their cognitive development. In E. H. Henderson & J. W. Beers (Eds.), *Developmental and cognitive aspects of learning to spell.* Newark, DE: International Reading Association.

Zweng, M. J., Garaghty, J., & Turner, J. (1979). *Children's strategies of solving verbal problems* (Final Report). Washington, DC: National Institute of Education. (ERIC Document Reproduction Service No. ED 178 359)

Index

Key: (*t*) indicates *table;* (*f*) indicates *figure.*

Notes

Notes

Notes

Notes

Notes

Notes

Notes

Notes